Mu

A Handbook for Care
of the Pregnant Patient

Accession no
36019293

KT-476-698

618`25NEW

BACHE EDUCATION CENTRE
LIBRARY
?21240

stamped
of

Multifetal Pregnancy

A Handbook for Care of the Pregnant Patient

Roger B. Newman, M.D.
Professor and Vice Chairman for Academic Affairs
Department of Obstetrics and Gynecology
Medical University of South Carolina;
Director, Department of Maternal and Fetal Medicine
Medical University of South Carolina Hospital
Charleston, South Carolina

Barbara Luke, Sc.D., M.P.H.
Professor, Department of Obstetrics and Gynecology
University of Michigan Medical School;
Director, Division of Health Services Research
University of Michigan Health System
Ann Arbor, Michigan

 LIPPINCOTT WILLIAMS & WILKINS
A **Wolters Kluwer** Company
Philadelphia · Baltimore · New York · London
Buenos Aires · Hong Kong · Sydney · Tokyo

Acquisitions Editor: Lisa McAllister
Developmental Editor: Kerry Barrett
Production Editor: Frank Aversa
Manufacturing Manager: Ben Rivera
Cover Designer: Patricia Gast
Compositor: Circle Graphics
Printer: RR Donnelley/Crawfordsville

© 2000 by **LIPPINCOTT WILLIAMS & WILKINS**
530 Walnut Street
Philadelphia, PA 19106 USA
LWW.com

All rights reserved. This book is protected by copyright. No part of
this book may be reproduced in any form or by any means, including
photocopying, or utilized by any information storage and retrieval
system without written permission from the copyright owner,
except for brief quotations embodied in critical articles and reviews.
Materials appearing in this book prepared by individuals as part of
their official duties as U.S. government employees are not covered
by the above-mentioned copyright.

Printed in the USA

Library of Congress Cataloging-in-Publication Data
Newman, Roger B.
  Multifetal pregnancy : a handbook for care of the pregnant
patient / authors, Roger B. Newman, Barbara Luke.
    p. ; cm.
  Includes bibliographical references and index.
  ISBN 0-7817-2217-9
  1. Multiple pregnancy. 2. Pregnant women—Care. 3. Prenatal
care. I. Luke, Barbara. II. Title.
  [DNLM: 1. Pregnancy, Multiple. 2. Pregnancy Complications—
therapy. 3. Prenatal Care. WQ 235 N554m 2000]
RG567 .N49 2000
618.2'5—dc   00-030145

Care has been taken to confirm the accuracy of the information
presented and to describe generally accepted practices. However,
the authors and publisher are not responsible for errors or omissions
or for any consequences from application of the information in this
book and make no warranty, expressed or implied, with respect
to the currency, completeness, or accuracy of the contents of the
publication. Application of this information in a particular situation
remains the professional responsibility of the practitioner.
  The authors and publisher have exerted every effort to ensure that
drug selection and dosage set forth in this text are in accordance with
current recommendations and practice at the time of publication.
However, in view of ongoing research, changes in government
regulations, and the constant flow of information relating to drug
therapy and drug reactions, the reader is urged to check the package
insert for each drug for any change in indications and dosage and for
added warnings and precautions. This is particularly important when
the recommended agent is a new or infrequently employed drug.
  Some drugs and medical devices presented in this publication
have Food and Drug Administration (FDA) clearance for limited use
in restricted research settings. It is the responsibility of the health
care provider to ascertain the FDA status of each drug or device
planned for use in their clinical practice.

10 9 8 7 6 5 4 3 2 1

To Diane, Bryan, Taylor, and Sarah,
whose love, support, and beauty inspire me.

ROGER NEWMAN

To Dr. Timothy R. B. Johnson
and Dr. Mary Jo O'Sullivan,
in recognition of the many lives they have influenced
during their long and caring careers
as teachers and obstetricians.

BARBARA LUKE

Contents

Contributing Authors

Roger B. Newman, M.D.
Professor and Vice Chairman for Academic Affairs
Department of Obstetrics and Gynecology
Medical University of South Carolina;
Director, Department of Maternal and Fetal Medicine
Medical University of South Carolina Hospital
96 Jonathan Lucas Street, Suite 634
Charleston, South Carolina 29425
Chapters 3, 5, 7, 8, 10, 11

Barbara Luke, Sc.D., M.P.H.
Professor, Department of Obstetrics and Gynecology
University of Michigan Medical School;
Director, Division of Health Services Research
University of Michigan Health System
1500 East Medical Center Drive, F4866 Mott
Ann Arbor, Michigan 48109-0264
Chapters 1, 2, 4, 6, 9, 12

Jill Mauldin, M.D.
Assistant Professor
Department of Obstetrics and Gynecology
Medical University of South Carolina
96 Jonathan Lucas Street, Suite 634
P.O. Box 250619
Charleston, South Carolina 29425
Chapter 5

Preface

Twinning has always fascinated us. The ancient Greeks placed the Gemini in the heavens and the ancient Romans attributed the birth of their city to the foundlings Romulus and Remus. A description of the twinning phenomena can be found in the writings of Hippocrates and has been part of every major obstetrical text. All of which begs the question: why a book on the care of the patient with a multifetal pregnancy? The answer is severalfold.

Although always considered an obstetrical challenge, the clinical concern for twins and higher order multiples was diminished by their relative rarity and their status as a sort of natural wonder. Geza Kurtz prefaced a 1958 review of 21 triplet sets with the following disclaimer, "Because of the rarity of triplet births, the human interest appeal of such an event is greater than its practical significance." It is obvious, however, that sociological changes and advances in reproductive science during the last two decades now require a reevaluation of that statement. More than 100,000 multiples are delivered yearly in the United States, representing approximately 3% of all live births in this country. Triplet and higher order births, which formerly were statistical improbabilities according to Hellin's hypothesis, now occur with a frequency approaching one in 500 live births. This national epidemic makes multifetal gestations more common than many of the classic obstetrical complications (pregestational diabetes, chronic hypertension, lupus erythematosus, placenta previa, placental abruption, breech presentation, and so on) that define the subspecialty of maternal fetal medicine.

This increased frequency of multifetal gestations serves to magnify the significant perinatal risks associated with these pregnancies. Despite phenomenal advances in maternal and neonatal care, the population-attributable fetal and newborn risks associated with multiple birth are compelling. Nationally, twins and triplets represent approximately 21% and 25% of all low birth weight and very low birth weight deliveries, respectively; 10% of all neonatal intensive care unit admissions; 16% of all neonatal deaths; and 15% of all cases of cerebral palsy.

Finally, reconsideration of the care of multifetal gestations is necessary because only in the last 20 to 25 years have we had the ability to make a reliable antepartum diagnosis. The advent of ultrasound has allowed the clinician to determine the normalcy of the gestation, follow its progress, assess the well-being of the fetuses, and plan for delivery. The question of what constitutes optimum prenatal care for multiples could not have been asked or answered until these technological innovations in obstetrics allowed us to consider the issue.

Multifetal Pregnancy: A Handbook for Care of the Pregnant Patient is dedicated to a discussion of the optimum antepartum and intrapartum management of multifetal gestations. This discussion includes the influence of placentation on pregnancy outcome, prenatal genetic diagnosis, multifetal pregnancy reduction and selective termination, appropriate nutritional intervention, and approaches to the prevention of preterm birth. There are also chapters discussing the obstetrical complications unique to multiple gestations, the increased risk of maternal morbidity associated with them, intrapartum management of multiples, and the care of triplet and higher order multiple birth.

This handbook is primarily for clinicians and clinicians in training but is also appropriate for certified nurse midwives, nurse practitioners, perinatal nurses, sonographers, nutritionists, and obstetrical care providers for women with multiples. Prenatal care for multifetal gestations is best provided by an experienced and multidisciplinary staff that can anticipate and manage the various and complex problems presented by multiple birth. This handbook summarizes the current state of understanding the varied problems. When available, the best scientific support for management recommendations is presented. Unfortunately, prenatal care is as individualized as any aspect of medicine, particularly in regard to multiple gestations. When convincing scientific support is unavailable, recommendations have been based on clinical experience, judgment, and philosophy. In these areas, we hope to point the direction for further research.

We have relied heavily on numerous colleagues within our university consortium for the study of multiple births. Dr. Mary Jo O'Sullivan at the University of Miami; Drs. Frank Witter and Mary Hediger at Johns Hopkins University; Drs. Clark Nugent and Tim Johnson at the University of Michigan; Dr. Peter Van Dorsten and Dr. Jill Mauldin (who co-authored Chapter 5: Role of Ultrasound in the Antepartum Management of Multiple Gestations) at the Medical University of South Carolina; and others have contributed to this text by collaborating with us to establish a database of over 3,000 multiple gestations, and by participating in the consortium's multifetal research efforts. We also greatly appreciate the support of Lisa McAllister, who had faith in this project, and Kerry Barrett, for shepherding the project to its completion. Finally, we must thank our patients; those mothers of two, three, or more who have trusted us to help them with this unexpected, thrilling, but terrifying complication of their pregnancy and have simultaneously taught us how to interpret their experiences for the benefit of others. We hope that this book helps to provide these mothers and their babies with the special care they deserve.

Roger B. Newman, M.D.
Barbara Luke, Sc.D.

Perinatal Significance of Multiple Gestations

RISING INCIDENCE OF MULTIPLE BIRTHS IN THE UNITED STATES

In 1998 there were 118,295 multiples born in the United States, the highest number ever recorded (1) (Fig. 1-1). This rise has been most dramatic in recent years, with increases between 1995 and 1996, 1996 and 1997, and 1997 and 1998, respectively, in the number of twin births by 4%, 3%, and 6%, and triplet and higher order multiple births by 19%, 16%, and 13% (1,2). Since 1980 the number of twins has risen by 62% (from 68,339 to 110,670) and the number of triplets and other higher-order multiple births has risen by 470% (from 1,337 to 7,625).

Another way to evaluate the frequency of multiple births is the number of multiple births per 1,000 or 100,000 live births, as the *twin birth rate* and the *higher-order multiple birth rate*. Since 1980, the twin birth rate (the number of twin births per 1,000 live births) has risen by 49% (from 18.9 to 28.1 per 1,000 live births). Since 1990 it has risen by 24% (from 22.6), including increases of 4%, 3%, and 6%, respectively, between 1995–1996, 1996–1997, and 1997–1998. The higher-order multiple birth rate (the number of triplet and higher-order births per 100,000 live births) has been rising even faster, increasing 20%, 14%, and 11%, respectively, during these same time periods. The higher order multiple rate has increased by 165% since 1990 (from 72.8 to 193.5 per 100,000 live births) and by 432% since 1980 (from 37.0 per 100,000 live births) (1,2).

In 1998, 1 in every 36 births was a twin and nearly 1 in every 500 births was a triplet or higher order birth, compared to 1 in 52 and 1 in 2,702, respectively, in 1980 (Table 1-1). These trends have also been noted in other industrialized nations, with the majority of the increase among primiparous women 30 years and older (3), and the most rapid rise among triplet and higher-order births since 1980 (4).

The dramatic rise in multiple births in the United States during the past 20 years has influenced measures of perinatal health at the state and national levels (5–8). Because infants of multiple births are much more likely to be premature (10% for singletons versus 55% for twins and 94% for triplets and higher-order multiples) and of low birth weight (5% for singletons versus 53% for twins and 92% for triplets and higher-order multiples), it has become increasingly more important to analyze trends in these perinatal measures by plurality (1).

Trend of Childbearing at Older Maternal Ages

It is estimated that one-fourth to one-third of the rise in multiple births is due to the trend in postponing childbearing, with multiple births occurring more frequently among older mothers (2,9). For example, between 1975 and 1998, among women 30 years and older the proportion of first births rose 330% (from 5.3% to 22.8%) and the proportion of all births rose 115% (from 16.5% to 35.5%).

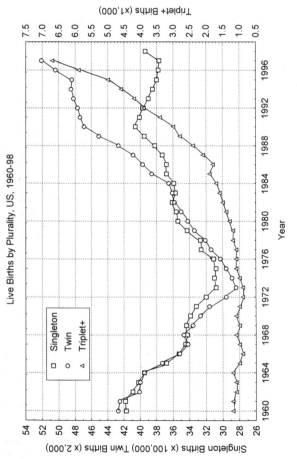

Figure 1-1. Live births by plurality, United States, 1960–1998.

Among women 40 years and older, this rise has been even more dramatic, the rate of first births increasing during this time period from 0.1% to 1.1% and of all births rising from 0.9% to 2.2% (Table 1-2). The birth rate has been relatively stable during the past 20 years for women in their twenties, but it has steadily risen for women in their thirties and forties (Table 1-3). As shown in Table 1-4, the proportion of multiple births is much higher among older mothers, and this percentage has risen dramatically since 1975. In 1998, 17.8% of births to mothers 45 years or older were multiple births. This rate was ten times higher than that among mothers younger than 20 years (1.5%) and more than four times higher than that among women in their thirties (4.1%) (1). In 1998 the multiple birth ratio was ten times higher for women 45 to 54 years (177.7 per 1,000 live births) compared to women 18 to 19 years (16.8), nearly seven times higher compared to women 20 to 29 years (25.9), and four times higher compared to women 30 to 39 years (40.6).

Infertility Treatments and Multiple Pregnancies

In the United States, an estimated 45% of women of childbearing age have impaired fecundity and would like to have children (or more children) (10,11). Fecundity problems increase with age, and after the age of 35 years rise sharply. According to data from the National Survey of Family Growth (12), the percentage of infertile women in the United States increased from 8.4% in 1982 and 1988 to 10.2% in 1995 (13). In absolute terms, there were an estimated 4.5 million infertile women in the United States in 1982, 4.9 million in 1988, and 6.2 million in 1995. Projected estimates are 6.3 million in 2000 and 6.5 million for 2010. This rise in infertility may be due to several factors, including a greater public awareness of infertility and an increase in pelvic inflammatory disease, secondary to subclinical cases of gonorrhea or chlamydial infection (13). Only about one-half of women with infertility problems seek medical help, and these women are more likely to be older, married, white, and wealthier than the overall population with infertility (10,14).

It is well known that infertility treatments increase the risk of multiple births (15–18). An estimated 25% to 26% of *in vitro* fertilization pregnancies are multiples (15,16); 38% of triplet and higher-order multiples are estimated to be the result of assisted reproductive technologies (ART) (19). Estimates from national surveys indicate that the use of ovulation-stimulating medications increased by 90% between 1973–1991 (19a). Monozygotic twinning has surprisingly increased due to the use of ART; with an increase between 4% to 10% (20–22). It has been suggested that the possibility of delay of developmental events, including premature and partial hatching of blastomeres from the zona pellucida, is the cause of this monozygotic twinning in infertility treatments (23–25).

The most recent annual summary of ART programs in the United States reported 65,863 cycles of ART treatment, 68% of which were with *in vitro* fertilization (IVF), 4% were with gamete intrafallopian transfer (GIFT), and 2% were with zygote intrafallopian transfer (ZIFT). These procedures resulted in 14,702 deliveries of 21,196 neonates (26). Of ART cycles resulting in clinical pregnancies,

Table 1-1. Frequency of live births by plurality, United States, 1960–1998

Year	All Liveborn Infants	Singletons	Twins	Triplet and Higher Order	Triplets	Quadruplets	Quintuplet
1960	4,257,850	4,171,166	1:50 (85,440)	1:3,423 (1,244)			
1961	4,268,326	4,182,226	1:50 (84,926)	1:3,636 (1,174)			
1962	4,167,362	4,086,056	1:52 (80,180)	1:3,701 (1,126)			
1963	4,098,020	4,016,662	1:51 (80,044)	1:3,679 (1,114)			
1964	4,027,490	3,947,334	1:51 (78,954)	1:3,351 (1,202)			
1965	3,760,358	3,684,752	1:50 (74,594)	1:3,716 (1,012)			
1966	3,606,274	3,534,962	1:51 (70,340)	1:3,710 (972)			
1967	3,520,959	3,451,594	1:52 (68,336)	1:3,422 (1,029)			
1968	3,501,564	3,431,156	1:51 (69,300)	1:3,160 (1,108)			
1969	3,600,206	—	—	—			
1970	3,731,386	—	—	—			
1971	3,555,970	3,491,638	1:56 (63,298)	1:3,439 (1,034)			
1972	3,258,411	3,198,382	1:55 (59,122)	1:3,593 (907)			
1973	3,136,965	3,079,244	1:55 (56,777)	1:3,323 (944)			
1974	3,159,958	3,101,117	1:54 (57,836)	1:3,144 (1,005)			
1975	3,144,198	3,083,940	1:53 (59,192)	1:2,950 (1,066)			
1976	3,167,788	3,106,038	1:52 (60,664)	1:2,917 (1,086)			
1977	3,326,632	3,262,676	1:52 (62,880)	1:3,092 (1,076)			
1978	3,333,279	3,267,931	1:52 (64,163)	1:2,813 (1,185)			

Year						
1979	3,494,398	1:52 (66,858)	1:2,907 (1,202)			
1980	3,612,258	1:52 (68,339)	1:2,702 (1,337)			
1981	3,629,238	1:51 (70,049)	1:2,620 (1,385)			
1982	3,680,537	1:51 (71,631)	1:2,480 (1,484)			
1983	3,638,933	1:50 (72,287)	1:2,310 (1,575)			
1984	3,669,141	1:50 (72,949)	1:2,220 (1,653)			
1985	3,760,561	1:48 (77,102)	1:1,912 (1,925)			
1986	3,756,547	1:47 (79,485)	1:2,071 (1,814)			
1987	3,809,394	1:46 (81,778)	1:1,781 (2,139)			
1988	3,909,510	1:46 (85,315)	1:1,639 (2,385)			
1989	4,040,958	1:45 (90,118)	1:1,444 (2,798)	1:1,598 (2,529)	1:17,646 (229)	1:101,024 (40)
1990	4,158,212	1:44 (93,865)	1:1,373 (3,028)	1:1,469 (2,830)	1:22,477 (185)	1:319,862 (13)
1991	4,110,907	1:43 (94,779)	1:1,225 (3,355)	1:1,317 (3,121)	1:20,252 (203)	1:186,859 (22)
1992	4,065,014	1:42 (95,372)	1:1,045 (3,891)	1:1,146 (3,547)	1:13,113 (310)	1:156,347 (26)
1993	4,000,240	1:41 (96,445)	1:960 (4,168)	1:1,043 (3,834)	1:14,441 (277)	1:70,180 (57)
1994	3,952,767	1:41 (97,064)	1:860 (4,594)	1:934 (4,233)	1:12,548 (315)	1:85,930 (46)
1995	3,899,589	1:40 (96,736)	1:784 (4,973)	1:857 (4,551)	1:10,684 (365)	1:68,414 (57)
1996	3,891,494	1:39 (100,750)	1:655 (5,939)	1:735 (5,298)	1:6,949 (560)	1:48,043 (81)
1997	3,880,894	1:37 (104,137)	1:576 (6,737)	1:631 (6,148)	1:7,610 (510)	1:49,125 (79)
1998	3,941,553	1:36 (110,670)	1:517 (7,625)	1:570 (6,919)	1:6,286 (627)	1:49,893 (79)

Numbers in parentheses are the actual number of infants of multiple births.

Table 1-2. Live births by birth order and maternal age, United States, 1975–1998

Birth Order and Year	Number of Births by Maternal Age (yr)							Percentage of Births by Maternal Age (yr)		
	All Ages	<20	20–24	25–29	30–34	35–39	≥40	≥30	≥35	≥40
First births										
1975	1,319,126	463,562	516,528	269,688	56,677	10,901	1,770	5.3	1.0	0.1
1980	1,545,604	435,333	605,183	371,859	112,964	18,241	2,024	8.6	1.3	0.1
1985	1,554,788	369,120	552,974	418,658	170,686	39,447	3,903	13.8	2.8	0.3
1990	1,689,118	401,900	515,455	465,458	230,612	66,541	9,152	18.1	4.5	0.5
1995	1,610,453	401,531	460,523	400,890	249,474	83,508	14,527	21.6	6.1	0.9
1998	1,576,478	384,397	437,632	394,268	248,986	93,428	17,767	22.8	7.1	1.1
All births										
1975	3,144,198	594,880	1,093,676	936,786	375,500	115,409	27,947	16.5	4.6	0.9
1980	3,612,258	562,330	1,226,200	1,108,291	550,354	140,793	24,290	19.8	4.6	0.7
1985	3,760,561	477,705	1,141,320	1,201,350	696,354	214,336	29,496	25.0	6.5	0.8
1990	4,158,212	533,483	1,093,730	1,277,108	886,063	317,583	50,245	30.2	8.8	1.2
1995	3,899,589	512,115	965,547	1,063,539	904,666	383,745	69,977	34.8	11.6	1.8
1998	3,941,553	494,357	965,122	1,083,010	889,365	424,890	84,809	35.5	12.9	2.2

Adapted from Ventura SJ, Martin JA, Curtin SC, et al. Births: final data for 1998. National Vital Statistics Report 2000, 48(3):1–100.

**Table 1-3. Birth rates by maternal age,
United States, 1975–1998**

Year	\<20	20–24	25–29	30–34	35–39	≥40
			Maternal Age (yr)			
1975	56.9	113.0	108.2	52.3	19.5	4.9
1980	54.1	115.1	112.9	61.9	19.8	4.1
1985	52.5	108.3	111.0	69.1	24.0	4.2
1990	61.3	116.5	120.2	80.8	31.7	5.7
1995	58.1	109.8	112.2	82.5	34.3	6.9
1998	52.1	111.2	115.9	87.4	37.4	7.7

Note: Birth rates are live births per 1,000 women in the specified age group.

39% of IVF, 34% of GIFT, and 36% of ZIFT resulted in multiples. There is debate over how many oocytes or embryos to transfer to minimize the risk of a multiple pregnancy, particularly a triplet of higher-order birth (27,28). While several authors advocate replacing only two oocytes or embryos (29–31) or three oocytes, zygotes, or embryos (32), others have demonstrated a high rate of spontaneous reduction (28% to 48%) (33,34) and the adverse effect of older maternal age (35,36). For example, a recent analysis of national ART data showed that with two embryos transferred, multiple birth rates were 23%, 20%, 12%, and 11%, respectively, for women 20 to 29 years of age, 30 to 34 years, 35 to 39 years, and 40 to 44 years (36). With three embryos transferred, the multiple birth rate was 46%, 40%, 29%, respectively, for women 20 to 29 years, 30 to 34 years, 35 to 39 years. For women 40 to 44 years, however, the multiple birth rate was less than 25% with as many as five embryos transferred.

RACIAL, ETHNIC, AND ENVIRONMENTAL FACTORS IN MULTIPLE GESTATIONS

Twinning rates have risen among the largest racial and ethnic groups in 1997–1998, but the twin birth ratio was highest for non-Hispanic white women (32.8 versus 32.2 for non-Hispanic black, and 21.2 for Hispanic women). In addition, non-Hispanic white women are more than twice as likely as non-Hispanic black women and more than three times as likely as Hispanic women to have a triplet or higher-order multiple birth. In 1998, the higher-order multiple birth ratio was 262.8 per 100,000 live births for non-Hispanic white women, compared with 87.3 for non-Hispanic black women and 75.3 for Hispanic women (1). Non-Hispanic white women are much more likely to seek infertility treatment, accounting for much of the disparity in the current higher-order multiple birth rates (10).

MATERNAL MORBIDITY ASSOCIATED WITH MULTIPLE GESTATIONS

Women pregnant with multiples are more likely to need intensive prenatal care (37), to need antenatal admission to the hospital

Table 1-4. Live births by plurality and maternal age, United States, 1975–1998

Plurality and Year	Number of Births by Maternal Age (yr)							Percentage of Births by Maternal Age (yr)		
	All Ages	<20	20–24	25–29	30–34	35–39	≥40	≥30	≥35	≥40
Singletons										
1975	3,083,940	587,265	1,074,099	916,778	366,114	112,376	27,308	16.4	4.5	0.9
1980	3,478,715	545,958	1,184,408	1,064,764	526,049	134,294	23,242	19.7	4.5	0.7
1985	3,681,534	471,427	1,119,989	1,174,584	678,108	208,548	28,878	24.9	6.4	0.8
1990	4,061,319	525,793	1,072,431	1,246,144	860,478	307,498	48,975	30.0	8.8	1.2
1995	3,797,880	504,752	945,971	1,035,896	875,002	368,957	67,302	34.5	11.5	1.8
1998	3,823,258	486,795	943,745	1,051,417	855,379	405,473	80,449	35.1	12.7	2.1
Twins										
1975	59,192	7,550	19,270	19,583	9,185	2,981	623	21.6	6.1	1.1
1980	68,339	7,212	21,374	22,712	12,944	3,559	538	24.9	6.0	0.8
1985	77,102	6,212	20,931	25,969	17,750	5,638	602	31.1	8.1	0.8
1990	93,865	7,605	20,945	30,020	24,466	9,587	1,242	37.6	11.5	1.3
1995	96,736	7,273	19,235	26,385	27,699	13,693	2,451	45.3	16.7	2.5
1998	110,670	7,475	20,916	29,901	30,781	17,676	3,921	47.3	19.5	3.5

Triplets and more[a]

Year										
1975	1,066	65	307	425	201	52	16	25.2	6.4	1.5
1980	1,337	83	385	474	321	67	7	29.5	5.5	0.5
1985	1,925	66	400	797	496	150	16	34.4	8.6	0.8
1990	3,028	85	354	944	1,119	498	28	54.3	17.4	0.9
1995	4,973	90	341	1,258	1,965	1,095	224	66.0	26.5	4.5
1998	7,625	87	461	1,692	3,205	1,741	439	70.6	28.6	5.8

All multiples

Year										
1975	60,258	7,615	19,577	20,008	9,386	3,033	639	21.7	6.1	1.1
1980	69,676	7,295	21,759	23,186	13,265	3,626	545	25.0	6.0	0.8
1985	79,027	6,278	21,331	26,766	18,246	5,788	618	31.2	8.1	0.8
1990	96,893	7,690	21,299	30,964	25,585	10,085	1,270	38.1	11.7	1.3
1995	101,709	7,363	19,576	27,643	29,664	14,788	2,675	46.3	17.2	2.6
1998	118,295	7,562	21,377	31,593	33,986	19,417	4,360	48.8	20.1	3.7

[a] Includes triplets, quadruplets, quintuplets, and other higher-order multiples.

Source: Adapted from Ventura SJ, Martin JA, Curtin SC, et al. Births: final data for 1998. National Vital Statistics Report 2000, 48(3):1–100.

(38), to have longer hospitalizations (39), and to experience significantly greater and more severe pregnancy-related morbidities (see Chapter 9). A portion of this risk is linked to maternal characteristics present at the onset of pregnancy, including older age, extremes of parity and pregravid weight, and conception with ART. The majority of this excess risk is due to higher plurality and an exaggeration of maternal adaptations to pregnancy and associated obstetric interventions. Even with multifetal pregnancy reduction (see Chapter 4), there is still residual higher risk of complications. In a recent case–control study of causes for admission of pregnant women to intensive care units, multiple pregnancy was found to be an independent risk factor, with an odds ratio of 2.3 (95% confidence interval [CI], 1.2–4.5) (40).

PERINATAL MORBIDITIES ASSOCIATED WITH MULTIPLE GESTATIONS

Multiple births are much more likely than singletons to be born prematurely (<37 weeks, 57% versus 10%) or with a low birth weight (LBW, <2,500 g, 56% versus 5%). Multiple births comprise only 3% of all births but account for 21% of all low birth weights, 19% to 24% of very low birth weights (VLBW, <1,500 g), and 20% of early preterm births (<32 weeks) (1,41,42). Multiple births account for 10% of stillbirths, 11% of intraventricular hemorrhages (grades 3 and 4), 10% of neonatal sepsis, and 14% of respiratory distress syndrome (2,43).

CHILDHOOD CONSEQUENCES OF MULTIPLE GESTATION

Because of their higher incidence of growth retardation and prematurity, infants of multiple births are at greater risk for neonatal morbidity, and fetal, neonatal, and postneonatal mortality than are singletons. Survivors are at continued higher risk of postneonatal morbidity and subsequent perinatally-related handicap (see Chapter 12). Admission to a neonatal intensive care unit (NICU) is necessary for about one-fourth of all twins and as many as three-fourths of all triplets and quadruplets, with an average length of stay of 18 days, 30 days, and 58 days, respectively. The incidence of respiratory distress syndrome, one of the most costly complications of prematurity, is reported to occur in as many as 14% of twins, 41% of triplets, and 64% of quadruplets. Infants of multiple gestation account for 20% of all NICU admissions, 16% of all neonatal deaths, and 26% of all perinatal deaths (41–43). Compared to singletons, the risk of dying before their first birthday is nearly seven times greater for twins, and nearly 20 times greater for triplets and higher-order multiples (39,44–46). Among survivors, the relative risk of severe handicap related to birth weight and gestational age is 1.7 (95% CI, 1.6–2.0) and 2.9 (95% CI, 1.5–5.5), respectively, for twins and triplets (47). Compared with singletons of the same gestational age, infants of multiple births have significantly lower physical and mental indices in early childhood (48), while cognitive outcome by school age has been related to medical complications, such as chronic lung disease, and social risk factors (49).

COST OF MULTIPLES

Hospital care accounts for the largest component of national health expenditures, which exceeded 1 trillion dollars in 1998 (50). Acute care, particularly in the NICU, is a major contributor to rising health care costs in the United States (51). For infants of multiple births, health care costs reflect their disproportionate morbidity. For twins, the predominant cost factor at birth is prematurity, and the cost is magnified in the presence of intrauterine growth retardation or congenital anomalies (39). For triplets and quadruplets, these factors remain equally important, but are exaggerated by the greater plurality. Analyses of inpatient costs of twin deliveries showed that birth weight and gestational age accounted fully for the increased use of NICU services among multiples (52). Effective prenatal interventions that could improve maternal nutritional status, fetal growth, and length of gestation would significantly reduce maternal and neonatal morbidity and the associated hospital charges of multifetal pregnancy.

CLINICAL CONSIDERATIONS AND KEY POINTS

- In 1998 there were 118,295 multiples born in the United States, the highest number ever recorded.
- Since 1980, the number of twin births has risen by 62% and the number of triplet and higher-order births has risen by 470%.
- It is estimated that one-fourth to one-third of the rise in multiple births is due to the trend in postponing childbearing, multiple births occurring more frequently among older mothers.
- Three-fourths of the rise in multiple births is estimated to be due to the use of ART, 25% to 38% of treatments resulting in multiple births.
- Debate exists regarding the number of oocytes, zygotes, or embryos (depending on the procedure) to transfer during ART; a higher number are needed to achieve clinical pregnancy among older women.
- Multifetal pregnancy is associated with significantly greater and more severe maternal morbidities, which occur in proportion to plurality, method of conception, and maternal age.
- Although multiple births comprise only 3% of all births, they account for 21% of all low birth weights, 19% to 24% of very low birth weights, 20% of early preterm births (<32 weeks), and 16% of neonatal deaths.
- Compared to singletons, the risk of dying before their first birthday is five times greater for twins and 14 times greater for triplets.
- Among survivors, the relative risk of severe handicap related to birth weight and gestational age is 1.7 (95% CI, 1.6–2.0) for twins and 2.9 (95% CI, 1.5–5.5) for triplets.
- For twins, the predominant cost factor at birth is prematurity. The cost is magnified in the presence of intrauterine growth retardation or congenital anomalies. For triplets and quadruplets, these factors remain equally important, but are exaggerated by their higher plurality.

REFERENCES

1. Ventura SJ, Martin JA, Curtin SC, et al. Births: final data for 1998. *Natl Vital Stat Rep* 2000;48(3):1–100.
2. Ventura SJ, Martin JA, Curtin SC, et al. Report of final natality statistics, 1996. *Mon Vital Stat Rep* 1998;46[11 Suppl]:1–99.
3. Westergaard T, Wohlfahrt J, Aaby P, et al. Population based study rates of multiple pregnancies in Denmark, 1980–94. *BMJ* 1997; 314:775–779.
4. Dunn A, Macfarlane A. Recent trends in the incidence of multiple births and associated mortality in England and Wales. *Arch Dis Child* 1996;75:F10–F19.
5. Centers for Disease Control and Prevention. State-specific variation in rates of twin births—United States, 1992–1994. *Morb Mortal Wkly Rep* 1997;46:121–125.
6. Centers for Disease Control and Prevention. Preterm singleton births—United States, 1989–1996. *Morb Mortal Wkly Rep* 1999; 48:185–189.
7. Centers for Disease Control and Prevention. Impact of multiple births on low birthweight—Massachusetts, 1989–1996. *Morb Mortal Wkly Rep* 1999;48:289–292.
8. Martin JA, Taffel SM. Current and future impact of rising multiple birth ratios on low birthweight. *Statistical Bulletin of the Metropolitan Life Insurance Co.* 1995;76:10–18.
9. Jewell SE, Yip R. Increasing trends in plural births in the United States. *Obstet Gynecol* 1995;85:229–232.
10. Chandra A, Stephen EH. Impaired fecundity in the United States: 1982–1995. *Fam Plann Perspect* 1998;30:34–42.
11. Abma JC, Chandra A, Mosher WD, et al. Fertility, family planning, and women's health: new data from the 1995 National Survey of Family Growth. National Center for Health Statistics. Vital Health Stat 23 1997;May:1–114.
12. National survey of family growth, 1982 and 1988. Hyattsville, MD: National Center for Health Statistics; 1989.
13. Stephen EH, Chandra A. Updated projections of infertility in the United States: 1995–2025. *Fertil Steril* 1998;70:30–34.
14. Kalmuss DS. The use of infertility services among fertility-impaired couples. *Demography* 1987;24:575–585.
15. Tan SL, Doyle P, Campbell S, et al. Obstetric outcome of in vitro fertilization pregnancies compared with normally conceived pregnancies. *Am J Obstet Gynecol* 1992;167:778–784.
16. Andrews MC, Muasher SJ, Levy DL, et al. An analysis of the obstetric outcome of 125 consecutive pregnancies conceived in vitro and resulting in 100 deliveries. *Am J Obstet Gynecol* 1986; 154:848–854.
17. Steptoe PC, Edwards RG, Walters DE. Observations on 767 clinical pregnancies and 500 births after human in vitro fertilization. *Hum Reprod* 1986;1:89–94.
18. Zimmerman R, Soor B, Braendle W, et al. Gonadotropin therapy of female infertility: analysis of results in 416 cases. *Gynecol Obstet Invest* 1982;14:1–18.
19. Wilcox LS, Kiely JL, Melvin CL, et al. Assisted reproductive technologies: estimates of their contribution to multiple births and newborn hospital days in the United States. *Fertil Steril* 1996; 65:361–366.

19a. Wysowski DK. Use of fertility drugs in the United States, 1973 through 1991. *Fertil Steril* 1993;60:1096–1098.

20. Luke B, Gillespie B, Min SJ, et al. Critical periods of maternal weight gain: effect on twin birth weight. *Am J Obstet Gynecol* 1997;177:1055–1062.

21. Luke B, Min SJ, Gillespie B, et al. The importance of early weight gain in the intrauterine growth and birth weight of twins. *Am J Obstet Gynecol* 1998;179:1155–1161.

22. Wenstrom KD, Syrop CH, Hammitt DG, et al. Increased risk of monochorionic twinning associated with assisted reproduction. *Fertil Steril* 1993;60:510–514.

23. Derom C, Derom R, Vlietnck R, et al. Increased monozygotic twinning rate after ovulation induction. *Lancet* 1987;1:1236–1238.

24. Edwards RG, Mettler L, Walters DE. Identical twins and in vitro fertilization. *J In Vitro Fert Embryo Transf* 1986;3:114–117.

25. Yovich JL, Stanger JD, Grauaug A, et al. Monozygotic twins from in vitro fertilization. *Fertil Steril* 1984;41:833–837.

26. SART/ASRM. Assisted reproductive technology in the United States: 1996 results generated from the American Society for Reproductive Medicine/Society for Assisted Reproductive Technology registry. *Fertil Steril* 1999;71:798–807.

27. Martin PM, Welch HG. Probabilities for singleton and multiple pregnancies after in vitro fertilization. *Fertil Steril* 1998;70:478–481.

28. Levene MI. Assisted reproduction and its implications for paediatrics. *Arch Dis Child* 1991;66:1–3.

29. Walters DE. Is it time to replace only two embryos? Can pregnancy rates by maintained when two embryos are replaced in in-vitro fertilization? *Hum Reprod* 1994;9:184–186.

30. Wang XJ, Warnes GM, Norman RJ, et al. Gamete intra-fallopian transfer: outcome following the elective or non-elective replacement of two, three or four oocytes. *Hum Reprod* 1993;8:1231–1234.

31. Nijs M, Geerts L, van Roosendaal E, et al. Prevention of multiple pregnancies in an in vitro fertilization program. *Fertil Steril* 1993;59:1245–1250.

32. Bollen N, Camus M, Staessen C, et al. The incidence of multiple pregnancy after in vitro fertilization and embryo transfer, gamete, or zygote intrafallopian transfer. *Fertil Steril* 1991;55:314–318.

33. Blumenfeld Z, Dirnfeld M, Abramovici H, et al. Spontaneous fetal reduction in multiple gestations assess by transvaginal ultrasound. *Br J Obstet Gynaecol* 1992;99:333–337.

34. Legro RS, Wong IL, Paulson RJ, et al. Multiple implantation after oocyte donation: a frequent but inefficient event. *Fertil Steril* 1995; 63:849–853.

35. Dickey RP, Olar TT, Curole DN, et al. The probability of multiple births when multiple gestational sacs or viable embryos are diagnosed at first trimester ultrasound. *Hum Reprod* 1990;5:880–882.

36. Schieve LA, Peterson HB, Meikle SF, et al. Live-birth rates and multiple-birth risk using in vitro fertilization. *JAMA* 1999;282:1832–1838.

37. Kogan MD, Martin JA, Alexander GR, et al. The changing pattern of prenatal care utilization in the United States, 1981–1995, using different prenatal care indices. *JAMA* 1998;279:1623–1628.

38. Haas JS, Berman S, Goldberg AB, et al. Prenatal hospitalization and compliance with guidelines for prenatal care. *Am J Public Health* 1996;86:815–819.
39. Luke B, Bigger H, Leurgans S, et al. The cost of prematurity: a case–control study of twins versus singletons. *Am J Public Health* 1996;86:809–814.
40. Bouvier Colle MH, Varnoux N, et al. Case–control study of risk factors for obstetric patients' admission to intensive care units. *Eur J Obstet Gynecol Reprod Biol* 1997;79:173–177.
41. Stevenson DK, Wright LL, Lemons JA, et al. Very low birth weight outcomes of the National Institute of Child Health and Human Development Neonatal Research Network, January 1993 through December 1994. *Am J Obstet Gynecol* 1998;179:1632–1639.
42. Donovan EF, Ehrenkranz RA, Shankaran S, et al. Outcomes of very low birth weight twins cared for in the National Institute of Child Health and Human Development Neonatal Research Network's intensive care units. *Am J Obstet Gynecol* 1998;179:742–749.
43. Gardner MO, Goldenberg RL, Cliver SP, et al. The origin and outcome of preterm twin pregnancies. *Obstet Gynecol* 1995;85:553–557.
44. Luke B, Minogue J. The contribution of gestational age and birthweight to perinatal viability in singletons versus twins. *J Matern Fetal Med* 1994;3:263–274.
45. Kiely JL, Kleinman JC, Kiely M. Triplets and higher-order multiple births: time trends and infant mortality. *Am J Dis Child* 1992;146:862–868.
46. Martin JA, Park MM. Trends in twin and triplet births: 1980–97. *Natl Vital Stat Rep* 1999;47(24):1–17.
47. Luke B, Keith LG. The contribution of singletons, twins, and triplets to low birth weight, infant mortality, and handicap in the United States. *J Reprod Med* 1992;37:661–666.
48. Brandes JM, Scher A, Itzkovits J, et al. Growth and development of children conceived by in vitro fertilization. *Pediatrics* 1992;90:424–429.
49. Leonard CH, Piecuch RE, Ballard RA, et al. Outcome of very low birth weight infants: multiple gestation versus singletons. *Pediatrics* 1994;93:611–615.
50. Highlights of the National Health Expenditures, 1998; http://www.hefa.gov/2000;June 5.
51. Office of Technology Assessment. Neonatal intensive care for low birthweight infants: costs and effectiveness. OTA-HCS-38. Washington, DC: US Government Printing Office, 1987.
52. Ettner SL, Christiansen CL, Callahan TL, et al. How low birthweight and gestational age contribute to increased inpatient costs for multiple births. *Inquiry* 1997;34:325–339.

Placentation, Zygosity, and Intrauterine Growth

BIOLOGY OF MULTIPLES

The Incidence of Twinning

The incidence of twinning around the world varies by a number of factors. Most of the fluctuations are in the rates of dizygotic, or fraternal twinning; whereas the rates of monozygotic or identical twinning are amazingly constant over time and among diverse populations. In the era prior to assisted reproductive technology, the incidence of monozygotic twinning was fairly constant around the world, typically about 3.2/1,000 live births. In contrast, dizygotic twinning ranged from a low of 1.3/1,000 live births among Asian populations to a high of 45/1,000 live births among the Yoruba in Nigeria, and varied during times of famine and war. The actual frequency of twinning may be much higher than any of these estimates, closer to 53.9/1,000 conceptions, but many twins are lost long before delivery, as the "vanishing twin" (see later) (1). Since the introduction and widespread use of assisted reproductive technologies in the 1980s, the incidence of multiple births has risen dramatically, particularly among industrialized nations. Surprisingly, the use of assisted reproductive technology also has caused the monozygotic twinning rate to increase, possibly due to the premature and partial hatching of blastomeres from the zona pellucida (2–7). An estimated one-third of all twins are identical, and two-thirds are fraternal. Among fraternal twins, approximately one-half are boy/girl, one-fourth are girl/girl, and one-fourth are boy/boy. Among triplets, an estimated 6% are identical; the others are a combination of identical and fraternal.

Monozygotic Twinning

Monozygotic twins occur from a single fertilized ovum and its subsequent division during development. The zygote divides one additional time, producing two separate and identical zygotes. Identical twins and triplets are monozygotic, indicating that they developed from a single zygote. The timing of this additional division determines the structure of the fetal membranes—the amnion or inner membrane and the chorion or outer membrane—and the placenta (Fig. 2-1). When the division occurs within 3 days after conception, when the original zygote has not yet implanted in the endometrium of the uterus, these identical twins have two separate placentas, two chorions, and two amnions—a diamnionic, dichorionic twin pregnancy. This type of placentation occurs in about 65% of monozygotic pregnancies. When the extra division occurs 4 to 7 days after conception, the twins have separate amnions but share a common chorion, and the placentas are fused—a diamnionic, monochorionic twin pregnancy. This type of placentation occurs in about 30% of monozygotic pregnancies. If the division occurs after the eighth day following conception, the identical twins share an amnion, chorion, and placenta—a monoamnionic, monochorionic

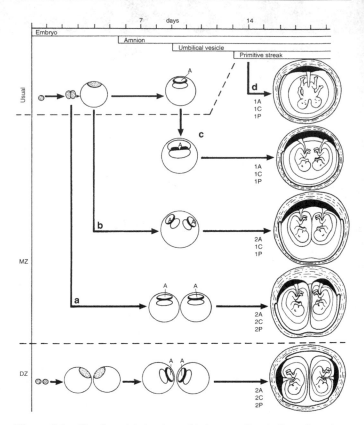

Figure 2-1. The placental structure of twins according to the embryonic timing of the additional division. The arrangement of the adnexa (fetal membranes) in twinning. **a–d:** Various forms of monozygotic (*MZ*) twins. **d:** Conjoined twins. *Top,* usual development, that is, singletons, with an approximate time scale. *A,* amnion and amniotic cavity; *C,* chorion; *P,* placenta. (From O'Rahilly R, Muller F. *Human embryology and teratology.* New York: Wiley–Liss, 1992, with permission.)

twin pregnancy. This is the rarest type of placentation, occurring in about 5% of monozygotic pregnancies. It is associated with the highest perinatal mortality. The rate of fetal demise is as high as 50%, mostly before 24 weeks' gestation. Demise is caused by entanglement of the umbilical cords due to fetal movement. When the additional division occurs after the eighth day following conception, conjoined twins can result. This is a rare condition (1:50,000 births) that often leads to fetal demise. Because of the higher incidence of malformations among monozygotic twins, there also is a higher rate of antenatal mortality compared with the rate among dizygotic twins. The rates of major and minor malformations among monozygotic twins compared to singletons are approximately 2.3% and 4.1% versus 1% and 2.5%, respectively.

Dizygotic Twinning

Dizygotic or fraternal twinning occurs after the release and fertilization of two separate ova by two different sperm. The blastocytes of each dizygotic twin implant within the uterus, and each developing fetus has its own amnion and chorion. If the blastocytes implant far apart in the uterus, the placenta of each twin is separate. If the blastocytes implant closely, the placentas may fuse but still contain separate amnions and chorions. Fraternal twins occur more frequently with advancing maternal age, by inheritance in some families through the maternal lineage, and with the administration of follicle-stimulating hormone (FSH) and clomiphene. The familial and racial incidence of dizygotic twinning is correlated with higher maternal levels of FSH and lutenizing hormone secretion (8–10). The higher incidence of dizygotic twinning with advancing maternal age also is caused by the higher levels of gonadotropin that occur naturally with aging.

Vanishing Twins

It is estimated that 21% of twins diagnosed in the first trimester, with two gestational sacs identified by ultrasound, are subsequently delivered as singletons (1). Among multiple pregnancies from *in vitro* fertilization, 46% of fetuses ascertained to be multiples at 12 weeks' gestation had spontaneously reduced to singletons by delivery (11). This phenomenon, termed the *vanishing twin*, probably occurs more frequently than previously believed and is associated with first-trimester bleeding in about 25% of cases. Careful pathologic examination of the placenta after delivery in these cases may reveal some embryonic remnants, such as irregular plaques or hemorrhages into the decidua capsularis.

Determination of Zygosity

Monochorionic placentation is analogous to monozygosity. The presence of twins of different sexes indicates dizygosity. For like-gender twins with diamniontic, dichorionic placentation, the differential diagnosis of zygosity can be determined using placental genetic markers, testing for blood groups, testing of restriction fragment length polymorphism (RFLP) of DNA fragments, or polymerase chain reaction (PCR) from very small samples of solid tissue (12,13).

PLACENTAL STRUCTURE

Growth and Aging of the Placenta

The growth of singleton placentas is fairly uniform throughout gestation, whereas in twins placental weight accelerates between 24 and 36 weeks, and plateaus after 37 weeks (14). Abnormally low placental weight is associated with congenital anomalies and maternal uteroplacental vascular insufficiency. Increased placental weight is associated with extensive villous edema, hydrops fetalis, fetal anemia, Rh factor incompatibility, maternal diabetes mellitus, maternal anemia, chronic intrauterine infection, intervillous thrombi, and subchorionic blood clots (14). Large-for-gestational age placentas have been associated acute antenatal hypoxia, neonatal death, high childhood blood pressure, and long-term neurologic sequelae (15–17).

Although both zygosity and placental membranes each exert a significant influence on twin birth weight, the latter may be a more

ortant determinant. Prenatal determination of placental cho-
nicity at the initial ultrasound examination is critical; there are
nplications regarding management, patient counseling, and perinatal outcome. The placental vasculature is a critical environmental factor influencing growth of multiple fetuses. Other morphologic
features of the placenta, such as infection and inflammation, and
the insertion and number of cord vessels also influence fetal
growth. Dizygotic and dichorionic twins are heavier than monozygotic and monochorionic twins. There is a strong correlation
between birth weight and placental weight ($r = 0.36-0.61$) (18).

Accelerated aging of the placenta in multiple gestation has been
reported (19). Grade III placentas are found earlier in gestation
and in significantly higher proportions than in singleton pregnancies at comparable gestational ages, as follows: 27% versus 4.5% at
32 to 34 weeks, 59% versus 26.5% at 35 to 37 weeks, and 76.2% versus 36.5% at 38 to 40 weeks. At the same gestational age, twin placentas are only about 69% heavier than those of singletons (14). In
addition, placental complications are more common in multiple
versus singleton pregnancies, including acute chorioamnionitis,
premature rupture of the fetal membranes, large placental infarction, and placental abruption (15,16).

Ultrasound Determination of Placental Membrane Structure

Determination of chorionicity by first-trimester transvaginal
ultrasound has been shown to be highly accurate (20–24). A wedge-
shaped junction, the *twin peak sign,* represents the fusion of two
chorionic membranes. A T-shaped junction represents the fusion of
two amnionic membranes. In triplet gestations, prenatal determination of chorionicity by ultrasound can be made by evaluating the
ipsilon zone, the junction of the three interfetal membranes (25).

Anomalies of the Placenta

Velamentous and Marginal Cord Insertions

Abnormal umbilical cord insertion (velamentous or marginal)
occurs in about 28% to 33% of monochorionic, 16% of dichorionic-
fused, and 13% of dichorionic-separate placentas. Velamentous insertion of the umbilical cord occurs in 7% to 8% of twin placentas
compared with about 1% in singleton placentas. Velamentous cord
insertion is associated with a higher risk of vasa previa, single
umbilical artery, twin transfusion syndrome, and congenital anomalies (26). Benirschke (27) suggested that this represents disturbed
placental growth caused by nutrient competition between closely
approximated twin embryos. Developing twin embryos that are
most closely approximated (monochorionic twins) therefore are subjected to the greatest peripheral growth of the placental mass
as placental expansion occurs away from a relatively nutrient-
deficient, central uterine zone. With this peripheral placental expansion, the body stalks are stretched, and the umbilical cords
develop a high frequency of velamentous insertion (28).

Single Umbilical Arteries

Monoarterial umbilical cord (single umbilical artery, SUA) occurs
among as many as 7% of twins versus 1% of singletons. SUA occurs
in only one of the cords of monozygotic twins, indicating that it

an acquired developmental anomaly. This theory is su[ ]
the finding of other malformations in placentas with S[ ]
Benirschke (27) suggested that the association of SUA wi[ ]
mentous insertion is a reflection of disturbed placental [ ]
tion. Such disturbed nutrition induces lateral placental gr[ ]
and therefore velamentous insertion, as well as secondary atro[ ]
of one of the two umbilical cord arteries. SUA is associated with a[ ]
increase in congenital anomalies (67%) (musculoskeletal, genitourinary, and cardiovascular) in the corresponding twin. The co-twin
often shows growth retardation, supporting the notion of disturbed
placental nutrition (29).

Anastomoses between Arteries and Veins

Vascular anastomoses can be found in nearly all monochorionic
placentas but are not found in dichorionic placentas, even when
the placentas are fused. Anastomoses most often occur in the central plane, where placental segments are joined, known as the
vascular equator. Deep anastomoses, which occur between arterial branches of one twin and venous branches of the co-twin
within a common cotyledon, are responsible for the flow between
siblings. It is believed that superficial anastomoses develop to
compensate for the deep placental anastomoses. Twin transfusion
syndrome (TTS), in which one twin transfuses blood to the other
via placental anastomoses, may occur in as many as 30% of all
monochorionic placentas. Anastomoses have a critical influence on
birth weight, the nature and severity of TTS, and survival. TTS
commonly presents during the second trimester with discordant
fetal growth and amniotic sacs (polyhydramnios and oligohydramnios), chronic malnutrition of the donor fetus, and high-out-
put heart failure in the recipient fetus caused by hypervolemia. In
pregnancies affected by severe TTS before 28 weeks' gestation, the
chances of survival are nil. Recently, a hemodynamic model of TTS
has been developed (30).

INTRAUTERINE GROWTH AND SURVIVAL
OF MULTIPLE FETUSES

Intrauterine Growth

Intrauterine growth has been observed to be independent of the
number of fetuses until the end of the second trimester, when the
rate slows for multiples (31). For twins, this is estimated to occur
at about 30 weeks, for triplets at 27 weeks, and for quadruplets at
26 weeks. Twins born at 40 weeks' gestation are actually lighter
than those born at 38 to 39 weeks, suggesting that intrauterine
growth for these infants stops after 39 weeks (32). The tenth percentile of growth for singletons is the mean for twins by 38 weeks,
for triplets by 36 weeks, and for quadruplets by 32 weeks (33–37).
Intrauterine growth of infants of multiple births peaks earlier
than for singletons; weight loss occurs at or before the singleton
range of maturity (38 to 41 weeks). This peak occurs earlier with
each additional fetus, and the risk of intrauterine growth retardation and subsequent fetal or neonatal death, or postnatal morbidity increases with advancing gestation (33,38–41).

Among twins, by 35 to 36 weeks 13% have birth weights below
the tenth percentile, increasing to 23% by 37 to 38 weeks, and

to 41 weeks (38,39). By 39 to 41 weeks, the odds ratio
retardation for the smaller and larger of the twin pair is
ed to be 5.23 (95% confidence interval [CI], 1.4–19.0) and
95% CI, 2.7–23.8), respectively (38,39). Among triplets, 12%
e birth weights less than the tenth percentile by 31 to 34 weeks,
creasing to 64% by 35 to 36 weeks (41). For quadruplets, this
ecline in birth weight occurs sooner and more dramatically.
Because the two strongest factors affecting perinatal survival
are gestational age and relative birth weight (42), adequacy of
intrauterine growth and optimal maturity for infants of multiple
births are central to their risk of morbidity and mortality, as
well as growth and development later in life (43).

Min et al. (44) developed a unique birth-weight reference based
on longitudinal measures of individual twins, and combining pre-
and postnatal measurements using ultrasound estimates and birth
weights (Tables 2-1 to 2-4). The difference between twin and *in
utero* estimates of singleton weight are shown in Figure 2-2. Twin
weights differed substantially (by 10% or more) from *in utero* singleton weights in the tenth percentile by 28 weeks, in the fiftieth percentile by 30 weeks, and in the ninetieth percentile by 34 weeks.
The difference between twins and *in utero* singletons at the fiftieth
percentile was 147 g (10%) at 30 weeks, 242 g (14%) at 32 weeks,
347 g (17%) at 34 weeks, 450 g (19%) at 36 weeks, 579 g (22%) at
38 weeks, and 772 g (27%) at 40 weeks. The difference between
twins and *in utero* singletons was greater at the tenth percentile
(15% at 30 weeks, increasing to 29% at 40 weeks), and less at the
ninetieth percentile (5% at 30 weeks increasing to 24% at 40 weeks).
According to this new twin growth reference, the peak rate of
growth occurs between 34 and 36 weeks (166.5 g/week) compared
with 36 to 38 weeks for singletons (225 g/week) (45).

Risk of Fetal Death

Based on preliminary studies on 183,562 twins, the birth weight
and gestational age associated with the lowest risk of intrauterine
growth retardation and fetal death has been estimated to be 2,500
to 2,800 g at 35 to 38 weeks (46). Subsequent studies with larger
study populations (352,629 twins) have confirmed this optimal birth-weight range and narrowed the gestational age to 36 to
37 weeks (33) (Figs. 2-3 through 2-5). More recent research has
estimated the optimal birth weight and gestation for triplets (based
on 9,523 infants) to be 1,900 to 2,100 g at 34 to 35 weeks (33).

Risk of Neonatal Death

The importance of birth weight, gestational age, and birth weight
for gestational age centers on the association of these measures
with subsequent morbidity and mortality. When the relative influences of birth weight and gestational age on perinatal morbidity and mortality are studied together, birth weight emerges
as the predominant factor (32,35,47,48). The intrauterine growth
of singletons and twins, as measured by birth weight, diverges
beginning at about 30 weeks' gestation (32,34,36,49). These differences increase from the 35th week of gestation to delivery.
Leroy et al. (34) reported differences of 150 g at 31 weeks that in-

(*text continues on page 30*)

Table 2-1.   Weight percentiles of twins by chorionicity

Week	n	Percentage Born	Mean	SD	Fifth	10th	25th	50th	75th	90th	95th
Monochorionic											
20	289	0	308.2	134.1	96	134	221	307	374	479	590
22	288	0	478.1	143.8	255	298	377	471	553	669	769
24	285	0	676.9	156.0	439	486	569	666	763	892	978
26	286	0	900.5	180.4	631	675	786	884	998	1,128	1,254
28	293	3	1,137.4	223.0	787	867	1,012	1,127	1,260	1,436	1,558
30	282	11	1,405.5	246.6	1,021	1,103	1,264	1,391	1,544	1,732	1,839
32	252	19	1,701.3	284.2	1,265	1,362	1,534	1,688	1,865	2,086	2,216
34	205	46	2,005.3	317.6	1,523	1,616	1,822	2,003	2,180	2,429	2,549
36	110	59	2,267.9	315.2	1,762	1,883	2,088	2,286	2,452	2,677	2,806
38	45	87	2,626.2	367.3	2,058	2,215	2,352	2,650	2,861	3,068	3,296
40	6	100	2,847.2	320.4	2,440	2,440	2,572	2,821	3,199	3,229	3,229
Dichorionic											
20	1,127	0	324.2	132.7	115	164	243	315	394	493	577
22	1,129	0	494.0	141.1	280	322	402	482	570	678	760
24	1,126	0	687.4	151.5	457	504	582	678	777	888	966
26	1,128	0	908.3	172.0	641	695	790	897	1,013	1,133	1,221
28	1,130	3	1,151.2	199.6	838	903	1,013	1,143	1,276	1,414	1,507
30	1,099	4	1,420.4	236.3	1,036	1,130	1,257	1,410	1,577	1,726	1,831
32	1,054	9	1,716.9	277.0	1,253	1,386	1,532	1,708	1,906	2,066	2,176
34	955	28	2,028.21	322.8	1,501	1,643	1,811	2,020	2,247	2,430	2,549
36	682	62	2,377.7	366.5	1,795	1,930	2,132	2,359	2,619	2,847	2,987
38	260	85	2,652.6	403.9	2,012	2,106	2,401	2,640	2,901	3,155	3,36
40	40	100	2,883.0	439.7	2,298	2,328	2,541	2,859	3,121	3,470	

From Min SJ, Luke B, Gillespie B, et al. Birthweight references for twins. *Am J Obstet Gynecol* 2000; 182:1250–1257, with permission.

Table 2-2. Weight percentiles of twins, all races, both sexes

Week	n	Percentage Born	Mean	SD	Fifth	10th	25th	50th	75th	90th	95th
Both sexes											
20	1,627	0	320.4	132.0	113	157	238	313	390	486	579
22	1,630	0	491.2	141.5	275	318	397	482	567	670	761
24	1,622	0	686.7	151.9	454	500	583	678	776	888	967
26	1,625	0	909.1	173.2	641	691	791	897	1,014	1,133	1,223
28	1,636	3	1,152.0	204.4	836	898	1,015	1,144	1,280	1,419	1,520
30	1,592	5	1,424.0	237.8	1,045	1,130	1,265	1,412	1,578	1,732	1,833
32	1,517	11	1,721.0	277.6	1,264	1,382	1,540	1,711	1,906	2,078	2,182
34	1,343	31	2,037.0	322.9	1,512	1,650	1,825	2,030	2,252	2,444	2,564
36	931	61	2,375.0	360.4	1,791	1,930	2,132	2,363	2,613	2,831	2,984
38	357	87	2,659.0	397.6	2,019	2,154	2,405	2,657	2,893	3,160	3,363
40	46	100	2,854.0	395.2	2,319	2,333	2,550	2,847	3,114	3,420	3,470
Girls											
20	783	0	312.4	126.5	114	155	234	304	382	472	546
22	783	0	480.2	136.3	277	306	389	472	557	657	719
24	781	0	672.8	149.6	452	489	570	664	762	860	949
26	783	0	890.1	171.7	376	631	772	882	995	1,116	1,188

28	789	3	1,130.5	203.6	811	879	1,001	1,123	1,257	1,398	1,484
30	767	4	1,397.2	237.4	1,018	1,093	1,239	1,387	1,556	1,707	1,796
32	734	10	1,690.5	271.7	1,253	1,335	1,504	1,681	1,868	2,050	2,149
34	659	30	2,001.3	316.6	1,489	1,593	1,792	2,001	2,209	2,408	2,539
36	460	58	2,328.5	351.3	1,755	1,882	2,088	2,316	2,557	2,788	2,890
38	191	89	2,620.7	392.2	1,973	2,079	2,352	2,616	2,868	3,101	3,359
40	21	100	2,823.3	392.2	2,319	2,345	2,531	2,779	3,128	3,300	3,390
Boys											
20	844	0	327.8	136.6	112	159	241	320	399	497	593
22	847	0	501.5	145.5	275	325	404	494	577	696	776
24	841	0	699.5	153.0	465	517	594	688	791	906	978
26	842	0	926.8	172.8	656	714	811	911	1,029	1,167	1,240
28	847	2	1,171.9	203.3	853	925	1,041	1,160	1,296	1,435	1,555
30	825	5	1,448.1	235.7	1,081	1,165	1,285	1,433	1,596	1,758	1,866
32	783	13	1,750.5	280.0	1,308	1,419	1,562	1,737	1,925	2,098	2,225
34	684	31	2,070.7	325.4	1,576	1,680	1,848	2,053	2,286	2,481	2,610
36	471	65	2,420.8	363.7	1,884	1,980	2,163	2,404	2,656	2,891	3,011
38	166	85	2,702.4	400.4	2,060	2,224	2,452	2,700	2,988	3,207	3,406
40	25	100	2,880.6	403.8	2,322	2,333	2,631	2,850	3,002	3,470	3,470

From Min SJ, Luke B, Gillespie B, et al. Birthweight references for twins. *Am J Obstet Gynecol* 2000; 182:1250–1257, with permission.

Table 2-3. Weight percentiles of white[a] twins by sex

Week	n	Percentage Born	Mean	SD	Fifth	10th	25th	50th	75th	90th	95th
Girls											
20	451	0	313.1	120.7	111	158	243	311	381	461	506
22	451	0	484.5	130.5	268	313	409	481	563	636	706
24	452	0	678.9	145.1	440	488	589	680	768	856	932
26	453	0	900.8	167.5	628	683	789	898	1,003	1,112	1,183
28	457	3	1,146.0	200.2	800	889	1,016	1,145	1,282	1,406	1,470
30	444	5	1,419.0	230.5	1,041	1,122	1,280	1,411	1,579	1,725	1,794
32	423	12	1,720.0	263.5	1,277	1,386	1,555	1,720	1,903	2,067	2,148
34	374	30	2,040.0	305.3	1,538	1,663	1,841	2,041	2,243	2,420	2,539
36	262	62	2,373.0	342.9	1,827	1,936	2,152	2,381	2,592	2,823	2,960
38	99	87	2,657.0	389.1	2,019	2,190	2,356	2,666	2,871	3,204	3,379
40	13	100	2,869.0	402.4	2,277	2,345	2,550	2,854	3,199	3,300	3,590
Boys											
20	533	0	334.6	130.1	130	178	252	327	406	497	586
22	535	0	510.7	139.3	293	341	423	506	586	689	771
24	530	0	711.0	145.7	474	531	615	706	797	907	974
26	532	0	940.9	167.5	660	730	830	935	1,045	1,168	1,239
28	536	1	1,190.0	201.6	852	936	1,067	1,187	1,316	1,438	1,555
30	526	5	1,471.0	233.3	1,082	1,177	1,326	1,474	1,616	1,766	1,871
32	500	15	1,781.0	276.7	1,318	1,436	1,601	1,779	1,958	2,106	2,225
34	426	31	2,115.0	317.5	1,607	1,709	1,903	2,123	2,323	2,492	2,593
36	292	63	2,466.0	348.1	1,886	2,000	2,211	2,477	2,701	2,891	2,995
38	106	82	2,769.0	396.5	2,154	2,240	2,482	2,788	3,045	3,290	3,464
40	19	100	2,883.0	419.1	2,123	2,333	2,572	2,850	3,089	3,470	3,803

[a] Hispanic and non-Hispanic.

From Min SJ, Luke B, Gillespie B, et al. Birthweight references for twins. Am J Obstet Gynecol 2000; 182:1250–1257, with permission.

Table 2-4. Weight percentiles of black twins by sex

Week	n	Percentage Born	Mean	SD	Fifth	10th	25th	50th	75th	90th	95th
Girls											
20	332	0	311.4	134.2	114	146	220	295	389	502	574
22	332	0	474.3	143.7	277	306	370	452	550	682	744
24	329	0	664.6	155.5	454	490	546	640	751	881	975
26	330	0	875.5	176.5	636	673	748	857	986	1,127	1,225
28	332	3	1,109.0	206.5	811	862	970	1,078	1,229	1,372	1,503
30	323	4	1,367.0	243.6	1,017	1,061	1,210	1,336	1,516	1,688	1,815
32	311	8	1,650.0	278.0	1,232	1,282	1,476	1,636	1,816	2,020	2,154
34	285	30	1,951.0	324.6	1,460	1,526	1,752	1,930	2,149	2,386	2,537
36	198	54	2,269.0	354.3	1,711	1,795	2,037	2,256	2,495	2,771	2,847
38	92	91	2,582.0	393.9	1,920	2,046	2,338	2,600	2,849	3,087	3,205
40	8	100	2,749.0	389.5	2,319	2,319	2,361	2,772	3,010	3,390	3,390
Boys											
20	311	0	316.2	146.6	92	139	222	303	387	518	621
22	312	0	485.7	154.5	256	314	383	471	551	700	793
24	311	0	679.9	163.0	451	498	570	660	752	903	1,016
26	310	0	902.5	179.2	654	699	787	873	993	1,152	1,255
28	311	4	1,140.0	202.7	860	914	1,008	1,117	1,250	1,421	1,555
30	299	6	1,408.0	234.9	1,069	1,152	1,252	1,383	1,540	1,737	1,861
32	283	9	1,696.0	278.0	1,301	1,400	1,521	1,670	1,853	2,073	2,227
34	258	30	1,998.0	325.9	1,512	1,655	1,800	1,956	2,167	2,442	2,645
36	179	66	2,348.0	377.4	1,804	1,943	2,103	2,293	2,539	2,904	3,0
38	60	90	2,585.0	382.9	1,948	2,100	2,383	2,542	2,797	3,117	
40	6	100	2,872.0	387.4	2,322	2,322	2,631	2,904	3,002	3,470	

From Min SJ, Luke B, Gillespie B, et al. Birthweight references for twins. *Am J Obstet Gynecol* 2000; 182:1250–1257, with permission.

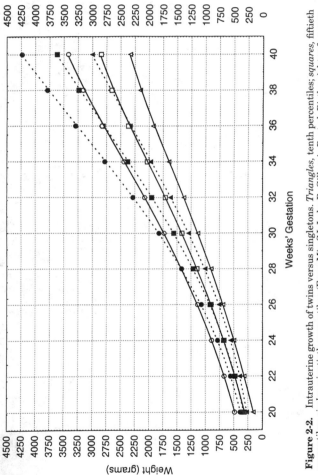

Figure 2-2. Intrauterine growth of twins versus singletons. *Triangles*, tenth percentiles; *squares*, fiftieth percentiles; *circles*, ninetieth percentiles. (From Min SJ, Luke B, Gillespie B, et al. Birthweight references for twins. *Am J Obstet Gynecol* 2000; 182:1250–1257, with permission.)

Weeks	24-5	26-7	28-9	30-1	32-3	34-5	36-7	38-9	40-1	>41	Weight
4900											4900
4600								3.9	2.1	2.3	4600
4300								1.9	1.3	1.8	4300
4000							3.3	1.2	1.0	1.4	4000
3700							2.4	0.9	1.0	1.5	3700
3400						3.2	2.4	1.1	1.1	1.6	3400
3100						5.5	2.8	1.4	1.5	2.0	3100
2800					7.0	9.6	3.9	2.2	2.4	2.8	2800
2500					13.2	15.4	7.1	4.4	4.9	5.2	2500
2200				23.3	21.2	30.2	15.1	11.2	12.2	13.1	2200
1900			53.6	40.4	32.3	67.3	33.9	28.6	26.5		1900
1600		75.1	78.5	47.6	54.3	138.6	78.8				1600
1300	163.6	108.0	72.0	74.5	112.4						1300
1000	210.4	101.8	103.5	155.6	231.4						1000
700	189.1	165.0	241.4	313.6	384.9						700
500	346.4	386.9	486.8	555.1							500
	24-5	26-7	28-9	30-1	32-3	34-5	36-7	38-9	40-1	>41	

Figure 2-3.   Relative risk of fetal death for singletons according to birth weight and gestational age. Double border, lowest risk birth weight–gestational age combination. Shaded area, higher risk birth weight–gestational age combinations. (Adapted from Luke B. Reducing fetal deaths in multiple births: optimal birthweights and gestational ages for infants of twin and triplet births. *Acta Genet Med Gemellol (Roma)* 1996;45:333–348, with permission.)

Weeks	24-5	26-7	28-9	30-1	32-3	34-5	36-7	38-9	40-1	>41	Weight
3400											3400
3100								1.8	2.3	4.1	3100
2800						2.7	2.3	1.7	1.7	3.5	2800
2500					3.3	1.8	1.3	1.4	1.7	2.9	2500
2200				6.7	2.8	1.3	1.0	1.2	2.3	3.4	2200
1900			9.1	6.0	2.8	1.5	1.8	2.7	3.7	5.3	1900
1600			6.8	5.3	2.8	2.7	3.7	5.9	6.7	9.2	1600
1300		17.5	7.3	7.9	4.3	5.2	10.1	13.1	18.4	24.5	1300
1000	49.4	18.1	12.8	18.3	11.0	18.9	29.6	35.0	23.6		1000
700	28.0	21.8	35.4	65.5	31.9	42.8					700
500	55.3	68.5	81.1	70.4	67.5						500
	24-5	26-7	28-9	30-1	32-3	34-5	36-7	38-9	40-1	>41	

Figure 2-4. Relative risk of fetal death for twins according to birth weight and gestational age. (Adapted from Luke B. Reducing fetal deaths in multiple births: optimal birthweights and gestational ages for infants of twin and triplet births. *Acta Genet Med Gemellol (Roma)* 1996;45:333–348, with permission.)

Weeks	24-5	26-7	28-9	30-1	32-3	34-5	36-7	38-9	40-1	>41	Weight
3400											3400
3100											3100
2800						5.3	4.2	7.4	22.5		2800
2500					8.0	2.7	1.8	6.1	15.1	38.2	2500
2200					2.9	1.3	1.7	3.6	11.4	24.9	2200
1900				3.2	1.3	1.0	1.5	3.0	7.8	19.1	1900
1600			4.3	2.1	1.3	1.4	4.2	8.8	14.7	23.9	1600
1300		5.6	3.0	2.2	2.3	4.7	10.4	11.6	17.9	52.1	1300
1000		7.1	3.0	4.6	6.6	10.5	15.3	25.5			1000
700	6.0	5.8	6.2	4.8	29.4	40.9					700
500	14.1	20.1	32.9								500
	24-5	26-7	28-9	30-1	32-3	34-5	36-7	38-9	40-1	>41	

Figure 2-5. Relative risk of fetal death for triplets and more according to birth weight and gestational age. (Adapted from Luke B. Reducing fetal deaths in multiple births: optimal birthweights and gestational ages for infants of twin and triplet births. *Acta Genet Med Gemellol (Roma)* 1996;45:333–348, with permission.)

eased to 420 g at 35 weeks and 610 g by 40 weeks. In describing ata on the 3,072 neonates in the Louisville Twin Study, Wilson (36) also found that from 31 weeks' gestation onward twin weight decreased progressively behind that of singletons so that by 38 weeks the singleton tenth percentile was equivalent to the twin fiftieth percentile, and the singleton fiftieth percentile was equivalent to the twin ninetieth percentile.

In a study of 15,902 twin births in New York City between 1978 and 1984, Kiely (32) found that twins born at 40 weeks' gestation and later were actually lighter than those born at 38 to 39 weeks, suggesting that for twins intrauterine growth stops after 39 weeks. In a study of all births in California between 1970 and 1976, Williams et al. (35) concluded that the peak growth rate in weight was about 250 g/week at 33 weeks for singletons compared to 175 g/week at 31 weeks for multiples.

Birth weight–specific mortality rates also vary widely between twins and singletons. Williams et al. (35) found that for birth weights of 1,251 to 2,500 g, the perinatal mortality rates for multiples were two to three times lower than for singletons, reversing above 2,750 g. Kiely (32) reported that for birth weights between 1,001 and 2,500 g, twins had birth weight–specific mortality rates equivalent to or substantially lower than those for singletons, even after adjusting for gestational age. Twins heavier than 3,000 g had much higher mortality rates. Among all twins in this study (32), perinatal mortality was 70% higher for infants with birth weights above 3,000 grams compared to infants with birth weights between 2,500 and 3,000 g.

Other investigators have reported similar findings. In a British study of 38,413 multiple births (of which 25,515 were twins), Botting et al. (50) found that for birth weights under 2,500 g, twins had significantly lower perinatal mortality rates than did singletons; between 2,500 and 3,499 g the rates were comparable, and for birth weights of 3,500 g and above, singletons had the survival advantage. Fabre et al. (51), in an analysis of the Spanish Perinatal Mortality National Survey, which included 1,956 twin births, also found lower perinatal mortality rates for twins compared to singletons at birth weights below 2,500 g.

Risk of Perinatal Morbidity and Mortality

Twin birth weights at or below the singleton tenth percentile for gestational age are associated with increased perinatal morbidity and mortality than are weights above the tenth percentile. Guaschino et al. (52), in a study of 194 pairs of twins born between 1974 and 1985 in Italy, found a relative risk of perinatal death of 4.8 for twins with birth weights below the singleton tenth percentile. In a Michigan study of 131 pairs of twins, Bronsteen et al. (53) found that birth weights at or below the singleton tenth percentile were associated with significantly higher morbidity, including the need for intensive postnatal therapy (umbilical artery catheterization), cardiovascular compromise (shock), and severe respiratory disease (days on greater than 40% oxygen). The financial costs of hospitalization of twins have been shown to increase geometrically with decreasing birth weight and gestational age (38,54).

The lower birth weight–specific mortality of twins with birth weights below 2,500 g, even after adjustment for gestational age may be due to the greater maturity of these infants com, singletons at equivalent weight. Several studies have s that the maturation process among twins is triggered earr among singletons. Using the lecithin to sphingomyelin (L/S, Leveno et al. (55) evaluated fetal lung maturation in 84 twir 137 singleton pregnancies. An L/S ratio exceeding 2, indicat maturity, was achieved between 34 and 36 weeks among singr tons compared to 31 to 32 weeks among twins. As discussed earlier, Ohel et al. (19) compared sonographically determined placental gradings of 158 twin and 474 singleton pregnancies at different gestational ages. Using a grading classification of I to III, these investigators found that at each gestational age from 29 weeks on, the proportion of grade III placentas was significantly greater among twins, suggesting different rates of maturation in these two groups.

CLINICAL CONSIDERATIONS AND KEY POINTS

- The actual incidence of twinning may be as high as 53.9/1,000 conceptions, but due to early losses ("vanishing twins"), the incidence of twin births is about 3.2/1,000 for monozygotic twins and 1.3 to 45/1,000 for dizygotic twins.
- An estimated one-third of twins are identical, and two-thirds are fraternal; among fraternal twins one-half are boy/girl, one-fourth girl/girl, and one-fourth boy/boy.
- Among monozygotic twin pregnancies, 65% have diamniotic, dichorionic placental membranes; 30% have diamniotic, monochorionic placental membranes; and 5% have monoamniotic, monochorionic placental membranes.
- Factors associated with dizygotic twinning include advancing maternal age (with higher levels of gonadotropins), genetic effects through the maternal lineage, and administration of FSH and clomiphene.
- Accelerated aging occurs in multiple pregnancies, as do a higher proportion of placental complications, including acute chorioamnionitis, premature rupture of membranes, large placental infarction, and placental abruption.
- Abnormal umbilical cord insertions occur more frequently in multiple pregnancies and are associated with a higher risk of vasa previa, TTS, and congenital anomalies.
- The intrauterine growth of twins diverges from that of singletons at the tenth percentile by 28 weeks, at the fiftieth percentile by 30 weeks, and at the ninetieth percentile by 34 weeks.
- The peak rate of growth of twins occurs between 34 and 36 weeks (166.5 g/week) compared with 36 to 38 weeks for singletons (225 g/week).
- The optimal combination of birth weight and gestation associated with the lowest risk of fetal death is 2,500 to 2,800 g at 36 to 37 weeks for twins and 1,900 to 2,100 g at 34 to 35 weeks for triplets.

REFERENCES

1. Landy HJ, Weiner S, Corson SL, et al. The "vanishing twin": ultrasonographic assessment of fetal disappearance in the first trimester. *Am J Obstet Gynecol* 1986;155:14–19.

3. Monozygous double inner cell masses in mouse blasto-following fertilization in vitro and in vivo. *J In Vitro Fert ryo Transf* 1990;7:177–179.
u YC. Monozygotic twin formation in mouse embryos in vitro. *cience* 1980;209:605–606.
Derom C, Derom R, Vlietinck R, et al. Increased monozygotic twinning rate after ovulation induction. *Lancet* 1987;1:1236–1238.

5. Edwards RG, Mettler L, Walters DE. Identical twins and in vitro fertilization. *J In Vitro Fert Embryo Transf* 1986;3:114–117.

6. Wenstrom KD, Syrop CH, Hammitt DG, et al. Increased risk of monochorionic twinning associated with assisted reproduction. *Fertil Steril* 1993;60:510–514.

7. Yovich JL, Stanger JD, Grauaug A, et al. Monozygotic twins from in vitro fertilization. *Fertil Steril* 1984;41:833–837.

8. Nylander PPS. Serum levels of gonadotrophins in relation to multiple pregnancy in Nigeria. *J Obstet Gynaecol Br Commonw* 1973;80:651–653.

9. Soma H, Takayama M, Kiyokawa T, et al. Serum gonadotropin levels in Japanese women. *Obstet Gynecol* 1975;46:311–312.

10. Martin NG, Olsen ME, Theile H, et al. Pituitary–ovarian function in mothers who have had two sets of dizygotic twins. *Fertil Steril* 1984;41:878–880.

11. Andrews MC, Muasher SJ, Levy DL, et al. An analysis of the obstetric outcome of 125 consecutive pregnancies conceived in vitro and resulting in 100 deliveries. *Am J Obstet Gynecol* 1986; 154:848–854.

12. Derom C, Bakker E, Vlietinck R, et al. Zygosity determination in newborn twins using DNA variants. *J Med Genet* 1985;22:279–282.

13. Kovacs B, Shahbahrami B, Platt LD, et al. Molecular genetic prenatal determination of twin zygosity. *Obstet Gynecol* 1988;72: 954–956.

14. Pinar H, Sung CJ, Oyer CE, et al. Reference values for singleton and twin placental weights. *Pediatr Pathol Lab Med* 1996;16: 901–907.

15. Naeye RL. Do placental weights have clinical significance? *Hum Pathol* 1987;18:387–391.

16. Naeye RL. Functionally important disorders of the placenta, umbilical cord, and fetal membranes. *Hum Pathol* 1987;18: 680–691.

17. Moore VM, Miller AG, Boulton TJC, et al. Placental weight, birth measurements, and blood pressure at age 8 years. *Arch Dis Child* 1996;74:538–541.

18. Falkner F. Twin growth in relationship to placentation. In: Falkner F, Tanner JM, eds. *Human growth: a comprehensive treatise,* 2d ed. Vol. 3. New York: Plenum Press, 1986:213–220.

19. Ohel G, Granat M, Zeevi D, et al. Advanced ultrasonic placental maturation in twin pregnancies. *Am J Obstet Gynecol* 1987; 156:76–78.

20. Barss VA, Benacerraf BR, Frigoletto FD. Ultrasonographic determination of chorion type in twin gestation. *Obstet Gynecol* 1985; 66:779–783.

21. D'Alton ME, Dudley DK. The ultrasonographic prediction of chorionicity in twin gestation. *Am J Obstet Gynecol* 1989;160:557–561.

22. Winn HN, Gabrielli S, Reece EA, et al. Ultrasonographic criteria for the prenatal diagnosis of placental chorionicity in twin gestations. *Am J Obstet Gynecol* 1989;161:1540–1542.

23. Monteagudo A, Timor-Tritsch IE, Sharma S. Early ar. determination of chorionic and amniotic type in multifeta tions in the first fourteen weeks by high-frequency transv ultrasonography. *Am J Obstet Gynecol* 1994;170:824–829.
24. Malinowski W. Very early and simple determination of choric and amniotic type in twin gestations by high-frequency trar. vaginal ultrasonography. *Acta Genet Med Gemellol (Roma)* 1997, 46:167–173.
25. Sepulveda W, Sebire NJ, Odibo A, et al. Prenatal determination of chorionicity in triplet pregnancy by ultrasonographic examination of the ipsilon zone. *Obstet Gynecol* 1996;88:855–858.
26. Robinson LK, Jones KL, Benirschke K. The nature of structural defects associated with velamentous and marginal insertion of the umbilical cord. *Am J Obstet Gynecol* 1983;146:191–193.
27. Benirschke K. Major pathologic features of the placenta, cord, and membranes. *Birth Defects* 1965;1:52–63.
28. Ramos-Arroyo MA, Ulbright TM, Yu PL, et al. Twin study: relationship between birth weight, zygosity, placentation, and pathologic placental changes. *Acta Genet Med Gemellol (Roma)* 1988; 37:229–238.
29. Heifetz SA. Single umbilical artery: a statistical analysis of 237 autopsy cases. *Lab Invest* 1983;48:6P(abst).
30. van Gemert MJC, Sterenborg HJCM. Haemodynamic model of twin–twin transfusion syndrome in monochorionic twin pregnancies. *Placenta* 1998;19:195–208.
31. McKeown T, Record R. Observations on fetal growth in multiple pregnancy. *J Endocrinol* 1952;8:386–401.
32. Kiely JL. The epidemiology of perinatal mortality in multiple births. *Bull NY Acad Med* 1990;66:618–637.
33. Luke B. Reducing fetal deaths in multiple births: optimal birthweights and gestational ages for infants of twin and triplet births. *Acta Genet Med Gemellol (Roma)* 1996;45:333–348.
34. Leroy B, Lefort F, Neveu P, et al. Intrauterine growth charts for twin fetuses. *Acta Genet Med Gemellol* 1982;31:199–206.
35. Williams R, Creasy RK, Cunningham GC, et al. Fetal growth and perinatal viability in California. *Obstet Gynecol* 1982;59:624–632.
36. Wilson RS. Growth and development of human twins. In: Falkner F, Tanner JM, eds. *Human growth: a comprehensive treatise,* 2d ed. Vol. 3. New York: Plenum Press, 1986:197–211.
37. Collins M, Bleyl J. Seventy-one quadruplet pregnancies. *Am J Obstet Gynecol* 1990;162:1384–1392.
38. Luke B, Minogue J, Witter FR. The role of fetal growth restriction and gestational age on length of hospital stay in twin infants. *Obstet Gynecol* 1993;81:949–953.
39. Luke B, Minogue J, Witter FR, et al. The ideal twin pregnancy: patterns of weight gain, discordancy, and length of gestation. *Am J Obstet Gynecol* 1993;169:588–597.
40. Fabris C, Licato D, Garzena E, et al. In-vitro fertilisation and intra-uterine growth retardation. *Paediatr Perinat Epidemiol* 1990;4:243–245.
41. Luke B, Bryan E, Sweetland C, et al. Prenatal weight gain and the birthweight of triplets. *Acta Genet Med Gemellol (Roma)* 1995;44:93–101.
42. Wilcox A, Skjoerven R. Birth weight and perinatal mortality: the effect of gestational age. *Am J Public Health* 1992;82:378–382.

...des J, Scher A, Itzkovits J, et al. Growth and development of ...dren conceived by in vitro fertilization. *Pediatrics* 1992;90: .4–429.

...Min SJ, Luke B, Gillespie B, et al. Birthweight references for twins. *Am J Obstet Gynecol* 2000;182:1250–1257.

.. Hadlock FP, Harrist RB, Martinez-Poyer J. In utero analysis of fetal growth: a sonographic weight standard. *Radiology* 1991;181: 129–133.

46. Luke B, Minogue J. Contribution of gestational age and birth weight to perinatal viability in singletons versus twins. *J Matern Fetal Med* 1994;3:263–274.

47. Hoffman HJ, Stark CR, Lundin FE, et al. Analysis of birth weight, gestational age, and fetal viability, US births, 1968. *Obstet Gynecol Surv* 1974;29:651–681.

48. Koops BL, Morgan LJ, Battaglia FC. Neonatal mortality risk in relation to birth weight and gestational age: update. *J Pediatr* 1982;101:969–977.

49. Luke B, Witter FR, Abbey H, et al. Gestational age–specific birth-weights of twins versus singletons. *Acta Genet Med Gemellol (Roma)* 1991;40:69–76.

50. Botting BJ, MacDonald Davies I, MacFarlane AJ. Recent trends in the incidence of multiple births and associated mortality. *Arch Dis Child* 1987;62:941–950.

51. Fabre E, Gonzalez de Aguero R, de Agustin JL, et al. Perinatal mortality in twin pregnancy: an analysis of birthweight-specific mortality rates and adjusted mortality rates for birth weight distributions. *J Perinat Med* 1988;16:85–91.

52. Guaschino S, Spinillo A, Stola E, et al. Growth retardation, size at birth and perinatal mortality in twin pregnancy. *Int J Gynaecol Obstet* 1987;25:399–403.

53. Bronsteen R, Goyert G, Bottoms S. Classification of twins and neonatal morbidity. *Obstet Gynecol* 1989;74:98–101.

54. Luke B, Bigger H, Leurgans S, et al. The costs of prematurity: a case–control study of twins versus singletons. *Am J Public Health* 1996;86:809–814.

55. Leveno KJ, Quirk JG, Whalley PJ, et al. Fetal lung maturation in twin gestation. *Am J Obstet Gynecol* 1984;148:405–411.

Genetic Diagnosis in Multiple Gestations

The increasing role of genetic diagnosis in both prenatal and general medicine is unquestioned. Genetic diagnosis will prove to be the medical frontier of the next millennium. Prenatal genetic diagnosis in multiple gestations presents numerous challenges because of the unique characteristics of these pregnancies. Genetic diagnosis in multiple gestations begins with experienced and professional genetic counseling. Specific issues of importance in the counseling of these couples include the impact of chorionicity and zygosity on prenatal diagnosis, the increased technical risks associated with prenatal diagnosis in multiples, the need for experienced operators and advanced ultrasound capabilities, and the qualitatively more difficult counseling associated with the discovery of discordant abnormal results including the consideration of selective termination.

Invasive prenatal diagnosis in twin gestations requires a technique that can reliably sample each fetus and provide accurate karyotypes and other genetic information. In addition, it must be acceptably safe. Safety is a major concern because of the inherently higher risks associated with multiple gestations and the greater operator skill required to evaluate two or more fetuses. The reliability and safety of invasive prenatal diagnosis are enhanced by the addition of skilled, high-resolution ultrasound guidance.

Successful prenatal genetic diagnosis also requires a genetic consultant who is experienced, fully informed, and confident in dealing with multiple gestation pregnancies. It requires counselors who are familiar with the testing techniques and can provide a supportive testing environment. Those working in this environment must be familiar with the psychological impact of a multiple pregnancy complicated by a genetic abnormality. Prenatal genetic diagnosis in multiple gestations should always include a consultation with an experienced and professional genetic counselor.

INDICATIONS FOR GENETIC DIAGNOSIS

Advanced Maternal Age

Approximately one-third of the increase in the frequency of multiple gestations in the United States has been attributed to the sociological phenomenon of delayed maternal childbearing. The peak of dizygotic twinning occurs at approximately 35 years of age, which also is the maternal age at which prenatal diagnostic testing has traditionally been offered due to the increased risk of age-related chromosomal nondisjunction.

Contrary to some previous reports, there is no convincing evidence that the risk of chromosomal aneuploidy is inherently increased in multiple gestations (1,2). These previous reports had failed to consider the differences in maternal age distribution between singleton and twin gestations. The apparent increase in the risk of chromosomal abnormality among multiples disappears when the association between dizygotic twinning and maternal age is considered.

zygotic gestations, all fetuses have the same karyotype,
...sk of aneuploidy is identical to the maternal age-related
. singleton gestation. There are rare reports of monozygotic
that have discordant karyotypes. This most commonly in-
...es the sex chromosomes and probably represents early mitotic
...disjunction followed by twinning (3–5).

In dizygotic gestations, each fetus has its own individual and independent risk of aneuploidy. The risk that at least one dizygotic twin fetus has a chromosomal abnormality is additive, that is, twice that of a singleton pregnancy. The probability that both fetuses are aneuploid, however, is the product of the individual risks. As a result, the likelihood that both dizygotic fetuses would be affected is extremely small. By far, the more common scenario is for one dizygotic fetus to be aneuploid while the other is normal.

Although zygosity can frequently be determined early in pregnancy, this is not always the case. On these occasions, counseling may be predicated on the assumption that in the United States about one-third of twin pregnancies are monozygotic and two-thirds are dizygotic. This ratio may vary somewhat based on population ethnicity, maternal age, and prevalence of use of assisted reproductive technology. The empiric risk of aneuploidy for a twin gestation of unknown zygosity is based on the maternal age-related risk of x and can be calculated as follows (6):

$$\frac{1}{3} x \left[\text{monozygotic}\right] + \frac{2}{3}(2x)\left[\text{dizygotic}\right]$$

According to this formula, the risk of aneuploidy in a twin gestation of unknown zygosity is approximately 5/3 that of the single-ton age-related risk. The practical significance of this calculation is that women older than 30 years with twins have approximately the same risk of aneuploidy as a woman 2 years older carrying a singleton gestation (Table 3-1). As a result, prenatal diagnosis is commonly offered to women carrying twins at the age of 33 years (7).

Table 3-1. **Quantitative risk of aneuploidy among dichorionic twins and twins of unknown zygosity compared with singletons, by maternal age**

Maternal Age (yr)	Risk of Aneuploidy		
	Singletons	Twin: Unknown Zygosity	Twin: Dichorionic
20	1/1,667	1/1,000	1/835
25	1/1,250	1/750	1/625
30	1/952	1/570	1/475
33	1/625	1/375	1/315
35	1/385	1/231	1/190
40	1/106	1/64	1/50

From Hook EB. Rates of chromosomal abnormalities of different maternal ages. *Obstet Gynecol* 1981;58:282–285, with permission.

Because ultrasonography allows determination of zygosity in a large percentage of cases, more specific estimates of aneuploid risk can be given to parents. For twins known to be monozygotic, the risk is the same as the maternal age-related risk (x). Twins known to be dizygotic have a 2x risk that either twin may be affected. The risk of both dizygotic twins being affected would be x^2. For example, a woman with an age-related risk of 1 in 150 for giving birth to a singleton Down syndrome infant would carry that same risk if she were pregnant with monozygotic twins. If she were pregnant with dizygotic twins, her risk of having at least one affected infant would be 1 in 75 $\left(\dfrac{1}{150} + \dfrac{1}{150} \right)$. While the risk of both dizygotic twins being affected would only be 1 in 22,500 $\left(\dfrac{1}{150} \times \dfrac{1}{150} \right)$.

Abnormal Maternal Serum α-Fetoprotein Screening

The role of maternal serum α-fetoprotein (MSAFP) screening in multiple gestations for the detection of fetal aneuploidy is best described as investigational. There have been no prospective studies of the sensitivity of Down syndrome screening with maternal age and multiple serum markers in multiple gestations. Several investigators have reported levels of α-fetoprotein, unconjugated estriol, and human chorionic gonadotropin in twins and have related them to singleton values. A composite of these studies suggests that the α-fetoprotein serum level in twins is 2.04 times that of a singleton, the unconjugated estriol level 1.64 times greater, and the human chorionic gonadotropin level 1.93 times greater (8). Theoretically, one could calculate an aneuploidy risk in twins by expressing the maternal serum analyte value for the twin gestation as a multiple of the singleton median and then divide that value by the respective multiple of the median for a normal twin, as described earlier. These derived twin multiples of the median could then be used to calculate a Down syndrome risk. With this theoretical construct, it is estimated that approximately 5% of twin pregnancies would screen positive and that almost one-half of the Down syndrome fetuses would be detected, which is similar to the current experience with multiple-marker Down syndrome screening of singletons (9,10). A retrospective review of maternal serum analyte values of 420 twins and 6,661 singleton pregnancies by Spencer et al. revealed a sensitivity for trisomy 21 of 51% with an "acceptable" 5% false-positive rate (11).

What constitutes an "acceptable" false-positive rate, however, has to be considered in the context of a number of other considerations that would not be issues in a singleton gestation. In the absence of a suggestive ultrasound finding, there is no way to target a specific fetus for invasive diagnostic testing. As a result, invasive testing will be required for both fetuses. Such testing is technically more involved and is associated with a greater risk, as will be discussed later. In addition, if the twins are discordant for chromosomal aneuploidy, difficult counseling would be required to determine continuing pregnancy management.

MSAFP screening has also been used to identify patients with fetal anomalies such as neural tube and abdominal wall defects.

In singleton gestations, an MSAFP value greater than 2.5 multiples of median (MOM) identifies approximately 80% of open neural tube defects with a false-positive rate between 2% and 3.5%. The normal MSAFP value for twins, however, is approximately double that of singletons as a result of the proportionately increased placental mass (12,13). Consequently, an MSAFP value of greater than 2.5 MOM in a twin gestation would identify 99% of anencephalic fetuses and 89% of open neural tube defects but with an unacceptable 30% false-positive rate (14).

Table 3-2 presents data collected by Cuckle et al. (14) describing the risk of an open neural tube defect, detection rates, and false-positive rates in twin gestations by multiples of the singleton median for α-fetoprotein. Setting the MSAFP cutoff at 5.0 MOM for twin gestations reduced the false-positive rate to 3.3% but the detection rates for open neural tube defects would be significantly reduced (39%). In order to maintain a sensitivity for open neural tube defects similar to that seen in singleton gestations (approximately 80%), an MSAFP cutoff greater than 3.0 MOM would have to be used. Unfortunately, this cutoff also is associated with a troublesome false-positive rate of 19%. Although there is no universally accepted standard, many centers have settled on an MSAFP cutoff of greater than 4.0 MOM which would detect almost 60% of open neural tube defects with an 8% false-positive rate. The California MSAFP screening program has been even more successful. Using an MSAFP cutoff greater than 4.5 MOM, more than 85% of open neural tube defects were detected with only a 5% false-positive rate (15).

The relatively high serum screening false-positive rates in multiple gestations is ameliorated somewhat by the continually improving reliability of diagnostic ultrasonography. Despite the presence of multiple fetuses, the sensitivity and the positive predictive value of ultrasound for anomaly detection in experienced

Table 3-2. Detection (DR) and false-positive (FPR) rates for open neural tube defects in singleton and twin gestations using singleton maternal serum α-fetoprotein (AFP) cutoff values

AFP Value (multiples of singleton median)	Open Neural Tube Defects			
	Singleton		Twin	
	DR (%)	FPR (%)	DR (%)	FPR (%)
>2.0	85	8.2	96	46
>2.5	75	3.3	89	30
>3.0	65	1.4	80	19
>4.0	47	0.3	58	7.8
>4.5	—	—	48	5.0
>5.0	—	—	39	3.3
>6.0	—	—	25	1.4

From Cuckle H, Wald N, Stevenson J, et al. Maternal serum alpha-fetoprotein screening for open neural tube defects in twin pregnancies. *Prenat Diagn* 1990;10:71–77, with permission.

operators should be greater than 80% and 90% respec
Targeted ultrasonography should have a diagnostic acc
open neural tube defects well over 95%. The decision to ,
to amniocentesis for definitive diagnosis will require a bal.
of the reliability of ultrasound against the risk of amniocentes
twin gestations. In many centers, a negative targeted ultrasou.
examination has replaced the previously routine performance c
diagnostic amniocentesis. Amniocentesis is usually reserved for
those cases where fetal anatomy is suspicious or poorly visualized
and in some cases to confirm an apparent abnormal scan.

Interpretation of amniotic fluid α-fetoprotein and acetylcholinesterase levels in twin gestations can be tricky. If one fetus is
affected with an open neural tube defect, many authorities would
recommend that the co-twin be assessed as well since the coexisting fetus has a 2% to 5% risk of concordance. In diamniotic/
dichorionic twin gestations with a thick dividing membrane,
the amniotic fluid α-fetoprotein and acetylcholinesterase values
are independent and reliable for each fetus (17). In diamniotic/
monochorionic twins, however, α-fetoprotein and acetylcholinesterase may diffuse across the thin dividing membrane from one
sac to the other, making assessment of the co-twin unreliable. This
unreliability again underscores the need for comprehensive ultrasonographic evaluation.

Parental Carriers of Single-Gene Disorders

Another indication for prenatal diagnostic testing may be pregnancies at increased risk of single-gene disorders such as cystic
fibrosis, Tay-Sachs disease, Duchenne's muscular dystrophy, sickle
cell disease, and thalassemia. As previously discussed, this risk is
affected by whether or not the twin gestation is monozygotic or
dizygotic. If the twins are known to be monozygotic, both or neither
of the twins is affected. The risk that both are affected is the same
as for a singleton gestation if both parents are known to be carri-
ers: 1 in 4. If the twins are known to be dizygotic, then the risk of
both being affected is much less, as follows:

$$\frac{1}{4} \times \frac{1}{4} = \frac{1}{16}$$

The risk that only one fetus is affected, however, is higher, as
follows:

$$\frac{1}{4}\left(\frac{3}{4}\right) + \frac{1}{4}\left(\frac{3}{4}\right) = \frac{6}{16}$$

The risk that at least one fetus is affected out of a dizygotic twin
pair is $\frac{1}{16} + \frac{6}{16} = \frac{7}{16}$.

Calculations can also be made when zygosity is unknown, again,
with the assumption that one-third of twin gestations in the United
States are monozygotic and two-thirds are dizygotic. In that scenario, the risk that at least one fetus is affected can be calculated
as follows:

$$\frac{1}{3}\left(\frac{1}{4}\right) + \frac{2}{3}\left(\frac{7}{16}\right) = \frac{3}{8}$$

...that both fetuses are affected in the scenario of unknown ...can be calculated as follows:

$$\Big) + \frac{2}{3}\left(\frac{1}{16}\right) = \frac{1}{8}$$

Thickened Nuchal Translucency

Measurement of nuchal translucency thickness in the first trimester by ultrasound is a promising technique for detection of aneuploidy in both singleton and multiple pregnancies. It holds particular promise for multiple pregnancies because it provides an ultrasound marker as to which fetus may be affected and can be used early enough in pregnancy to allow selective termination of an affected fetus.

In singleton pregnancies, first-trimester nuchal translucency thickness combined with maternal age can be used to identify more than 80% of aneuploid fetuses with an acceptable false-positive rate of 5% (18). In 448 twin pregnancies scanned between 10 and 14 weeks by Sebire et al. (19), the fetal nuchal translucency measurement was greater than the ninety-fifth percentile of gestational age-specific singleton norms (based on fetal crown rump length) for 7.3% of twin fetuses, including 88% of twins with Down syndrome (19). The false-positive rate was higher for monochorionic fetuses (8.4%) than for dichorionic pregnancies (5.4%). Because a false-positive screening test result typically leads to an invasive diagnostic procedure with attendant risk, it is important to note that increased fetal nuchal translucency thickness was present in at least one fetus among 13.7% of monochorionic and 9% of dichorionic twin pairs (19).

Although the results of these investigations of fetal nuchal translucency thickness screening in twins are promising, the relatively high false-positive rates are concerning. Perhaps with larger sample sizes, particularly for monochorionic twins, better sensitivities and false-positive rates can be defined for potential use in general screening. Until results of such studies are available, general screening of twins for fetal nuchal translucency thickness remains investigational. Many centers use this technique to help guide decisions regarding multifetal pregnancy reduction in high-order multiples. An increased nuchal translucency measurement at the time of multifetal pregnancy reduction may help identify which fetus or fetuses should be targeted for the procedure. Although it does not eliminate the risk of leaving a fetus with chromosomal aneuploidy, this screening tool should reduce the risk substantially.

Other Indications

Other indications for prenatal diagnosis in multiple gestations are essentially the same as those for singleton pregnancies. These include a previous pregnancy with a chromosomal abnormality, a parental structural chromosomal rearrangement, known fetal anomalies, and in some cases, parental anxiety.

AMNIOCENTESIS

Traditional Technique

Prior to any prenatal diagnostic test, a detailed ultrasound evaluation should be performed by an experienced sonographer

Regardless of the trimester, the scan should include fetal bio try and a thorough anatomic survey of all fetuses. This anatom survey should include a measurement of the fetal nuchal transl cency in the first trimester and fetal sexing in the second tr mester as they may prove useful as fetal markers if aneuploidy is detected later. The position of each fetus, the number and location of each placenta, and the presence, location, and characteristics of the dividing membrane should be described. A conclusion as to the likely amnionicity, chorionicity, and zygosity should be drawn using the ultrasound characteristics described in Chapter 5. It is recommended that the operator draw a picture outlining the spatial relations between the fetus and the mother (right side or left side), the fetal presentation, and respective placental locations. Such a drawing may prove important because the relative positions of the twins are likely to change after the first or early second trimester.

Genetic amniocentesis is traditionally performed between 15 and 18 weeks of gestation using the technique initially described by Elias et al. (20). With this technique, a 20- or 22-gauge spinal needle is inserted under continuous ultrasound guidance into one of the twin sacs. Twenty milliliters of amnionic fluid is aspirated and labeled as to the corresponding twin. After aspiration of the first amniotic fluid sample, 1 to 2 cc of an inert dye (usually indigo carmine) diluted in 10 cc of sterile water is injected into the first sac followed by removal of the spinal needle. Using a second needle, the second amniotic fluid sac is entered, and a fluid sample is obtained, also under continuous ultrasound guidance. Aspiration of a clear amniotic fluid specimen from the second sac confirms sampling of the second fetus. Alternatively, aspiration of a dye-tinged amniotic fluid specimen suggests the inadvertent second sampling of the first sac. It is important to note however, that this may also be the result of a monoamniotic twin gestation, which should be reassessed ultrasonically in this situation. Another caution is that use of a large volume of undiluted dye may result in light blue coloration of the fluid in the second sac, particularly in monochorionic/diamniotic twins. With high concentrations, there may be transmembranous passage of dye after placement into the initial sac. With the normally employed small volumes (1 to 2 cc) of diluted dye, this has not been a clinical problem. Another caution that may allay a great deal of anxiety is to warn mothers that on rare occasion they may notice a blue tinge to their urine after intrauterine instillation of indigo carmine. Some investigators have suggested adding a small amount of air to the dye. When the dye is injected into the amnionic sac, microbubbles appear on the ultrasound scan and outline the sac. This technique may prove useful in confirming a suspected monoamniotic gestation because the microbubbles surround both fetuses (21).

Methylene blue was previously used by many clinicians as the amniotic fluid dye of choice. However, in the early 1990's, this practice was called into question with a series of reports noting an increased risk of fetal small bowel atresia following intraamniotic instillation of this dye. Nicolini and Monni reported that four (19%) of 21 twin amniocenteses performed between 15 and 17 weeks where methylene blue was used resulted in the birth of a child with small bowel atresia (22). Van der Pol et al. (23) reported on 86 twin gestations in The Netherlands in which methylene blue had been

during genetic amniocentesis. In 17 (19.8%) of the 86 twin
s, an infant was born with jejunal atresia. In 15 of the 17 cases,
e sac into which methylene blue was injected could be retrospec-
ively identified, and in each case that was the affected fetus. Van
der Pol et al. (23) also reviewed the obstetrical records of the 67 infants born with jejunal atresia in The Netherlands between 1986
and 1991. Of these 67, 20 (30%) were twins, and 19 of them had
undergone genetic amniocentesis. In these 19 genetic amniocenteses, methylene blue was used in 18 cases and indigo carmine in 1.
The effect on the small bowel may be a localized vasoconstriction
mediated by a methylene blue-induced increase in norepinephrine
and dopamine release from sympathetic nerves supplying the
mesentery and small bowel vessels (24). Another plausible expla-
nation may involve endothelial effects on the fetal small bowel from
exposure to swallowed methylene blue.

Other concerns associated with intraamniotic injection of methylene blue have been the occurrence of neonatal hemolytic anemia
and hyperbilirubinemia when the dye is used in the third trimester
(25,26). Third-trimester use of methylene blue to confirm rupture
of membranes also may cause fetal skin staining that is difficult to
discern from persistent neonatal cyanosis.

Indigo carmine is now the preferred dye for use in twin amniocentesis. Jejunal atresia in association with use of indigo carmine
has been reported in only one single case (23). Studies by Cragan
et al. (27) and Pruggmayer et al. (28) on 78 and 298 twin amniocenteses, respectively, in which indigo carmine was used also identified only one instance of small bowel atresia and no other cluster-
ing of congenital anomalies. Despite the apparent safety of indigo
carmine dye as a marker in twin amniocenteses, continued surveillance for fetal malformations is recommended because indigo
carmine does exhibit a mild vasoconstrictive effect when injected
intravenously (29).

Dye-free Techniques

Dye-free techniques have been proposed in order to avoid any
potential chemical or teratogenic risk. Because of the constantly
improving imaging capabilities of ultrasonography, some operators
choose to forego dye injection and rely entirely on ultrasound guidance to ensure that both sacs are separately sampled. Although
this approach is successful in the vast majority of cases, virtually
all operators have experienced the return of blue-tinged amniotic
fluid after feeling confident they had successfully entered the second sac. In the study by Van der Pol et al. (23), experienced operators aspirated dye-stained amniotic fluid in 3.5% of the attempts to
obtain fluid for the second twin. With a dye-free technique, this
repeated sampling of the first sac would be undetected, and genetic
evaluation of the second twin would not be performed.

Other proposed dye-free techniques include single needle insertion, dual needle simultaneous insertion, and the use of non-dye
amniotic fluid markers. The single needle technique involves insertion of a single spinal needle into the proximal sac near the insertion of the dividing membrane. Amniotic fluid is aspirated under
real-time ultrasound visualization, the stylet is reinserted, and the
needle is advanced until tenting of the dividing membrane is seen
The spinal needle is then further advanced until it pops throug

the dividing membrane and enters the second sac (30). D alization of the spinal needle's popping through the divid. brane confirms placement into the second sac.

In some cases the anatomic arrangement of the sacs m allow insertion of a single needle in proximity to the dividing n brane. Another limitation is potential contamination of the sec sample with cells from the first sac. Such contamination could the retically lead to an incorrect diagnosis of mosaicism in the second twin. Replacing the stylet after the first sampling and before advancing the needle minimizes this risk. A final concern is that puncture of the dividing membrane could result in a pseudomonoamniotic twin gestation. Progressive enlargement of the membrane defect may allow entanglement of the umbilical cords and the possibility of fetal loss. Such a case has been described after percutaneous umbilical blood sampling of a dichorionic twin with disruption of the dividing membrane in the second trimester (31). Although both twins survived, at birth there was a large defect in the dividing membrane between the sacs and extensive intertwining of the umbilical cords.

Bahado Singh et al. (32) described a dual needle technique with simultaneous insertion. With ultrasound, the dividing membrane is visualized, and with continuous ultrasound guidance a spinal needle is inserted into one sac and amniotic fluid is aspirated. While the first needle is left in place, a second needle is inserted into the second sac. Simultaneous visualization of both needle tips in separate sacs is believed to be satisfactory evidence that both amniotic sacs have been sampled. Disadvantages of this technique include the fact that multiple operators are required, it depends on occasionally confusing ultrasound visualization, and simultaneous needle insertion may be more than some women are prepared to tolerate.

The third approach entails use of a non-dye amniotic fluid marker. One such marker is the microbubble previously described. Another non-dye marker is a membrane-free hemolysate of maternal blood. Unfortunately, preparation of the latter marker is time consuming and complex. It involves sonication of red blood cells, centrifugation, and purification to remove the red blood cell membranes (33).

Efficacy and Reliability

The efficacy of twin amniocentesis approaches 100% with continuous ultrasound guidance. In a large multicenter European experience, successful sampling of both fetuses was achieved with dye instillation in 100% of 529 amniocenteses (28). Two U.S. studies showed 100% successful sampling in 73 and 101 twin pregnancies respectively (34,35). It is important to note that in monochorionic (monozygotic) twin gestations, sampling of both twins is still required even though both originate from the same zygote and should be genetically identical. Despite highly reliable ultrasound findings, it is impossible to be certain that a pregnancy is monozygotic. For example, what appears to be a single monochorionic placentation may prove to be a fused dichorionic placenta. In addition, early mitotic nondisjunction can result in monozygotic fetuses with discordant karyotypes. One of the more common scenarios is when an initially 46,XY monozygotic twin loses

osome during early mitotic replication. The monozygotic
d up being genetically and phenotypically different—one
male and the other a 45,X female (36).

other concern with interpretation of amniocentesis results
rs in monochorionic gestations with elevated amniotic fluid
fetoprotein values. The presence of an open fetal neural tube
defect is associated with an elevated amniotic fluid α-fetoprotein
level and a positive acetylcholinesterase. Typically, fewer than 10%
of twins are concordant for neural tube defects even if monozygotic.
In most cases, ultrasound examination allows adequate evaluation
of the co-twin's anatomy. Occasionally however, ultrasound may not
be sufficiently reliable, and evaluation of the second twin's amniotic
fluid α-fetoprotein may be required. In dichorionic twins, the intervening membrane is thicker, and both amniotic fluid α-fetoprotein
and acetylcholinesterase levels are reliable (17). However, for monochorionic twins, the thinner diamniotic membrane allows equili-
bration of the amniotic fluid α-fetoprotein and acetylcholinesterase
levels, resulting in false-positive values in the sac of the unaffected
co-twin.

Safety

The risk of genetic amniocentesis of twins is believed to be higher
than that of singleton amniocentesis. Perinatal mortality rates
associated with a singleton amniocentesis were reported in multicenter comparison of amniocentesis and chorionic villus sampling
(CVS) sponsored by the National Institute of Child Health and
Human Development (37). In this trial, the perinatal mortality
rate after singleton amniocentesis was 7.9/1,000, somewhat lower
than the 17.0/1,000 reported by Tabor et al. in the largest single-
center experience reported in the literature (38). In another large
single-center experience, reported by Anderson et al. (39), 330 twin
gestations were sampled with a corresponding perinatal loss rate
of 3.6% up to 28 weeks' gestation. However, the operators did not
routinely employ continuous ultrasound guidance.

In six reports of genetic amniocentesis of twin gestations (Table
3-3) in which continuous ultrasound guidance was routinely
employed, the success rate was 100% in every experience. The loss
rates prior to 20 weeks ranged between 0 and 6.1%, whereas the
loss rates prior to 28 weeks ranged from 2.3% to 8.1% (28,34,35,
40–42). The composite loss rate by 20 weeks' gestation was 2.3%
and 4.1% by 28 weeks. In all the studies cited, the fetal loss rate by
28 weeks appears to be several times higher than that experienced
by singleton gestations undergoing amniocentesis. It is difficult to
determine, however, whether this increased loss rate is procedure
related or reflects the inherently increased risk of very early preterm delivery in multifetal gestations.

No results of randomized, controlled trials of twin amniocentesis have been reported, so it is impossible to accurately determine the procedure-related versus background loss rates. Reported
loss rates for twins prior to 28 weeks' gestation after normal results
of a second-trimester ultrasound examination without amniocentesis range between 4.5% and 7.2%. These rates are very similar to the 28-week loss rates reported after twin amniocentesis
(43–45). Although the sample was not randomized, Ghidini et al.
(35) included an unsampled control group with a normal second-

Table 3-3. Efficacy and safety of twin amniocentesis performed with the use of continuous ultrasound guidance

Reference	Years of Procedure	n	Success Rate (%)	Loss Rate to 20 Weeks (%)	Loss Rate to 28 Weeks (%)
Pruggmayer et al. (40)	1982–89	98	100	6.1	8.1
Pruggmayer et al. (28)	1981–90	529	100	2.4	3.7
Wapner et al. (34)	1984–90	73	100	1.8	2.9
Ghidini et al. (35)	1987–92	101	100	0.0	3.0
Buscaglia et al. (41)	1985–95	55	100	—	4.4
Sebire et al. (42)	1987–95	176	100	1.1	2.3
Total		1,032	100	2.3	4.1

trimester ultrasound findings which they compared to their 101 twin amniocenteses (35). The two groups were similar with the exception of the amniocentesis group being older. Both groups had a fetal loss rate of 2% at 25 weeks' gestation and there were no significant differences in the loss rates at 28 weeks (3.5% versus 3.2%, respectively) (35).

Palle et al. (46) were able to relate the post-amniocentesis loss rate to the number of needle insertions. They reported a 22% loss rate for twins with at least two punctures in one or more sacs, 15% with one puncture of each sac, 6% when only one sac was punctured because of an undetected twin pregnancy, and 3% for singletons undergoing amniocentesis (47).

Despite the limitations and uncertainties in the available literature, we currently counsel patients undergoing twin amniocentesis that the procedure-related risk may be slightly higher than that of singleton amniocentesis. We tell patients the procedure-related risk is approximately 1%, which is superimposed on an increased background loss rate prior to 28 weeks' gestation. Although there are relatively few data, it seems likely that postprocedure loss rates would be even higher following early amniocentesis. For singleton gestations, amniocentesis performed before 13 weeks' gestation is associated with an increased risk of amniotic fluid leakage, clubbed feet, and fetal loss. It is anticipated that these risks would be magnified for multiple gestation.

CHORIONIC VILLUS SAMPLING

Technique

Another alternative for prenatal genetic diagnosis in twins is chorionic villus sampling. Chorionic villus sampling (CVS) has proven to be an efficacious and safe alternative to amniocentesis

LIBRARY, UNIVERSITY OF CHEST

in singletons and has the added advantage of being a first-trimester procedure. Centers experienced in the performance of CVS in singletons have successfully expanded this technique to prenatal diagnosis for twins.

As with amniocentesis, a preliminary ultrasound should be performed to confirm the viability of each fetus and to assess gestational age by means of measurement of fetal crown-rump length. The number and location of each placenta should be identified and carefully documented, as well as the location and thickness of the dividing membrane. CVS is performed between 10.0 and 12.9 weeks and can be performed with either a transcervical or transabdominal approach. Selective sampling of the chorion frondosum of each fetus will often require the combination of both aspiration methods. In one study of 101 twins, CVS was performed transcervically on both fetuses in 36 pregnancies (35%), transabdominally on both fetuses in 28 pregnancies (23%), and required a combined approach in 44 pregnancies (42%) (47).

CVS is most reliably performed when separate placental sites can be identified. As the procedure is performed, the location of the catheter or needle tip must be meticulously followed by means of ultrasound to ensure that each chorion frondosum is individually sampled. In those cases where the placentas are not anatomically separate, CVS becomes more problematic with no technique available to ensure that both fetuses are sampled separately. When the placentas are fused or the twins are identical with a single placenta, the CVS catheter or needle tip should be placed in close proximity to the umbilical cord insertion sites prior to aspiration. When the umbilical cord insertion sites are in close proximity or cannot be identified, opposite ends of the placenta should be sampled. Another approach is to take only a single sample if it is strongly believed that the placentation is monochorionic and therefore monozygotic.

Each alternative technique runs an increasing risk of failure to sample each fetus separately. With some of these latter approaches as well as in the case of chromosomal mosaicism, a second-trimester amniocentesis may be necessary to clarify the findings. If the presence of same-sex dichorionic twins is diagnosed from two different chorionic tissue specimens and no polymorphic markers exist that allow differentiation of the samples, then later confirmation by means of amniocentesis may be advisable. Because of the earlier gestational age at which CVS is performed, there is also a greater risk of fetal aneuploidy. In a study by Wapner et al. (34), fetal aneuploidy occurred among 3.1% of fetuses and 5.7% of pregnancies. Because of the possibility of discordant results, it is imperative that the location and characteristics of each fetus be described and documented for future reference.

Efficacy and Reliability

A significant limitation of CVS for twins is the potential contamination of one sample with villi from the other twin. This can occur when sampling is performed from a location near the dividing membrane, which may contain villi from the chorion frondosum of each twin. For this reason, the optimal sampling site is believed to be at the umbilical cord insertion site and away from the membranous interface. Contamination can also occur when the cath-

LIBRARY, UNIVERSITY OF CHEST

eter or needle must pass through one placenta in order to sample the other. An admixture of chorionic villi from the more proximal lying chorion frondosum can occur during aspiration of the more distal placenta. The complementary use of both transcervical and transabdominal CVS can obviate traversing one placenta to sample the other in some cases.

Twin-twin contamination during CVS complicates approximately 4% of samples (48). To avoid diagnostic errors, the laboratory needs to be aware of this potential for twin-twin contamination. Even with a mixed sample, aneuploidy can obviously still be identified. When a mixture of XX and XY cells occurs, the situation can often be clarified by follow-up ultrasound examination rather than requiring a second-trimester amniocentesis. However, cases of complete twin-twin cell contamination in which one twin is sampled twice and the co-twin is not sampled at all remains a risk that is substantially higher with CVS than with twin amniocentesis. Diagnostic errors occurred in 2 of 161, 2 of 256, and 2 of 104 multiple gestations undergoing CVS in the series of Wapner et al. (34), DeCatte et al. (47), and Pergament et al. (48), respectively. It should also be noted that a mixed cell culture will invalidate a biochemical analysis because cells from the unaffected fetus may normalize the biochemical results obtained from the cells of the affected fetus.

Due to the inability in some cases to be certain that both placentas have been sampled separately, the procedure of choice for fetal karyotyping in twin pregnancies remains second-trimester amniocentesis. However, when the risk of chromosomal aneuploidy may be unusually high (maternal age 40 years or older, parental chromosomal translocation, abnormal fetal nuchal translucency measurements), CVS may be preferable in that earlier diagnosis may allow for a safer selective termination if an abnormality is found (49). Selective termination after 16 weeks of gestation is associated with a threefold increased risk of fetal loss compared with selective termination prior to 16 weeks (50). There also is a significant inverse correlation between the gestational age at which selective termination is performed and the gestational age at delivery (50).

Safety

Groups led by Wapner (34), DeCatte (47), and Pergament (48) have published reviews of their experience with twin CVS (Table 3-4). Both Wapner and Pergament report a post-CVS loss rate prior to 28 weeks of less than 3%, which compares favorably with the loss rates reported after twin amniocentesis.

The overall fetal loss rate reported by DeCatte et al. was slightly higher than that reported by Wapner et al. (3.7%) and Pergament et al. (4.9%). The losses reported by DeCatte et al., however, included two congenitally malformed fetuses, the spontaneous abortion of a 45X fetus, and a pregnancy complicated by severe twin-twin transfusion (47). Exclusion of these cases reduces the fetal loss rate to 4.8%, which is more consistent with the other reports.

Although not a randomized control group, DeCatte et al. (47) compared the outcomes of 104 women with twin pregnancies undergoing CVS with those of 101 consecutively enrolled women with twin pregnancies who did not undergo prenatal diagnosis.

Table 3-4.   Risk of fetal loss after twin chorionic villus sampling

Variable	Wapner et al., 1993 (34)	Pergament et al., 1992 (48)	DeCatte et al., 1996 (47)
Pregnancies sampled	244	126	104
Fetuses sampled	488	252	208
Elective abortion			
Both fetuses	3	2	0
Selective termination	10	4	2
Lost to follow-up study	1	0	0
Delivery cohort			
Pregnancies	240	124	104
Fetuses	470	244	206
Fetal loss <28 wk	7 (2.9%)	3 (2.4%)	15 (7.3%)[a]

[a] Total fetal loss rate including two selective reductions, seven spontaneous abortions (<500 g), and six late-pregnancy losses.

The rate of spontaneous abortion (less than 500 g) of twins after first-trimester CVS (7 of 206; 3.4%) was comparable with that of the control group (14 of 202; 6.9%). The perinatal mortality rates (exclusive of losses less than 500 g) were also similar between the CVS group (12 of 197; 6.1%) and the control twins (10 of 188; 5.3%). DeCatte et al. (47) also analyzed perinatal outcome and did not find any significant differences in mean birth weight, rate of low birth weight, mean gestational age at delivery, or preterm delivery rate between the first-trimester CVS and control twin groups.

The results of limited studies of CVS in multiple gestations suggest a fairly equivalent risk of fetal loss compared to twin amniocentesis but a higher risk of diagnostic error and twin-twin cell contamination. These limitations can be minimized but not eliminated with increasing experience with the procedure and a mastery of both transabdominal and transcervical CVS techniques. Proficiency with transcervical CVS in singleton pregnancies is only achieved after performing several hundred procedures for most operators (51). As a result, few centers are proficient at performing this procedure for multiple gestations.

The main advantage of CVS is that it can be performed in the first trimester. Both elective termination and selective termination when discordant results are obtained are medically safer and psychologically easier in the first trimester than in the second. The option of first-trimester prenatal diagnosis allows the patient's privacy to be respected.

SUMMARY

The presence of more than one fetus complicates prenatal genetic diagnosis as it does most of the other aspects of prenatal care. However, genetic diagnosis can be effectively and safely performed as long as the unique requirements of multiple gestations are appreciated. Genetic counseling must address issues such as calculation of specific genetic risks for multiples, the unique procedural risks imposed by multiples, and the options available should fetal abnormalities be detected.

Sonographers must be able to assess amnionicity, chorionicity, and zygosity. Sonographers must be proficient in fetal anatomic scanning and in guiding invasive diagnostic procedures. Finally, operators need to be aware of the special challenges presented by multiples and should have a wide breadth of experience in the performance of both amniocentesis and CVS in singleton gestations. They also should be experienced in the performance of these procedures for multiple gestations, which is technically more demanding. These procedures need to be performed in such a way as to ensure that both fetuses are reliably sampled and documented so that in follow-up care any abnormalities can be correctly identified.

Although test results are usually reassuring for most couples, the operator must be prepared to deal with disappointing results. The most difficult of these situations may be when the results are discordant for fetal abnormality. In these cases, the normality of the co-twin must be confirmed as well as the identity of the abnormal twin. Decisions regarding selective termination must take into consideration the fetal and neonatal natural history of the abnormality and its likely effect on the long-term health and survival of the normal co-twin. Sebire et al. (52) reported on 19 twin pregnancies discordant for fetal trisomy. Selective termination was chosen in 13 of 14 cases of trisomy 21 but in only 1 of 5 cases of trisomy 18. This decision making appears to reflect an appreciation of the relative survivability associated with these two aneuploidies and a desire not to threaten the normal co-twin when fetal or neonatal demise is the naturally expected outcome. All pregnancies managed by means of selective termination resulted in live birth of the chromosomally normal co-twin. Among the expectantly managed trisomy 18 pregnancies, the chromosomally normal infant survived in each case and the abnormal twin died in either the antepartum or the early neonatal period (52).

REFERENCES

1. Lubs HA, Ruddle FH. Chromosomal abnormalities in the human population: estimate of rates based on New Haven Newborn Study. *Science* 1970;169:495–497.
2. Rodis JF, Egan JFX, Craffet A, et al. Calculated risk of chromosomal abnormalities in twin gestations. *Obstet Gynecol* 1990;76: 1037–1041.
3. Flannery DB, Brown JA, Redwine FO, et al. Antenatally detected Kleinfelter syndrome in twins. *Acta Genet Med Gemellol (Roma)* 1984;29:529–531.
4. Dallapiccola B, Stomeo C, Ferranti B, et al. Discordant sex in one of three monozygotic triplets. *J Med Genet* 1985;22:6–11.
5. Perlman EJ, Stetten G, Tuck-Muller CM, et al. Sexual discordance in monozygotic twins. *Am J Obstet Gynecol* 1990;37:551–557.
6. Myrianthopoulos N. An epidemiologic survey of twins in a large prospectively studied population. *Am J Hum Genet* 1970;22: 611–617.

7. Hook EB. Rates of chromosomal abnormalities of different maternal ages. *Obstet Gynecol* 1981;58:282–285.
8. Wapner RJ. Genetic diagnosis in multiple pregnancies. *Semin Perinatol* 1995;19:351–362.
9. Neveux LM, Palomaki GE, Knight GJ, et al. Multiple marker screening for Down syndrome in twin pregnancies. *Prenat Diagn* 1996;16:29–34.
10. Wald N, Cuckle H, Wu TS, George L. Maternal serum unconjugated oestriol and human chorionic gonadotropin levels in twin pregnancies: implications for screening for Downs syndrome. *Br J Obstet Gynaecol* 1991;98:905–908.
11. Spencer K, Salonen R, Muller F. Down syndrome screening in multiple pregnancies using alpha-fetoprotein and free beta-hCG. *Prenat Diagn* 1994;14:537–542.
12. Thom H, Buckland C, Campbell A, et al. Maternal serum α-fetal protein in monozygotic and dizygotic twin pregnancies. *Prenat Diagn* 1984;4:341–346.
13. Ghaosh A, Woo J, Rawlinson H, et al. Prognostic significance of maternal serum α-fetoprotein levels in twin pregnancies. *Br J Obstet Gynecol* 1982;89:718–721.
14. Cuckle H, Wald N, Stevenson J, et al. Maternal serum alpha-fetoprotein screening for open neural tube defects in twin pregnancies. *Prenat Diagn* 1990;10:71–77.
15. Lustig L, Feuchtbaum L, Cunningham G. MSAFP screening for open neural tube defects in twin pregnancies. In: *Proceedings of the Eighth International Congress on Human Genetics,* Washington Convention Center, Washington, D.C. October 6–11, 1991:49(4).
16. Edwards MS, Ellings JM, Newman RB, et al. Predictive value of antepartum ultrasound examination for anomalies in twin gestations. *Ultrasound Obstet Gynecol* 1995;6:43–49.
17. Stiller R, Lockwood C, Belanger K, et al. Amniotic fluid α-fetoprotein concentrations in twin gestations: dependence on placental membrane anatomy. *Am J Obstet Gynecol* 1988;158:1088–1092.
18. Snijders RJM, Johnson S, Sebire NJ, et al. First trimester ultrasound screening for chromosomal defects. *Ultrasound Obstet Gynecol* 1996;7:216–226.
19. Sebire NJ, Snijders RJM, Hughes K, et al. Screening for trisomy 21 in twin pregnancies by maternal age and fetal nuchal translucency thickness at 10–14 weeks of gestation. *Br J Obstet Gynaecol* 1996;103:999–1003.
20. Elias S, Gerbie A, Simpson JL, et al. Genetic amniocentesis in twin gestations. *Am J Obstet Gynecol* 1980;138:169–173.
21. Tabsch K. Genetic amniocentesis in multiple gestation: a new technique to diagnose monoamniotic twins. *Obstet Gynecol* 1990;75:296–298.
22. Nicolini U, Monni G. Intestinal obstruction in babies exposed in utero to methylene blue. *Lancet* 1990;336:1258–1259.
23. Van der Pol SG, Wolf H, Boer K, et al. Jejunal atresia related to the use of methylene blue in genetic amniocentesis in twins. *Br J Obstet Gynaecol* 1992;22:141–143.
24. Soares-da Silva P, Caramona M. Effects of methylene blue on the uptake, release, and metabolism of noradrenaline in mesenteric artery vessels. *J Pharm Pharmacol* 1988;40:534–538.
25. Crooks J. Haemolytic jaundice in the neonate after intraamniotic injection of methylene blue. *Arch Dis Child* 1982;57:822–823.

26. Kirsch IR, Cohen HJ. Heinz body hemolytic anemia from the use of methylene blue in neonates. *J Pediatr* 1980;96:276–278.
27. Cragan JD, Martin ML, Khoury MJ, et al. Dye used during amniocentesis and birth defects. *Lancet* 1993;340:1352.
28. Pruggmayer MR, Jahoda MG, Van der Pol JG, et al. Genetic amniocentesis in twin pregnancies: results of a multicenter study of 529 cases. *Ultrasound Obstet Gynecol* 1992;2:6–10.
29. Erickson JC, Widmer BA. The vasopressor effect of indigo carmine. *Anesthesiology* 1968;29:188–189.
30. Jeanty P, Shah D, Roussis P. Single needle insertion in twin amniocentesis. *J Ultrasound Med* 1990;9:511–517.
31. Megory E, Weiner E, Shalev E, et al. Pseudomonoamniotic twins with cord entanglement following genetic funipuncture. *Obstet Gynecol* 1991;78:915–917.
32. Bahado Singh R, Schmitt R, et al. New technique for genetic amniocentesis in twins. *Obstet Gynecol* 1992;79:304–306.
33. Beekhuis JR, DeBrulin HW, Van Lith JM, et al. Second trimester amniocenteses in twin pregnancies: maternal haemoglobin as a dye marker to differentiate diamniotic twins. *Br J Obstet Gynaecol* 1992;99:126–127.
34. Wapner RJ, Johnson A, Davis G. Prenatal diagnosis in twin gestations: a comparison between second trimester amniocentesis and first trimester chorionic villus sampling. *Obstet Gynecol* 1993;82:49–56.
35. Ghidini A, Lynch L, Hicks C, et al. The risk of second trimester amniocentesis in twin gestations: a case-controlled study. *Am J Obstet Gynecol* 1993;169:1013–1016.
36. Gonsoulin W, Copeland K, Carpenter R, et al. Fetal blood sampling demonstrating chimerism in monozygotic twins discordant for sex and tissue karyotype (46,XY and 45,X). *Prenat Diagn* 1990;10:25–28.
37. Rhoads GG, Jackson LG, Schlesselman SE, et al. The safety and efficacy of chorionic villus sampling for early prenatal diagnosis of cytogenetic abnormalities. *N Engl J Med* 1989;320:609–617.
38. Tabor A, Phillip J, Madser M, et al. Randomized controlled trial of genetic amniocenteses in 4,606 low-risk women. *Lancet* 1986;1:1287–1289.
39. Anderson RL, Goldberg JD, Golbus MS. Prenatal diagnosis in multiple gestation: 20 years' experience with amniocentesis. *Prenat Diagn* 1991;11:263–270.
40. Pruggmayer M, Baumann P, Schutte H, et al. Incidence of abortion after genetic amniocentesis in twin pregnancies. *Prenat Diagn* 1991;11:637–640.
41. Buscaglia M, Ghisoni L, Bellotti AM, et al. Genetic amniocenteses in twin pregnancies by a single trans-abdominal insertion of the needle. *Prenat Diagn* 1995;15:17–19.
42. Sebire NJ, Noble PL, Psarra A, et al. Single uterine entry for genetic amniocentesis in twin pregnancies. *Ultrasound Obstet Gynecol* 1996;7:26–31.
43. Prompelan HJ, Madjam H, Schillinger H. Prognose von sonographisch fruhdiagnostizierter Zwillingsschwangerschafter. *Geburtshilfe Frauenheilkd* 1989;49:715–719.
44. Coleman BG, Grumbach K, Arger PH, et al. Twin gestations: monitoring of complications and anomalies with ultrasound. *Radiology* 1987;165:449–453.

45. Pretorious D, Budorick N, Sciosia A, et al. Twin pregnancies in the second trimester in an α-fetoprotein screening program: sonographic evaluation and outcome. *AJR Am J Roentgenol* 1993;12: 1007–1013.
46. Palle C, Andersen JW, Tabor A, et al. Increased risk of abortion after genetic amniocentesis in twin pregnancies. *Prenat Diagn* 1983;3:83–89.
47. DeCatte L, Liebaers I, Foulon W, et al. First trimester chorionic villus sampling in twin gestations. *Am J Perinatol* 1996;13:413–417.
48. Pergament E, Schulman J, Copeland K, et al. The risk and efficacy of chorionic villus sampling in multiple gestations. *Prenat Diagn* 1992;12:377–384.
49. Sebire NJ, Noble PL, Psarra A, et al. Fetal karyotyping in twin pregnancies: selection of techniques by measurement of fetal nuchal translucency. *Br J Obstet Gynaecol* 1996;103:887–890.
50. Evans MI, Goldberg JD, Dommergues M, et al. Efficacy of second trimester selective termination for fetal abnormalities: international collaborative experience among the world's largest centers. *Am J Obstet Gynecol* 1994;171:90–94.
51. Report of a WHO consultation on first trimester diagnosis: risk evaluation in CVS. *Prenat Diagn* 1986;6:451.
52. Sebire NJ, Snijders RJM, Santiago C, et al. Management of twin pregnancies with fetal trisomies. *Br J Obstet Gynaecol* 1997;104: 220–223.

4

Multifetal Pregnancy Reduction and Spontaneous Fetal Death

MULTIFETAL PREGNANCY REDUCTION

History of Multifetal Pregnancy Reduction

Since the 1970's, the rate of multifetal pregnancies has risen dramatically in the United States, due primarily to infertility treatments. The use of assisted reproductive technologies carries a 25% to 40% risk of resulting in pregnancies of three or more fetuses, depending on the medications and techniques used. Gestational age and birth weight are the two most important factors affecting perinatal morbidity and mortality; with each additional fetus, both of these factors are reduced. The length of gestation and birth weight of infants from multifetal pregnancies are inversely proportional to the number of fetuses present. According to U.S. vital statistics, the average birth weight and gestational age of singletons is 3,358 g at 39.3 weeks, compared with 2,500 g at 36.2 weeks for twins, and 1,698 g at 32.2 weeks for triplets (1,2). Published series show that the average birth weight and gestational age are about 1,455 g at 30.5 weeks for quadruplets and 980 g at 29 weeks for quintuplets.

Once a multifetal pregnancy has occurred, there are three options, each with potential benefits and harms: abort the entire pregnancy; continue the pregnancy; or abort some of the embryos. For many couples who have endured months or years of infertility treatment to achieve the current pregnancy, the first option may not be acceptable. The risks of maternal and neonatal morbidity and mortality with the second option increase directly with the number of embryos (3). In addition to exponentially increased risks of fetal, neonatal, or infant death, the survivors of a multifetal pregnancy remain at continued higher risk of permanent disability (4). In a recent study investigators estimated the risk of there being at least one disabled child per sibship to be 7.4% for twins, 21.6% for triplets, and 50% for quadruplets and quintuplets (5).

The third option, to abort some of the embryos (termed **multifetal pregnancy reduction** or **nonselective embryo reduction**), has emerged as a method of improving the chances of survival and health (6–8). Originally introduced as a method of selectively terminating a fetus affected by a genetic disorder without aborting the unaffected co-twin (9), it is now widely used to terminate one or more presumably normal fetuses to improve survival rates for the remaining fetuses and to decrease maternal morbidity (10). This procedure has also been extended to use in prenatal diagnosis in order to avoid repeated elective abortions. Couples at risk of Mendelian disease are offered the option of undergoing superovulation and assisted fertilization, genetic diagnosis in the first trimester, and selective termination of affected fetuses (11). Although this approach may not be morally acceptable to some, acceptance among patients has been high despite the significant cost, invasiveness of assisted reproductive techniques (ART), and the emotional trauma of multifetal pregnancy reduction (12).

Multifetal embryo reduction is not an optimal solution to the problems associated with multifetal pregnancy. Although it is understood that the production of multifetal pregnancies may not be completely avoidable for patients undergoing infertility treatments, many experts strongly believe these procedures should not be considered a safety net for infertility clinics (13). In a recent editorial (14) the guidelines of the Ethics Committee of the American Society for Reproductive Medicine were cited, indicating that "the Committee condemns the practice of transferring excessive numbers of preembryos with the intention of using selective reduction in the event of multiple pregnancies." Many practitioners who currently perform multifetal pregnancy reductions strongly favor prevention of these situations and consider reduction a temporary solution until such time as infertility treatments are improved (13,15–17).

To better advise patients regarding the risks of the procedure in terms of pregnancy loss and early preterm birth, Evans et al. (18–20) published a series of summaries based on a consortium of national and international centers. The first collaborative report was based on 183 cases from seven centers in the United States, the United Kingdom, and France from 1986 to 1991, the second and third reports were based on data from nine centers in the United States, the United Kingdom, France, and Italy on 463 cases from 1991 to 1993 and 1,789 cases from 1993 and 1994, respectively. These reports indicate an improvement in the pregnancy loss rate at 24 weeks' gestation or sooner from 16.5% in 1988 to 1991, 13% transcervically and transvaginally, and 8% transabdominally in 1991 to 1993, to 11.7% in 1993 and 1994. A higher starting number of fetuses is associated with a greater pregnancy loss rate, but between 1986 to 1991 and 1993 and 1994 there were improvements for every plurality. There also was a decline in the pregnancy loss rate for reductions of quintuplets or higher from 32.5% to 19.2%, for quadruplets from 16.1% to 13.0%, for triplets from 9.1% to 7.6%, and for twins from 16.7% to 9.0% (18,20). Although this loss rate may seem high, it compares very favorably with the spontaneous loss rate from assisted reproductive technology of 16.1% (ranging from 13.3% to 21.9%, depending on the procedure) (21). Possible causes of pregnancy loss after reduction include procedure-related trauma or infection or uterine contractions due to an inflammatory response to the resorbing dead fetoplacental tissue (22). Women with a prior history of spontaneous abortion are at significantly higher risk of pregnancy loss after reduction than are other women (23).

These investigators reported higher pregnancy loss rates with the use of air than with potassium chloride, among procedures performed for structural malformations than among those performed because of chromosomal anomalies, and when the procedure is performed at 17 weeks' gestation or later versus 16 weeks or earlier (14.4% versus 5.4%) (19). In addition, the gestational age at delivery correlates inversely with the starting number, finishing number, and the gestational age at the time of the procedure (Table 4-1). A major concern with this procedure is not to do damage to the surviving fetus or fetuses. Loss occurred in all pregnancies with a

Table 4-1. Pregnancy losses and deliveries as a function of finishing number

Finishing Number	n	Losses ≤24 wk		Deliveries								Mean Weeks' Gestation
				25–28 wk		29–32 wk		33–36 wk		≥37 wk		
		n	%	n	%	n	%	n	%	n	%	
1986–91 data[a]												
Triplets	26	7	26.9	3	11.5	4	15.4	9	34.6	3	11.5	33.3
Twins	380	54	14.2	20	5.2	30	7.9	121	31.8	157	41.3	35.6
Singletons	57	14	24.6	3	5.3	3	5.3	10	17.5	28	49.1	37.1
Overall	463	75	16.2	26	5.6	37	8.0	188	40.6	188	40.6	
1986–94 data[b]												
Triplets	68	12	17.6	5	7.4	21	30.9	23	33.8	7	10.3	32.9
Twins	1,437	156	10.9	66	4.6	127	8.8	528	36.7	560	39.0	35.3
Singletons	284	39	13.7	8	2.8	11	3.9	33	11.6	193	68.0	37.6
Overall	1,789	207	11.6	79	4.4	159	8.9	584	32.6	760	42.5	

Adapted from [a]Evans MI, Dommergues M, Wapner RJ, et al. Efficacy of transabdominal multifetal pregnancy reduction: collaborative experience among the world's largest centers. *Obstet Gynecol* 1993;82:61–66 and [b]Evans MI, Dommergues M, Wapner RJ, et al. International collaborative experience of 1789 patients having multifetal reduction: a plateauing of risks and outcomes. *J Soc Gynecol Investig* 1996;3:23–26, with permission.

monochorial placenta, presumably caused by passage of the injected toxin through placental vascular shunts or because acute hemodynamic changes occurred in the survivor (19).

The Question of Reducing Triplets to Twins

Berkowitz et al. (24) suggested that women pregnant with four or more fetuses were the ideal candidates for nonselective embryo reduction. Subsequent studies have supported this recommendation, including higher birth weights and longer gestations (Tables 4-2 and 4-3). The real debate concerns reducing triplets to twins (24–28). More than 40% of multiple pregnancies reduced are triplets, and more than 80% of triplets are reduced to twins (19). In addition to being born 4 weeks earlier in gestation and 800 g lighter in average birth weight, triplets have a greater than twofold higher risk of disability (5).

Several investigators have reported a significant reduction in early preterm births (24 to 32 weeks) of triplets reduced to twins compared with nonreduced triplets (7% versus 16% [29]; 10% versus 24% [30]; 7% versus 21% [22]). Because of this dramatic reduction in a known risk factor for handicap, reduction of triplets to twins may not improve the chances of survival, but may reduce the rate of handicap and improve the quality of life for those remaining (22,31). Haning et al. (32) showed that triplets are delivered about 3.7 weeks earlier than are reduced twins and 4.9 weeks earlier than are nonreduced twins. Santema et al. (33) reported more than a threefold higher rate of stillbirths (8.5% versus 2.5%), twofold higher rate of early neonatal death (10.2% versus 4.5%), and 1.5 times higher rate of late neonatal death (4.1% versus 2.7%) for triplets compared with twins. The majority of neonatal mortality and severe morbidity (patent ductus arteriosus and intraventricular hemorrhage) among triplet gestations have been reported at gestations of less than 30 weeks (34,35).

Maternal factors also should be taken into consideration in reducing triplets to twins. These factors include serious heart disease, uterine malformations, and prior early preterm births. As discussed in Chapter 9, maternal complications can occur earlier and be more severe, particularly with triplet and higher-order pregnancies. Last, but certainly of central importance, are the overwhelming social and financial concerns of the parents.

The Question of Reducing Twins to Singletons

The diagnosis of a twin pregnancy with one abnormal fetus is a complex medical and ethical situation. Prior to the use of reduction, parents had only two choices—abort both fetuses, including the normal one, or continue the pregnancy knowing that one fetus is affected. The risk of a major congenital defect is approximately twice as high among twins as it is among singletons, with rates approaching 10% among monozygotic twins (36). The reduction of twin pregnancy to a singleton for maternal medical, psychological, or socioeconomic reasons (termed **elective reduction**) is re controversial and less frequently performed than reduction use of fetal abnormalities. In some centers, reduction of twins gletons is not performed (37) or is performed only in the case

(*text continues on page 62*)

Table 4-2. Meta-analysis of the effect of multifetal pregnancy reduction on pregnancy outcomes

Outcome	Nonreduced Twins vs Medically Reduced to Twins		Nonreduced Triplets vs Medically Reduced to Twins	
	Odds Ratio and 95% Confidence Interval	Significance	Odds Ratio and 95% Confidence Interval	Significance
Length of gestation (wk)				
24–28	1.12 (0.34–3.71)	NS	2.38 (0.68–8.33)	NS
28–32	2.49 (0.95–6.47)	NS	4.90 (1.85–13.00)	$p = .0002$
32–36	0.48 (0.29–0.78)	$p = .002$	2.90 (1.11–7.58)	$p < .00001$
>36	1.65 (1.14–2.39)	$p = .009$	0.09 (0.04–0.20)	$p < .00001$
Birthweight (g)				
<1,500	0.48 (0.21–1.11)	NS	4.73 (2.12–10.55)	$p < .00001$
1,500–2,500	0.86 (0.53–1.40)	NS	1.99 (1.28–3.09)	$p = .002$
>2,500	1.92 (1.04–3.53)	$p = .002$	0.07 (0.01–0.45)	$p < .00001$
<10th%ile	0.36 (0.18–0.72)	$p = .002$	0.84 (0.56–1.28)	NS
Complications				
Preeclampsia	1.25 (0.77–2.03)	NS	2.38 (1.20–4.74)	$p = .01$
Premature rupture of the membranes	0.62 (0.36–1.06)	NS	1.79 (0.91–3.52)	NS
...ncy loss ≤24 wk as a function ... number ≥4 versus ≥3			2.24 (1.51–3.33)	$p < .00001$

...fetal reduction and pregnancy outcomes: a meta-analysis. Am J Obstet Gynecol 1998;178(2):S124, with permission.

Table 4-3. Birth weight and gestation outcomes by plurality and reduction status

Reference	Study Years and Location	Pregnancies and Percentage ART		No. of Singletons	No. of Medically Reduced Singletons	No. of Nonreduced Twins	No. Spontaneously Reduced to Twins[b]	No. Medically Reduced to Twins[b]	No. of Nonreduced Triplets[b]	No. Medically Reduced to Triplets[b]
		No.	%							
Mean birthweight (g)										
Sassoon et al., 1990 (92)	1981–89 Los Angeles	30	57 (case–control)			15 (2,475)			15 (1,720)	2 (1,449)
Donner et al., 1990 (93)	1985–89 Brussels	18	100		4 (2,996)			12 (2,249)		
Porreco et al., 1991 (94)	Not stated Denver	24	100					13 (2,227)	11 (2,239)	
Boulot et al., 1993 (29)	1985–91 Montpellier, France	80	95					32 (2,340)	48 (1,870)	
Bollen et al., 1993 (31)	1987–92 Brussels	72	100				7 (2,465)	17 (2,512)[a] 14 (2,329)[b]	32 (1,668)	
Macones et al., 1993 (43)	1988–92 Philadelphia	124	Not stated			63 (2,293)		47 (2,279)	14 (1,593)	
Lipitz et al., 1994 (30)	1984–92 Tel Aviv	140	94					31 (2,350)	84 (1,780)	
Santema et al., 1995 (33)	1981–91 Rotterdam, The Netherlands	120	52 (case–control)			80 (2,030)			40 (1,478)	
Alexander et al., 1995 (44)	1988–93 Birmingham, AL	74	100			42 (2,512)		32 (2,038)		

		N	% singleton				
Tallo et al., 1995 (95)	1988–93 Providence, RI	202	50 (case–control)	62 (3,594)[c] 62 (3,268)[d]	68 (2,571)[c] 68 (2,212)[d]		6 (1,950)[c] 7 (895)[d]
Groutz et al., 1996 (96)	Not stated Tel Aviv	40	100	30 (2,361)	30 (2,210)[e] 10 (1,844)[f]		
Smith-Levitan et al., 1996 (45)	1990–94 Manhasset, NY	201	100	88 (2,507)	59 (2,338)	12 (2,407)	54 (1,906)
Silver et al., 1997 (97)	1990–94 Evanston, IL	126	57 (case–control)	54 (2,062)[c] 54 (2,429)[d]	18 (1,837)		
Fitzsimmons et al., 1998 (98)	1985–96 Vancouver, Canada	196	37 (case–control)	108 (2,166)[c] 56 (2,374)[d]			16 (1,683)[c] 16 (1,695)[d]
Yaron et al., 1999(78)	1987–96 Detroit	967	Not stated	195 (2,254)[g] 565 (2,123)[h]	134 (2,381)		9 (1,636)
Mean Gestation (wk)							
Sassoon et al., 1990 (92)	1981–89 Los Angeles	30	57 (case–control)	15 (36.6)			15 (35.0)
Donner et al., 1990 (93)	1985–89 Brussels	18	100	4 (38.3)	12 (36.0)		2 (33.0)
…t al.,	Not stated Denver	24	100		13 (35.5)		11 (35.7)

continued

Table 4-3. Continued

Study Years and Location	Pregnancies and Percentage ART No.	%	No. of Singletons	No. of Medically Reduced Singletons	No. of Nonreduced Twins	No. Spontaneously Reduced to Twins[b]	No. Medically Reduced to Twins[b]	No. of Nonreduced Triplets[b]	No. Medically Reduced to Triplets[b]
Sommergues et al., 1991 (25), 1983–88 Strasbourg and Paris	58	98		10 (37.7)			24 (34.9)		6 (34.3)
Boulot et al., 1993 (29), 1985–91 Montpellier, France	80	95					32 (36.7)	48 (34.4)	
Boulot et al., 1993 (99), 1986–91 Montpellier, France	61	97					24 (37.7)		
Bollen et al., 1993 (31), 1987–92 Brussels	72	100				7 (37.5)	17 (36.9)[a] 14 (34.0)[b]	32 (32.5)	
Macones et al., 1993 (43), 1988–92 Philadelphia	124	Not stated			63 (34.8)		47 (35.6)	14 (31.2)	
Lipitz et al., 1994 (30), 1984–92 Tel Aviv	140	94					31 (36.7)	84 (33.5)	
Santema et al., 1995 (33), 1981–91 Rotterdam, The Netherlands	120	52 (case–control)			80 (35.5)			40 (32.0)	
Tallo et al., 1995 (95), 1988–93 Providence, RI	202	50 (case–control)	62 (40.0)[c] 62 (39.0)[d]		68 (37.0)[c] 68 (35.0)[d]			6 (34.0)[c] 7 (27.0)[d]	

Source	Years	Location	No. of pregnancies	%					
Alexander et al., 1995 (44)	1988–93	Birmingham, AL	74	100		42 (35.4)		32 (33.8)	
Groutz et al., 1996 (96)	Not stated	Tel Aviv	40	100	30 (36.9)			30 (35.9)[e] 10 (33.3)[f]	
Haning et al., 1996 (32)	1988–93	Providence, RI	260	100	132 (37.9)	64 (34.6)	25 (33.4)		9 (29.7)
Smith-Levitan et al., 1996 (45)	1990–94	Manhasset, NY	201	100	88 (35.0)	12 (35.2)	59 (35.5)		54 (32.8)
Silver et al., 1997 (97)	1990–94	Evanston, IL	126	57	54 (33.6)[c] 54 (36.0)[d] 108 (34.6)[e]		18 (32.6)		16 (32.6)[c]
Fitzsimmons et al., 1998 (98)	1985–96	Vancouver, Canada	196	37 (case–control)	56 (35.4)[d]				16 (32.4)[d]
Sebire et al., 1997 (22)	1986–96	London, UK	113	Not stated	66 (36.0)		66 (36.0)		47 (34.0)
Yaron et al., 1999 (78)	1987–96 Detroit		967	Not stated	195 (35.8)[a] 565 (24.4)[h]		134 (35.6)		9 (32.9)

Note: Number of pregnancies in the study versus subtotals within categories may not add because of pregnancy losses at 24 or fewer weeks' gestation.
[a] Reduction performed transvaginally.
[b] Reduction performed transcervically.
[c] Spontaneously conceived.
conceived with infertility treatment.
reduced to twins.
ts reduced to twins.
ins from the Quest Diagnostics Database.
from Wayne State University Perinatal Database.
ve technology.

of monoamniotic twins or a lethal anomaly of one twin (31). Others have advocated the opposite viewpoint, that a woman should not be forced to accept the "side effect" of current reproductive technology (38). This reasoning emphasizes that if assisted reproductive technology could be refined to provide the option of conceiving a singleton or a multiple gestation and the woman chose a singleton, reduction would not be viewed as abnormal or excessive. Likewise, a woman should not be forced into having multiples if she does not want more than one baby, because a therapeutic option is available (termed **selective reduction** in the case of a normal fetus).

Reduction was originally reported in 1978 as the selective termination of an abnormal twin diagnosed with Hurler's syndrome (9), and in 1981 it was used on a twin fetus with Down syndrome (39). Initial attempts to perform selective reduction failed, most likely because of monozygosity and a shared placenta. In such cases, demise of the remaining twin occurs because of disseminated intravascular coagulation. Selective reduction currently can be performed on monozygotic twins by means of umbilical cord ligation under ultrasound guidance or with fiber optic fetoscopy (40). Outcomes are better for dizygotic twin reductions, resulting in liveborn singletons in 85% of cases (19). There is actually a greater risk of pregnancy loss at 24 weeks or earlier for reduction to singletons than there is for reduction to twins (13.7% versus 10.9%) (20). There also may be residual adverse effects on intrauterine growth and length of gestation compared with nonreduced singletons.

A recent summary of 10 years of experience with 82 reductions to singletons (23 elective reductions and 59 selective terminations due to fetal chromosomal or structural abnormalities) showed an overall pregnancy loss rate of 8.5%; and of the remaining 75 cases, the preterm delivery rate was 20% (41). Procedures performed at 14 weeks or sooner had a longer procedure-to-loss interval (4.1 weeks versus 1.2 weeks), lower preterm delivery rate (7.1% versus 27.6%), longer mean gestation (38.4 weeks versus 35.7 weeks) and higher mean birth weight (3,299 g versus 2,577 g). The investigators suggested that the difference in procedure-to-loss interval in the two groups reflects differing etiologies, with the latter group more likely to be procedure related. The investigators emphasized, however, that to diagnose abnormalities in twin pregnancies prior to 14 weeks, it is necessary to use transvaginal ultrasonography and chorionic villus sampling.

Residual Perinatal Effects

Although reduction to twins or even singletons narrows the differences in length of gestation and average birth weight to be closer to that of nonreduced twins or singletons, there often remain some residual adverse effects, particularly with a higher starting number of fetuses (Fig. 4-1). Most investigators have reported shorter length of gestation and lower birth weights among pregnancies reduced to twins than for nonreduced twins (19,42–44), although some have shown no significant differences (45,46) (Table 4-3). Some studies, though, have failed to consider maternal anthropometric factors known to influence birth weight and gestation (height, prepregnancy weight, and gestational weight gain), as well as lifestyle factors such as maternal iron status, parity, smoking, maternal age and race. In addition, many studies lack

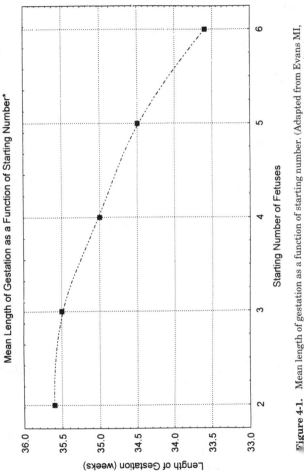

Mean Length of Gestation as a Function of Starting Number*

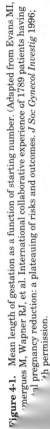

Figure 4-1. Mean length of gestation as a function of starting number. (Adapted from Evans MI, ~mergues M, Wapner RJ, et al. International collaborative experience of 1789 patients having ~al pregnancy reduction: a plateauing of risks and outcomes. *J Soc Gynecol Investig* 1996; ~h permission.

the statistical power to demonstrate a reliable difference. Because women who undergo multifetal pregnancy reduction are much more likely to be pregnant with multiples because of infertility treatments, there may be baseline differences between them and women who have conceived multiples spontaneously, which would help explain some of the differences in outcomes (47). There also is evidence of reduced hormonal support after reduction, resulting in a higher incidence of prematurity and growth retardation independent of other factors (see later).

Parental Concerns and Psychological Effects

Contrary to medical opinion, patient surveys have indicated an overall positive attitude toward conceiving twins or triplets and an increased willingness to consider multifetal pregnancy reduction for quadruplet and higher-order pregnancies (48,49). In a recent survey of patients undergoing infertility treatments (48), 67% of respondents expressed a desire to conceive twins and 50% to conceive triplets; both significantly correlated with increasing maternal age. An understanding of the risk of conceiving multiples was significantly correlated with the length of infertility, indicating that patients became better educated the longer they received treatment. An understanding of the risk associated with multifetal pregnancy reduction was not associated with gravidity or length of infertility treatment, but an increased willingness to consider the procedure correlated with increasing maternal age. Evans et al. (16) reported that most couples considering multifetal pregnancy reduction were more concerned with permanent morbidity from prematurity than with fetal mortality. Concerns over caring for so many infants, the costs, associated stress, and the effect on older siblings all factor into a couples' decision to choose reduction (23,50). Religious beliefs play an important role in couples' decision to decline reduction (50).

Attitudes regarding reduction may change once faced with the reality of a multiple pregnancy. In a survey of women undergoing infertility treatment, Leiblum et al. (51) found that fewer than 8% would consider aborting all but one fetus if they conceived quadruplets. In contrast, in a questionnaire given to 20 reduction patients and their husbands postpartum, 20% of couples indicated that they would have preferred to reduce to a single fetus rather than twins, and that they generally viewed the reduction as a "normal and necessary procedure" (37).

There are also reported attitudinal differences to reduction ong men versus women. In a survey of patients undergoing rtility treatment, although a nearly equal number of men and indicated that they would never consider multifetal pregeduction (26% versus 28%), more than twice as many men answered that they would consider multifetal pregction for triplets (18% versus 7%) (49). In this survey, their preference in regard to a higher-order prego pregnancy, 95% of women and 88% of men would but 68% of women and 61% of men would choose rly three times as many men as women choose tion procedure on a television monitor (58% venty-five percent of couples reported that icate openly with each other about their thoughts and emotions regarding the reduction during the first week after delivery (53).

Compared with women who spontaneously or electively lose their pregnancies, women who have undergone reduction express a briefer period of mourning, and fewer remember having anniversary grief reactions (52). This may be because the feelings of acute pain and grief are buffered by the relief and attachment to the remaining children and the realization of a long-standing goal of giving birth. Understandably, women who undergo reduction and subsequently lose the pregnancy experience significantly more depressive symptoms than their pregnant or postpartum peers (23,52). In a study of women who had undergone reduction conducted up to 5 years after the procedure (52), mourning for the reduced fetuses was remembered by 70% of the women. Grieving had lasted an average of about a month, and there were current lingering feelings of sadness and guilt. An anniversary grief reaction to the loss of the reduced fetuses was experienced by 37% of women. About 20% of women recalled more stress during the reduction procedure and continued to mourn their fetal loss longer. These women tended to be younger, more religious, and from larger families, and had viewed their fetuses more frequently at ultrasonography before the procedure. Ninety-three percent of patients who gave birth would choose to undergo reduction again, 5% were ambivalent, and 2% would not have undergone the reduction. Of the women who had miscarriages, 70% to 75% indicated that they would have elected to undergo reduction again (23,52). It has been recommended that the provision of psychological support both before and after the reduction would facilitate the emotional recovery of women and their husbands (52).

The Reduction Procedure

Of the three different technical procedures for reduction reported (transcervical, transvaginal, and transabdominal), the latter is now used most commonly (13,54). Several methods have been used for reduction with varying results. The most common method of reduction currently is ultrasound-guided fetal intracardiac injection of potassium chloride through a 20- or 22-gauge needle. The transabdominal approach is generally performed between 10 and 13 weeks' gestation. Prior to 10 weeks, the procedure is technically more difficult because of smaller fetal size, the larger distance between the fetus and the maternal abdominal wall, and the limitations in the resolution of transabdominal ultrasound. By waiting until 10 to 13 weeks, there may be spontaneous loss of one or more embryos, thereby alleviating the need for reduction altogether. Spontaneous loss of one or more fetuses has been reported in 14% to 30% of triplet pregnancies (32,55). At the end of the twelfth week of gestation, evidence of growth delay is more frequent. Because fetuses with growth delay are at increased risk of spontaneous death and chromosomal abnormalities, they may be targeted for reduction (56). After 12 weeks, the risk of spontaneous loss of one or more fetuses is small, and the risk of disseminated intravascular coagulopathy from a larger mass of degenerating fetal tissue may be increased.

The selection of fetuses to be terminated depends on the technical ease with which the procedure can there is evidence of significant size discrepancies (i.e., fetuses with smaller crown-rump length), increased nuchal translucency (57–60), or gross anomalies. In addition, the fetus in the sac over the internal os is left alone (61). In the case of reduction due to an abnormality, proper identification of the abnormal fetus, chorionicity, and severity or lethality of the diagnosis is essential. When the abnormality is morphologic, the targeted fetus can be readily identified with ultrasound examination, but in the case of a chromosomal abnormality, accurate visual identification may not be possible. In this situation, it is recommended that the karyotypically abnormal fetus be identified with certainty by means of amniocentesis, placental biopsy, or fetal blood sampling prior to the procedure (61). A confirmatory specimen of either amniotic fluid or fetal blood should be subjected to genetic analysis after the reduction to verify that the correct fetus was targeted.

Biochemical Values

After first-trimester selective reduction, levels of maternal α-fetoprotein increase in the second trimester (62,63). It is suggested that this elevation is probably caused by the release of tissue or serum from the dead fetus or fetuses and is positively correlated with the number of reduced fetuses. The routine use of maternal α-fetoprotein levels in the second trimester to screen for neural tube defects is therefore not reliable in the care of these patients, and a comprehensive ultrasonographic structural survey should be conducted instead.

With the demise of one or more fetuses, either spontaneously or iatrogenically, there is a small risk to the mother of developing disseminated intravascular coagulopathy (61). This complication is believed to be caused by the release of thromboplastic material into the maternal circulation. Because of the potential risk to the mother, periodic coagulation profiles are recommended to detect the early development of this complication. Reports of bimonthly coagulation studies performed throughout pregnancy after reductions have shown this to be a rare complication (19,64).

Total residual endometrial function decreases after multifetal reduction, as reflected by a decline in the levels of insulin-like growth factor binding protein-1 (IGFBP-1), placental protein 14 (PP14), human chorionic gonadotropin, estradiol, and progesterone (65,66). This decline in maternal serum concentrations of placental hormones, which occurs within 2 weeks after reduction and persists for several months, may be largely responsible for the higher incidence of growth retardation and early preterm births among these pregnancies (67).

SPONTANEOUS FETAL DEATH AND THE VANISHING TWIN

Incidence

It is estimated that no more than 1 in 4 natural conceptions, and no more than 1 in 50 natural twin conceptions survive to term. If 1 in 8 spontaneous pregnancies begins as twins, for each born twin pair, 10 to 12 twin pregnancies result. According to these estimates, 12% to 15% of all adults may be the result of twin conceptions. The excess fetal mortality among twins is not confined to monozygotic twins but occurs among like-sexed twin pregnancies (68).

It is estimated that about 20% to 50% of fetuses in multiple pregnancies identified by ultrasound during the first trimester are spontaneously lost (69–71). The spontaneous loss of one twin is most common in the first trimester. Usually associated with some vaginal spotting, early fetal loss does not have an adverse effect on the surviving twin (69,72). An estimated 28% of implantations from *in vitro* fertilization are lost spontaneously; the probability of pregnancy loss after visualization of fetal heart motion is about 5.7% (73).

Spontaneous fetal loss after the first trimester occurs in about 2% to 5% of twin pregnancies (74–76). This estimate increases threefold to fourfold for monochorionic versus dichorionic twins (76,77). Fetal death also is more common when a structural abnormality is present. Pregnancy loss rates at 24 weeks or earlier for triplet pregnancies have been reported to range from 3.5% (22), 6% (29), and 8% (55), to 25% (30,78). Reported rates of spontaneous reduction from triplets to twins or singletons range from 14% to 18% (31,32,79,80) to 30% (55). In a study of 302 pregnancies resulting from *in vitro* fertilization using either three embryos, three oocytes, or three zygotes, triplet pregnancies occurred in only 8.3% of cases, twin pregnancies in 23.2%, and singleton pregnancies in 68.5% (81).

Fetal Loss Due to Older Maternal Age

In the United States in 1997, 35%, 48%, and 68% of singleton, twin, and triplet and higher-order births, respectively, were to women ages (30 years and older (see Chapter 1). Older maternal age is associated with intrinsically reduced fecundity and a higher risk of fetal loss (82–84). For this reason, a higher number of embryos may be transferred (particularly in women over age 40) to achieve a pregnancy and in view of the higher known loss rate (83,84). In a prospective study of first-trimester ultrasound findings, Dickey et al. (82) estimated that when two gestational sacs were present, the probability of delivering twins was 63% for maternal ages less than 30 years versus 52% for maternal ages of 30 or older. With three gestational sacs present, the probability of a triplet birth was 45% for maternal ages younger than 30 years versus 18% for maternal ages of 30 years or older. These investigators estimated the probability of a twin birth when two viable embryos were present to be 90% for maternal ages less than 30 years versus 84% for maternal ages of 30 years or older. With three viable embryos, they estimated the probability of a triplet birth to be 90% for maternal ages less than 30 years versus 44% for maternal ages 30 years or older.

Perinatal and Postneonatal Risks

Although it has been suggested that first-trimester reductions do not have an adverse effect on the surviving fetuses, significant morbidity has been reported. et al. (85) reported neurologic damage to the survivor in four twin pregnancies with fetal demise occurring and 21 weeks. In monochorionic pregnancies, twin may have devastating repercussions for such as central nervous system abnormalities compromise, renal impairment, or even death of a normal outcome in a monozygotic pregnancy mise is only about 17%.

As described for the mother, one mechanism of injury may be the embolization of tissue thromboplastin through placental anastomoses to the surviving twin (77,88). Other mechanisms of neurologic injury may include fetal hypotension with hypoxemia and fetal exsanguination into the low pressure system created by the dead twin. In dichorionic twin pregnancies, fetal demise increases the risk of prematurity (72,74,75).

Neurologic abnormality of the surviving twin has been reported with fetal demise as early as 18 weeks. Neurologic damage has been reported in 5% to 19% of surviving twins, with an increased risk of cerebral palsy (74,75,89). The neurologic morbidity of the surviving co-twin includes cerebellar necrosis, hydranencephaly, hydrocephalus, hemorrhagic infarct, microcephaly, multicystic encephalomalacia, porencephaly, and spastic quadriplegia.

Few long-term studies have been conducted to evaluate the effect of multifetal pregnancy reduction on the development of the surviving children. Brandes et al. (90) reported on seven children (two sets of twins and one set of triplets) born after multifetal pregnancy reduction compared with controls matched for age, sex, birth weight, gestation, mode of delivery, and plurality. The investigators found no significant differences up to 38 months of age. There is a need for more research on the long-term effects of reduction and fetal loss on growth and development during childhood.

CLINICAL CONSIDERATIONS AND KEY POINTS

- Multifetal pregnancy reduction is associated with an 8% risk of losing the entire pregnancy prior to 24 weeks' gestation.
- The incidence of maternal or antenatal hospitalization, preterm labor, and cesarean birth decreases with multifetal pregnancy reduction.
- The incidence of preeclampsia, gestational diabetes, and other pregnancy complications does not decrease with multifetal pregnancy reduction.
- Multifetal pregnancy reduction to twins is associated with longer gestation, higher birth weights, and lower rates of admission to neonatal intensive care.

REFERENCES

1. Taffel SM. Health and demographic characteristics of twin births: United States, 1988. National Center for Health Statistics. *Vital Health Stat 21* 1992;(50):1–17.
2. Martin JA, MacDorman MF, Mathews TJ. Triplet births: Trends and outcomes, 1971–94. National Center for Health Statistics. *Vital Health Stat 21* 1997;(55):1–20.
   trikoversusky BM, Vintzileos AM. Management and outcome ultiple pregnancies of higher fetal order: literature review. *Gynecol Surv* 1989;44:578–584.
   Keith LG. The contribution of singletons, twins, and low birth weight, infant mortality, and handicap in the es. *J Reprod Med* 1992;37:661–665.
   Shimizu T, Hayakawa K. Incidence of handicaps in and associated factors. *Acta Genet Med Gemellol* 81–91.
   ch L. Selective reduction: an unfortunate mis-ol 1990;75:873–874.

7. ACOG Committee Opinion. Committee on Ethics. Multifetal pregnancy reduction and selective fetal termination. No. 94. Washington, DC: American College of Obstetricians and Gynecologists, 1991.
8. ACOG Committee Opinion. Committee on Ethics. Nonselective embryo reduction: ethical guidance for the obstetrician-gynecologist. No. 215. Washington, DC: American College of Obstetricians and Gynecologists, 1999.
9. Aberg A, Mitelman F, Cantz M, et al. Cardiac puncture of fetus with Hurler's disease avoiding abortion of unaffected co-twin. Lancet 1978;ii:990–991.
10. Dumez Y, Oury JF. Method for first trimester selective abortion in multiple pregnancy. Contrib Gynecol Obstet 1986;15:50–53.
11. Brambati B, Formigli L, et al. Selective reduction of quadruplet pregnancy at risk of beta thalassaemia. Lancet 1990;2:1325–1326.
12. Brambati B, Tului L, Baldi M, et al. Genetic analysis prior to selective fetal reduction in multiple pregnancy: technical aspects and clinical outcome. Hum Reprod 1995;10:818–825.
13. Berkowitz RL, Lynch L, Stone J, et al. The current status of multifetal pregnancy reduction. Am J Obstet Gynecol 1996;174:1265–1272.
14. Jones HW. Twins or more (Editorial). Fertil Steril 1995;63:701–702.
15. Hobbins JC. Selective reduction: a perinatal necessity? (Editorial.) N Engl J Med 1988;318:1062–1063.
16. Evans MI, Littmann L, King M, et al. Multiple gestation: the role of multifetal pregnancy reduction and selective termination. Clin Perinatol 1992;19:345–357.
17. Evans MI, Littmann L, St. Louis L, et al. Evolving patterns of iatrogenic multifetal pregnancy generation: implications for aggressiveness of infertility treatments. Am J Obstet Gynecol 1995;172:1750–1755.
18. Evans MI, Dommergues M, Wapner RJ, et al. Efficacy of transabdominal multifetal pregnancy reduction: collaborative experience among the world's largest centers. Obstet Gynecol 1993;82:61–66.
19. Evans MI, Dommergues M, Timor-Tritsch I, et al. Transabdominal versus transcervical and transvaginal multifetal pregnancy reduction: international collaborative experience of more than one thousand cases. Am J Obstet Gynecol 1994;170:902–909.
20. Evans MI, Dommergues M, Wapner RJ, et al. International collaborative experience of 1789 patients having multifetal pregnancy reduction: a plateauing of risks and outcomes. J Soc Gynec Investig 1996;3:23–26.
21. Society for Assisted Reproductive Technology, American So for Reproductive Medicine. Assisted reproductive technolog United States: 1996 results generated from the American for Reproductive Medicine/Society for Assisted Reproduc nology Registry. Fertil Steril 1999;71:798–807.
22. Sebire NJ, D'Ercole C, Sepulveda W, et al. Effec reduction from trichorionic triplets to twins. Br J C 1997;104:1201–1203.
23. McKinney M, Downey J, Timor-Tritsch I. The ps of multifetal pregnancy reduction. Fertil Steri
24. Berkowitz RL, Lynch L, Chitkara U, et al. f multifetal pregnancies in the first trimest 318:1043–1047.

25. Dommergues M, Nisand I, Mandelbrot L, et al. Embryo reduction in multifetal pregnancies after infertility therapy: obstetrical risks and perinatal benefits are related to operative strategy. *Fertil Steril* 1991;55:805–811.

26. Benshushan A, Lewin A, Schenker JG. Multifetal pregnancy reduction: is it always justified? *Fetal Diagn Ther* 1993;8:214–220.

27. Souter I, Goodwin TM. Decision making in multifetal pregnancy reduction for triplets. *Am J Perinatol* 1998;15:63–71.

28. Craigo SD. Triplet pregnancy and multifetal reduction: a rational review of the data. *Contemp Ob/Gyn* 1999;April:78–80,83–84, 89–91,95.

29. Boulot P, Hedon B, Pelliccia G, et al. Effects of selective reduction in triplet gestation: a comparative study of 80 cases managed with or without this procedure. *Fertil Steril* 1993;60:497–503.

30. Lipitz S, Reichman B, Uval J, et al. A prospective comparison of the outcome of triplet pregnancies managed expectantly or by multifetal reduction to twins. *Am J Obstet Gynecol* 1994;170:874–879.

31. Bollen N, Camus M, Tournaye H, et al. Embryo reduction in triplet pregnancies after assisted procreation: a comparative study. *Fertil Steril* 1993;60:504–509.

32. Haning RV Jr, Seifer DB, Wheeler CA, et al. Effects of fetal number and multifetal reduction on length of in vitro fertilization pregnancies. *Obstet Gynecol* 1996;87:964–968.

33. Santema JG, Bourdrez P, Wallenburg HCS. Maternal and perinatal complications in triplet compared with twin pregnancy. *Eur J Obstet Gynecol Reprod Biol* 1995;60:143–147.

34. Creinin M, Katz M, Laros R. Triplet pregnancy: changes in morbidity and mortality. *J Perinatol* 1991;11:207–212.

35. Holcberg G, Biale Y, Lewenthal H, et al. Outcome of pregnancy in 31 triplet gestations. *Obstet Gynecol* 1982;59:472–476.

36. Luke B, Keith LG. Monozygotic twinning as a congenital defect and congenital defects in monozygotic twins. *Fetal Diagn Ther* 1990;5:61–69.

37. Vauthier-Brouzes D, Lefebvre G. Selective reduction in multifetal pregnancies: technical and psychological aspects. *Fertil Steril* 1992; 57:1012–1016.

38. Craparo FJ. Selective reduction: is there a limit? *Int J Fertil Menopausal Stud* 1995;40:62–66.

39. Kerenyi T, Chitkara U. Selective birth in twin pregnancy with discordancy for Down's syndrome. *N Engl J Med* 1981;304:1525–1527.

40. Quintero RA, Reich H, Puder KS. Umbilical-cord ligation of an acardiac twin by fetoscopy at 19 weeks of gestation. *N Engl J Med* 1994;330:469–471.

    ⁷aron Y, Johnson KD, Bryant-Greenwood PK, et al. Selective ter-
    ⁻nation and elective reduction in twin pregnancies: 10 years'
    ⁻rience at a single center. *Hum Reprod* 1998;13:2301–2304.

        r CA, Rosenfeld DL, Rawlinson K, et al. Perinatal outcome
        ⁻ltifetal reduction to twins compared with nonreduced
        ⁻estations. *Obstet Gynecol* 1991;78:763–767.

        ⁻A, Schemmer G, Pritts E, et al. Multifetal reduction of
        ⁻ns improves perinatal outcome. *Am J Obstet Gynecol*
        ⁻986.

        ⁻ammond KR, Steinkampf MP. Multifetal reduc-
        ⁻ multiple pregnancy: comparison of obstetrical
        ⁻duced twin gestations. *Fertil Steril* 1995;64:

45. Smith-Levitan M, Kowalik A, Birnholz J, et al. Selective reduction of multifetal pregnancies to twins improves outcome over non-reduced triplet gestations. *Am J Obstet Gynecol* 1996;175:878–882.

46. Lipitz S, Uval J, Achiron R, et al. Outcome of twin pregnancies reduced from triplets compared with nonreduced twin gestations. *Obstet Gynecol* 1996;87:511–514.

47. Luke B, Keith LG, Damewood MD. Maternal characteristics of women delivered of twins: natural versus induced. *Int J Fertil* 1993;38:12–15.

48. Gleicher N, Campbell DP, Chan CL, et al. The desire for multiple births in couples with infertility problems contradicts present practice patterns. *Hum Reprod* 1995;10:1079–1084.

49. Goldfarb J, Kinzer DJ, Boyle M, et al. Attitudes of in vitro fertil-ization and intrauterine insemination couples toward multiple gestation pregnancy and multifetal pregnancy reduction. *Fertil Steril* 1996;65:815–820.

50. Porreco RP, Harmon RJ, Murrow NS, et al. Parental choices in grand multiple gestation: psychological considerations. *J Matern Fetal Med* 1995;4:111–114.

51. Leiblum SR, Kemmann E, Taska L. Attitudes toward multiple births and pregnancy concerns in infertile and non-infertile women. *J Psychosom Obstet Gynecol* 1990;11:197–210.

52. Schreiner-Engel P, Walther VN, Mindes J, et al. First-trimester multifetal pregnancy reduction: acute and persistent psychologic reactions. *Am J Obstet Gynecol* 1995;172:541–547.

53. Kanhai HHH, de Haan M, van Zanten LA, et al. Follow-up of pregnancies, infants, and families after multifetal pregnancy reduction. *Fertil Steril* 1994;62:955–959.

54. Dechaud H, Picot MC, Hedon B, et al. First-trimester multifetal pregnancy reduction: evaluation of technical aspects and risks from 2,756 cases in the literature. *Fetal Diagn Ther* 1998;13: 261–265.

55. Seoud MAF, Toner JP, Kruithoff C, et al. Outcome of twin, triplet, and quadruplet in vitro fertilization pregnancies: the Norfolk experience. *Fertil Steril* 1992;57:825–834.

56. Nazari A, Check JH, Epstein RH, et al. Relationship of small-for-dates sac size to crown-rump length and spontaneous abortion in patients with a known date of ovulation. *Obstet Gynecol* 1991;78:369–373.

57. Taipale P, Hiilesmaa V, Salonen R, et al. Increased nuchal translucency as a marker for fetal chromosomal defects. *N Eng J Med* 1997;337:1654–1658.

58. Hyett J, Perdu M, Sharland G, et al. Using fetal nuchal tr' lucency to screen for major congenital cardiac defects at ' weeks of gestation: population based cohort study. *BM* 318:81–85.

59. Pandya PP, Brizot ML, Kuhn P, et al. First-trimester f' translucency thickness and risk for trisomies. *Ob* 1994;84:420–423.

60. Nicolaides KH, Brizot ML, Snijders RJ. Fetal nuch' ultrasound screening for fetal trisomy in the first nancy. *Br J Obstet Gynaecol* 1994;101:782–78(

61. Stone J, Berkowitz RL. Multifetal pregnancy tive termination. *Semin Perinatol* 1995;19

62. Wapner RJ, Davis GH, Johnson A, et a' multifetal pregnancies. *Lancet* 1990;33

63. Lynch L, Berkowitz RL. Maternal serum α-fetoprotein and coagulation profiles after multifetal pregnancy reduction. *Am J Obstet Gynecol* 1993;169:987–990.

64. Chitkara U, Berkowitz RL, Wilkins IA, et al. Selective second-trimester termination of the anomalous fetus in twin pregnancies. *Obstet Gynecol* 1989;690–694.

65. Johnson MR, Abbas A, Nicolaides KH. Maternal plasma levels of human chorionic gonadotropin, oestradiol and progesterone before and after fetal reduction. *J Endocrinol* 1994;143:309–312.

66. Abbas A, Johnson M, Chard T, et al. Maternal plasma concentrations of insulin-like growth factor binding protein-1 and placental protein 14 in multifetal pregnancies before and after fetal reduction. *Hum Reprod* 1995;10:207–210.

67. Sebire NJ, Sherod C, Abbas A, et al. Preterm delivery and growth restriction in multifetal pregnancies reduced to twins. *Hum Reprod* 1997;12:173–175.

68. Boklage CE. The frequency and survival probability of natural twin conceptions. In: Keith LG, Papiernik E, Keith DM, et al., eds. *Multiple pregnancy: Epidemiology, gestation, and perinatal outcome.* London: Parthenon, 1995:41–50.

69. Landy HJ, Weiner S, Corson SL, et al. The "vanishing twin:" ultrasonographic assessment of fetal disappearance in the first trimester. *Am J Obstet Gynecol* 1986;155:14–19.

70. Samuels P. Ultrasound in the management of the twin gestation. *Clin Obstet Gynecol* 1988;31:110–122.

71. Blumfeld Z, Dirfeld M, Abramovici H, et al. Spontaneous fetal reduction in multiple gestations assessed by transvaginal ultrasound. *Br J Obstet Gynaecol* 1992;99:333–337.

72. Prompeler HJ, Madjar H, Klosa W, et al. Twin pregnancy with single fetal death. *Acta Obstet Gynecol Scand* 1994;73:205–208.

73. Legro RS, Wong IL, Paulson RJ, et al. Multiple implantation after oocyte donation: a frequent but inefficient event. *Fertil Steril* 1995;63:849–853.

74. Fusi L, Gordon H. Twin pregnancy complicated by single intrauterine death: problems and outcome with conservative management. *Br J Obstet Gynecol* 1990;97:511–516.

75. Eglowstein M, D'Alton ME. Intrauterine demise in multiple gestation: theory and management. *J Matern Fetal Med* 1993;2:272–275.

76. Kilby MD, Govind A, O'Brien PM. Outcome of twin pregnancies complicated by a single intrauterine death: a comparison with viable twin pregnancies. *Obstet Gynecol* 1994;84:107–109.

Burke MS. Single fetal demise in twin gestation. *Clin Obstet Gynecol* 1990;33:69–78.

on Y, Bryant-Greenwood PK, Dave N, et al. Multifetal pregnancy reductions of triplets to twins: comparison with non-reduced triplets and twins. *Am J Obstet Gynecol* 1999;180:71.

Heyman E, Asztalos EV, et al. The outcome of triplet, and quintuplet pregnancies managed in a perinatal neonatal, and follow-up data. *Am J Obstet Gynecol* 59.

d-trimester fetal death in triplet pregnancies. 1;77:6–9.

81. Bollen N, Camus M, Staessen C, et al. The incidence of multiple pregnancy after in vitro fertilization and embryo transfer, gamete, or zygote intrafallopian transfer. *Fertil Steril* 1991;55:314–318.

82. Dickey RP, Olar TT, Curole DN, et al. The probability of multiple births when multiple gestational sacs or viable embryos are diagnosed at first trimester ultrasound. *Hum Reprod* 1990;5:880–882.

83. Qasim SM, Karacan GH, Sheldon R, et al. High-order oocyte transfer in gamete intrafallopian transfer patients 40 or more years of age. *Fertil Steril* 1995;64:107–110.

84. Widra EA, Gindoff PR, Smotrich DB, et al. Achieving multiple-order embryo transfer identifies women over 40 years of age with improved in vitro fertilization outcome. *Fertil Steril* 1996;65: 103–108.

85. Anderson RL, Golbus MS, Curry CJR, et al. Central nervous system damage and other anomalies in surviving fetus following second trimester antenatal death of co-twin. *Prenat Diagn* 1990; 10:513–518.

86. Szymonowicz Q, Preston M, Yu VVM. The surviving monozygotic twin. *Arch Dis Child* 1986;61:454–458.

87. Enbom JA. Twin pregnancy with intrauterine death of one twin. *Am J Obstet Gynecol* 1985;152:424–429.

88. Gonen R, Heyman E, Asztalos E, et al. The outcome of triplet gestations complicated by fetal death. *Obstet Gynecol* 1990;75:175–178.

89. Rydhstrom H, Ingemarsson I. Prognosis and long-term follow-up of a twin after antenatal death of the co-twin. *J Reprod Med* 1993;38:142–146.

90. Brandes JM, Itskovitz J, Scher A, et al. The physical and mental development of co-sibs surviving selective reduction of multifetal pregnancies. *Hum Reprod* 1990;5:1014–1017.

91. Avni M, Luke B. Multifetal reduction and pregnancy outcomes: a meta-analysis. *Am J Obstet Gynecol* 1998;178:S124.

92. Sassoon DA, Castro LC, Davis JL, et al. Perinatal outcome in triplet versus twin gestations. *Obstet Gynecol* 1990;75:817–820.

93. Donner C, McGinnis JA, Simon P, et al. Multifetal pregnancy reduction: a Belgian experience. *Eur J Obstet Gynecol Reprod Biol* 1990;38:183–187.

94. Porreco RP, Burke MS, Hendrix ML. Multifetal reduction of triplets and pregnancy outcome. *Obstet Gynecol* 1991;78:335–339.

95. Tallo CP, Vohr B, Oh W, et al. Maternal and neonatal morbidity associated with in vitro fertilization. *J Pediatr* 1995;127:794–800.

96. Groutz A, Yovel I, Amit A, et al. Pregnancy outcome after multifetal pregnancy reduction to twins compared with spontaneously conceived twins. *Hum Reprod* 1996;11:1334–1336.

97. Silver RK, Helfand BT, Russell TL, et al. Multifetal reducti* increases the risk of preterm delivery and fetal growth restric* in twins: a case–control study. *Fertil Steril* 1997;67:30–33.

98. Fitzsimmons BP, Bebbington MW, Fluker MR. Perinat* neonatal outcomes in multiple gestations: assisted repr* versus spontaneous conception. *Am J Obstet Gynecol* ˅ 1162–1167.

99. Boulot P, Hedon B, Pelliccia G, et al. Multifetal pregr* tion: a consecutive series of 61 cases. *Br J Obstet C* 100:63–68.

Role of Ultrasound in the Antepartum Management of Multiple Gestations

Rates of perinatal death in multiple gestations have decreased dramatically in the past 20 years (1). However, perinatal morbidity and mortality remain substantially higher for twin pregnancies than for singletons. Fetal death is three times more common and neonatal mortality is nearly ten times greater among twin than singleton pregnancies. At all gestational ages, the increased complication rates among twin and higher-order multiple gestations are largely due to an increased incidence of preterm delivery, fetal growth restriction, and congenital anomalies. Ultrasound has an enormous potential to detect these complications and decrease the morbidity and mortality associated with them in multiple gestations (2). Ultrasonography allows for the early and accurate detection of multiple fetuses. In addition, it is extremely effective in determining both chorionicity and amnionicity during the first trimester and in the detection of anomalies during the second trimester. Mid-trimester cervical length measurement has also begun to help identify pregnancies likely to be complicated by early preterm labor and delivery. Finally, by using ultrasound to describe interval growth patterns of multiple fetuses, obstetricians may modify, and preferably, minimize the effect of intrauterine growth restriction on perinatal outcome.

FIRST-TRIMESTER ULTRASONOGRAPHY

The role of ultrasonography in the assessment of multiple gestations begins in the first trimester by: 1) making the correct diagnosis of multiple gestational sacs; 2) measuring crown-rump length for accurate gestational age dating; and 3) identifying the type of placentation.

Diagnosis of Multiple Gestation

In most instances, first-trimester ultrasound allows early diagnosis of multifetal gestation. Patients at high risk of multiple gestation should undergo scanning soon after the diagnosis of pregnancy. This includes patients undergoing assisted reproductive techniques and those with a uterine size greater than dates, hyperemesis gravidarum, or a family history of twins.

The accuracy of ultrasound in diagnosing twin and higher-order multiple gestations increases markedly between the fifth and sixth week of pregnancy. In the investigation by Doubilet and Benson, 8% of 325 multiple gestations were undercounted with respect to the number of fetuses. The undercounting was significantly higher for monochorionic rather than for dichorionic twins or higher-order gestations. Undercounting also occurred significantly more frequently on sonograms obtained between 5.0 and 5.4 weeks than at 5.5 to 5.9 weeks, 19% versus 9%, respectively. This may be explained in part by the sonographic appearance of the yolk sac at 5.5 weeks of pregnancy. Certainly, after 6 weeks' gestational age, determination of fetal number is more easily achieved by counting fetal poles with cardiac activity within each gestational sac. Use of transvaginal sonography allows definitive diagnosis at least 1 week earlier in most cases, depending on maternal size and uterine positioning.

A definitive diagnosis of multiple gestation should not be made unless specific embryos or embryonic parts can be identified within each gestational sac. Numerous sonographic findings can mimic a second anembryonic cavity or sac. These confusing sonographic findings may include a ghost artifact due to refraction error, a subchorionic blood clot, a chorioamniotic separation, a decidual pseudosac in the contralateral horn of a bicornuate or didelphic uterus, or excessive transducer pressure in a thin woman producing an hourglass effect on a single gestational sac. The vanishing twin phenomenon is a relatively frequent occurrence, reported among as many as 20% of twin gestations diagnosed in the first trimester (4). This high rate should not be artificially inflated by misidentification of a twin gestation based on visualization of an anembryonic cavity. From the patient's perspective, the diagnosis of a vanishing twin will always be remembered as the loss of a "child," the "surviving co-twin" may be affected by the loss of its "sibling."

The RADIUS study group confirmed that routine prenatal ultrasound is valuable in the detection of multiple gestations at an early gestational age (5). The RADIUS study was a randomized controlled trial involving 15,530 women, 7,812 of whom were assigned to a routine screening group and 7,718 to a control group. The screened group underwent two ultrasound examinations, one at 18 to 20 weeks' gestation and the second at 31 to 33 weeks' gestation. All but one of the multiple pregnancies in the screened group were diagnosed prior to 26 weeks' gestation. Twenty-three multiple pregnancies (37%) in the control group were not identified until after 26 weeks, and 8 were not diagnosed until the patient was admitted for delivery. Other studies (6–8), although none as large as the RADIUS trial, have confirmed that routine ultrasound screening allows for the reliable diagnosis of multiple gestations early in pregnancy. When routine screening was not used, a large number of multiples went undetected until the third trimester, and sometimes until delivery. It is intuitive that only after the early diagnosis of a multifetal gestation has been made can interventions be initiated to reduce the maternal and perinatal morbidity associated with this condition.

After institution of a policy of performing routine second-trimester ultrasonography, Persson et al. (9) identified 98% of 254 twin gestations among women undergoing obstetric care a' Malmo General Hospital, Sweden. In a subsequent analysis of th outcomes of these pregnancies, the authors reported that the av age gestational age at detection decreased from 33 to 19 we Multiples in the routine ultrasound screening group had a l perinatal mortality rate, a higher gestational age at delivery. low birth weight infants, and no cases of very low birth deliveries (less than 1,500 g) compared to a historical contr of twins from the preceding decade (10). Although the s a secondary analysis with an insufficient sample size ' statistical significance, the multiple gestations in the RADIUS trial in the routine ultrasound screening group had a rate of adverse perinatal outcome of 25% compared with 37.7% for the unscreened control group (relative risk, 0.7; 95% confidence interval [CI], 0.39–1.11; p = .13) (11).

Accurate Gestational Age Dating

The first trimester is the ideal time to confirm or establish accurate gestational age dating. This is especially important considering the high rate of premature labor that occurs among multiple gestations. In the latter half of the first trimester, measurement of the fetal crown-rump length is the most accurate way to determine gestational age. The estimated gestational age based on the last menstrual period is confirmed if the crown-rump length agrees within 5 to 7 days. If the fetal crown-rump length does not agree, new gestational age estimates can be established with an anticipated accuracy of 5 to 7 days greater or less. On many occasions, twins or higher-order multiples may be the result of assisted reproductive technology such as *in vitro* fertilization or gamete intrafallopian transfer, and in those cases gestational age can be accurately determined from the date of extrauterine fertilization.

Fetal crown-rump length standards are the same for singleton and twin gestations and should be equally reliable. If the diagnosis of twins is delayed until the second trimester, measurements of biparietal diameter, abdominal circumference, and femur length are also as reliable for assessing the gestational age of twins as they are for singletons (12). It is only in the third trimester that these biometric measurements become uncertain. Although abdominal circumference measurements are generally smaller in twin gestations by the third trimester, there are conflicting results regarding the relationship between biparietal diameter of singletons and twins. For the most part, femur lengths of twin fetuses are similar to those of singletons.

Determination of Amnionicity and Chorionicity

Determination of amnionicity is based on visualization of an intertwin membrane. The importance of this membrane is underscored by the markedly different antenatal management schemes for a monoamnionic versus diamniotic gestation (see Chapter 8). Risks associated with monoamnionicity include high rates of twin-twin transfusion, cord entanglement, shared organs, and fetal death. As pregnancy progresses, the detection and evaluation of this membrane becomes increasingly difficult because of uterine crowding and progressive thinning of the membrane. Evaluation also is limited when the pregnancy is complicated by oligohydramnios in one or more of the fetal compartments.

The diagnosis of chorionicity is important because of the perinatal implications associated with a monochorionic placentation such as high rates of growth retardation, growth discordancy, congenital anomaly, and perinatal mortality compared to dichorionic gestations (13). Sonographic determination of chorionicity should be attempted in all multiple gestations and is best performed in the first and early second trimesters. Approximately 20% of gestations have a single chorion, and virtually all of these have some component of shared circulation. The ante-

natal diagnosis of chorionicity is helpful in differentiating intrauterine growth restriction related to insufficient uteroplacental
perfusion and twin-twin transfusion syndrome resulting from un-
balanced arteriovenous shunting within a monochorionic placenta.
Knowledge of chorionicity significantly impacts genetic counseling. The risk of prenatal diagnosis in multiple gestations is discussed in Chapter 3. Vascular communication within a monochorionic placenta allows the occurrence of hemodynamic instability or
transplacental embolization of thromboplastic material associated
with the spontaneous or induced demise of one fetus. Because the
diagnosis of a monochorionic twin gestation may alter subsequent
diagnosis and management, establishing the placentation early in
the pregnancy is crucial to the appropriate management of multiple gestations.

When two placentas are visualized or the fetuses are discordant
for gender, the gestation is dichorionic and diamniotic. In the
absence of these findings, monochorionicity is possible, and further assessment is necessary. A single placental site is characteristic of a monochorionic twin gestation, although a single placental
site also can represent a fused dichorionic placenta. Several techniques have been described for the sonographic assessment of chorionicity. D'Alton and Dudley (14) described counting the number of
layers present in the intertwin membrane. In a monochorionic
gestation, only the two layers of juxtaposed amnion are detected.
In a dichorionic pregnancy, the intertwin membrane consists of
amnion and chorion from each gestational sac, and therefore three
or four layers are seen. If only three layers are seen, the two chorionic membranes are fused and visualized as a single layer. In
D'Alton and Dudley's series, chorionicity was accurately determined in 100% of dichorionic gestations and 94% of monochorionic
gestations. Vayssiere et al. (15) confirmed the use of this method
when they were 95% accurate in determining chorionicity in their
investigation.

Townsend et al. (16) subjectively described the intertwin membrane as thick or thin to differentiate chorionicity. Membranes
were described as thin (monochorionicity) when they were "fine
and hairlike." Often the membrane was visible only in short segments. Thick membranes (dichorionicity) had a definable thickness
and could be visualized over longer courses. With this method, 89%
of dichorionic pregnancies were correctly identified during the second trimester. Although their sonographic description of the membrane was subjective, the authors found the results to be consistent
and easily reproducible between sonographers (91% interobserver
concordance).

The dividing membrane becomes progressively thinner throughout the third trimester, so the accuracy of ultrasound determination
decreases. The result is a 52% detection rate for dichorionic gestations in the third trimester. Oligohydramnios also complicates
categorization of chorionicity late in pregnancy. After 28 weeks
gestation, D'Alton and Dudley (14) were only able to accurately
determine placentation in one out of six patients who presented
with discordant twin growth and oligohydramnios.

The use of a membrane thickness cutoff value of 2 mm has been
used by some investigators to correctly assign chorionicity in more
than 80% of the cases (17). A value greater than 2 mm measured

near the placental insertion site suggests the presence of a "thick" dichorionic, diamniotic membrane. Unfortunately, the reproducibility of this measurement has been questioned (18).

Visualization of a twin peak or lambda sign is useful in the diagnosis of a dichorionic gestation (19). In this situation, the placenta develops a triangular projection of chronic villi between the layers of the dividing membrane at the junction of the fused placentas. Regardless of the gestational age at which this sign is visualized, the pregnancy is considered dichorionic (Fig. 5-1). In monochorionic placentations, the membranes approach the chorionic plate in a perpendicular manner without intervening chorionic villi. At 10 to 14 weeks' gestation, twin pregnancies without the lambda sign can accurately be classified as monochorionic. Unfortunately, the absence of the lambda sign after 16 weeks does not accurately identify monochorionicity. Other authors have confirmed this lack of reliability in diagnosing monochorionicity as pregnancy progresses (20).

Babinski et al. (21) described the use of three-dimensional vaginal ultrasonography in the first trimester to accurately determine amnionicity. In this case, two-dimensional vaginal ultrasound detected two closely positioned embryos with only one yolk sac visualized. No amniotic membrane could be seen. Because amnionicity could not be determined and conjoined twinning could not be excluded, three-dimensional ultrasonography was used and clearly depicted two yolk sacs and two separate fetal poles, thereby making the diagnosis of a monochorionic, diamnionic pregnancy. The authors encouraged the use of three-dimensional technology in selected high-risk cases.

Prenatal determination of zygosity by means of DNA analysis has been reported in pregnancies complicated by discordancy in growth or for anomalies (22). This technique involves evaluation of highly polymorphic markers on multiple chromosomes. Exclusion of monozygosity requires demonstration of differences in at least two markers, preferably on different chromosomes. DNA testing for zygosity may require both polymerase chain reaction and Southern blot technique in order to evaluate multiple chromosomal markers; complete evaluation takes as long as a week or longer. Norton et al. (22) have recommended DNA studies for cases in which management would be altered by clear demonstration of dizygosity or monozygosity.

In summary, the diagnosis of amnionicity and chorionicity can be accurately made by means of ultrasound examination. Consistent findings of dichorionicity include separate placentas, different genders, a thick intertwin membrane, and a prominent twin peak sign. Counting layers of the dividing membrane is easier in the late first and early second trimesters, as is the subjective evaluation of the sonographic appearance of the intertwin membrane. A composite of ultrasonographic findings (fetal sex, placental number, membrane thickness, and twin peak sign), allows the prediction of amnionicity and chorionicity with excellent reliability (Table 5-1). The sensitivity for detection of dichorionicity and monochorionicity was 97.3% and 91.7%, respectively (23). In the same report, monoamnionicity was diagnosed with 100% accuracy. On rare occasions, when traditional sonographic determination of chorionicity is inconclusive, circumstances of discordant growth or

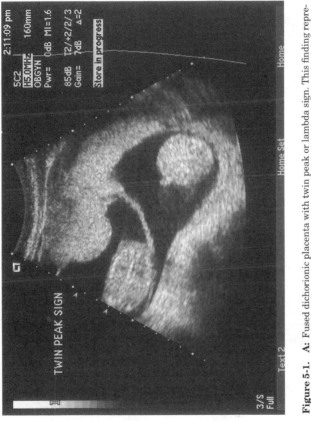

Figure 5-1. A: Fused dichorionic placenta with twin peak or lambda sign. This finding represents the projection of chorionic villous tissue between the layers of the dividing membranes at the junction of the fused placenta.

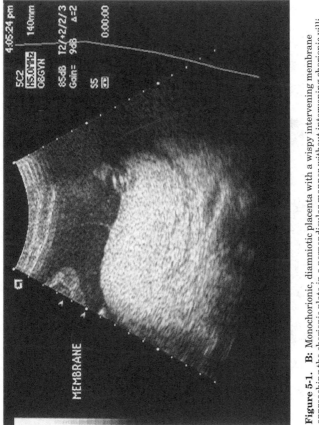

Figure 5-1. B: Monochorionic, diamniotic placenta with a wispy intervening membrane approaching the chorionic plate in a perpendicular manner without intervening chorionic villi.

Table 5-1. Ultrasonographic prediction of amnionicity and chorionicity

Variable	Accuracy	Reference
Membrane		
Thickness		
Quantitative (≥ 2 mm)	89%	Townsend et al., 1988 (16)
Subjective (thick/thin)	80%	Winn et al., 1989 (17)
Layers counted	100% dichorionic	D'Alton and Dudley, 1989 (14)
	94% monochorionic	Vayssiere et al., 1996 (15)
Placenta		
Insertion site, lambda sign		
Present 10–14 wk	93% dichorionic	Sepulveda et al., 1997 (19)
Absent 20 wk	100% monochorionic	
Composite evaluation		
Fetal sex, placental number, membrane thickness, lambda sign	97.3% dichorionic	Scardo et al., 1995 (23)
	91.7% monochorionic	

structural integrity may warrant evaluation by means of DNA analysis. Three-dimensional ultrasound may also be used to clarify amnionicity in unusual circumstances when the diagnosis of a single gestational sac or conjoined twins is a possibility.

Typically, the same criteria described above will be used in the assessment of placentation for triplet pregnancies. The knowledge that the pregnancy was achieved through the use of assisted reproductive technology makes trichorionicity most likely. It is important to remember, however, that monozygotic splitting is more common with assisted fertility than it is with spontaneous conception (24). Visualization of the "ipsilon zone" also helps identify placentation in triplet pregnancies (Fig. 5-2). The upsilon zone is the junction of the three intrafetal membranes. Chorionicity can frequently be determined by examining the relative membrane thicknesses at the ipsilon zone (25).

SECOND-TRIMESTER ULTRASONOGRAPHY

Detection of Anomalies

As the maternal population ages, the prevalence of multifetal pregnancies increases. These fetuses consequently are at increased risk of chromosomal aneuploidy associated with advanced maternal age (26). In addition, epidemiological studies show a 1.5- to threefold increase in the incidence of fetal anomalies among twin and higher-order gestations (27–29). Monozygotic twins have a

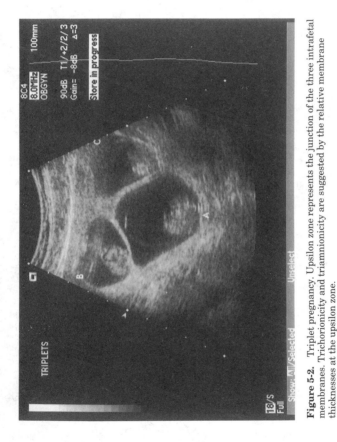

Figure 5-2. Triplet pregnancy. Upsilon zone represents the junction of the three intrafetal membranes. Trichorionicity and triamnionicity are suggested by the relative membrane thicknesses at the upsilon zone.

substantially higher risk of congenital anomalies compared with either singletons or dizygotic twins (12,30). As a consequence, ultrasound scanning for fetal anomalies in multiple gestations is clearly justifiable and best performed between 18 and 20 weeks' gestation.

Discordant findings for dizygotic twins usually are due to differences in genetic predisposition. However, discordance found in monozygotic gestations may be a result of the underlying stimulus to zygote splitting, variation in gene expression, or symmetry and laterality defects during zygote splitting. They also can occur as a consequence of abnormal placentation (31).

When Baldwin (27) reviewed the literature on 112,384 twin pregnancies, it was clear that the highest prevalence of anomalous fetuses occurred among monochorionic twins. For any given defect, the pregnancy may be concordant or discordant between fetuses in terms of the presence of abnormality or its severity. Most structural abnormalities (80% to 90%) in a multifetal gestation are discordant among fetuses (31). However, when the abnormality is concordant, monozygotic twins are more commonly affected (27). The most common structural defects are cardiac abnormalities, central nervous system defects, including neural tube defects, facial clefting, and gastrointestinal defects. Congenital anomalies of twins can be grouped into those specific to the twinning process itself, such as conjoined twins, sirenomelia, holoprosencephaly, neural tube defects, and cloacal exstrophy, and those resulting from vascular interchange, such as the acardiac monster, microcephaly, renal dysplasia, intestinal atresia, and aplasia cutis. Finally, some defects in multifetal gestations are the result of intrauterine crowding, such as foot deformities, hip dislocation, and asymmetry of the skull.

The ability of ultrasound to depict congenital anomalies in multiple gestations has not been adequately studied by in a large, prospective, multicenter trial. There have been several smaller series from single centers, the largest of which was a report of 245 twin gestations with a 4.9% incidence of anomalies. In that series, there was an 88% sensitivity for the detection of fetal anomaly (21 of 24 affected fetuses were properly identified). The specificity was 100% with no false-positive diagnoses (29).

Some families choose to continue a multiple gestation in which the fetuses are discordant for fetal anomalies. Others choose termination of the entire pregnancy or selective termination of the affected twin. Naturally, this management plan necessitates knowledge of chorionicity and consideration of the risk to the unaffected fetus. After counseling, the burden is ultimately left with the family to determine the degree of risk that is acceptable in regard to losing the normal twin as a complication of the selective termination procedure.

Sonographic Assessment of the Cervix

Preterm birth is the most significant contributor to perinatal morbidity and mortality in twin and higher-order multiple births. In singleton pregnancies, the rate of preterm delivery at or before 32 weeks is 1% to 2%. For twin gestations, 5% to 10% are born prior to 32 weeks. The rate for triplet gestations is double or triple that of twin gestations. Programs aimed at the prevention of early

:livery of multiple gestations have included components of
▸atient education, restriction of maternal activity, frequent contact with health care providers, and serial cervical examination.
Recent findings have suggested that transvaginal ultrasound for
the measurement of cervical length may be useful in the prediction of preterm delivery (32–34).

In a large, multicenter, prospective investigation (32), cervical
length was measured by means of transvaginal sonography between 22 and 24 weeks' gestation in 147 twin pregnancies. A cervical length of 25 mm or less was detected in 18% of the cases, of
which 27% delivered prior to 32 weeks of pregnancy and 54% were
delivered before 35 weeks (Table 5-2). Overall, when screening
examinations were performed at 24 weeks, a cervical length of
25 mm or less was associated with a sevenfold increase in risk of
preterm delivery prior to 32 weeks.

In a European observational study of 215 twin pregnancies
(33), transvaginal cervical lengths were measured between 22
and 24 weeks' gestation. The distribution of cervical lengths was
skewed to the left when compared with a similar distribution of cervical lengths for singletons. The mean cervical length was 36.8 mm
for twin gestations in this study. Twenty-three patients (11%) had
a cervical length of 25 mm or less at 23 weeks. That group included
80% of the women who delivered at or before 30 weeks and 45% of
those who delivered prior to 32 weeks. The authors found that a
cervical length less than 30 mm was associated with 30% risk of
preterm delivery and that the risk escalated to 70% with a cervix
10 mm or shorter. In summary, the risk of preterm delivery increases exponentially as the cervix shortens.

Imseis et al. (34) showed that a transvaginal ultrasonographic
cervical length measurement greater than 35 mm between 24 and
26 weeks for twin gestations is predictive of low risk of delivery
before 34 weeks' gestation. In the sample of 85 women with twins,
the mean cervical length for those delivering at or after 34 weeks'
gestation was 36.4 mm, significantly greater than the mean cervical length of patients who delivered prior to 34 weeks' gestation

Table 5-2. Cervical length and risk of spontaneous preterm birth

Cervical Length	Study Cohort	Spontaneous Preterm Birth		
		<32 wk	<35 wk	<37 wk
Number	147	13	47	80
>25 mm	82%	5%	27%	49%
≤25 mm	18%	27%	54%	73%
Odds ratio		6.9	3.2	2.8
95% confidence interval		2.0–24.2	1.3–8.0	1.1–7.7
p Value		.002	.01	.03

From Goldenberg RL, Iams JD, Miodovnik M, et al. The preterm predictic
study: risk factors in twin gestations. *Am J Obstet Gynecol* 1996; 175:1047–10⁵

(27.7 mm). Only 3% of the twins with a cervical length of more than 35 mm was delivered before 34 weeks' gestation (34).

Amniotic Fluid Volume

Assessment of amniotic fluid volume is an important method of determining fetal well-being. Volumes determined to be outside the range of normal are associated with higher rates of adverse perinatal outcome (35,36). Amniotic fluid volume is assessed in a semiquantitative manner by means of either measurement of the deepest vertical pocket (DVP) or determination of the amniotic fluid index (AFI). The AFI is a sum of the largest vertical pocket in each of the four uterine quadrants. Investigators have shown the AFI to be reproducible in singleton pregnancies (37,38). Moore (39) found that the AFI method was superior to the deepest vertical pocket (DVP) method for amniotic fluid assessment in singleton pregnancies.

Abnormalities of amniotic fluid volume in multiple gestations occur more frequently than in singleton pregnancies, yet there has been relatively little published on the assessment of amniotic fluid in multiple gestation. Most of what has been published regarding the assessment of amniotic fluid volume in multiple pregnancies has been based on qualitative estimation of fluid volume rather than the semiquantitative techniques popular for evaluation of singleton pregnancies.

Studies of amniotic fluid volume in twin gestations have included the assessment of an overall AFI, evaluation of the DVP in each gestational sac, and measurement of a two-diameter pocket of each twin's largest fluid pocket (40–42). The overall AFI for multiple gestations is measured without regard to the intervening membrane. The uterus is divided into four quadrants along the sagittal midline and midway on the fundus. The vertical depth of the largest fluid pocket in each of four quadrants is measured in centimeters, and the sum of the measurements is the AFI. Other authors have recommended evaluation of the DVP of each twin sac to assess the adequacy of the amniotic fluid volume. Chau et al. (42) advised using the two-diameter pocket, which is obtained by multiplying the maximum depth by the horizontal width of the largest amniotic fluid pocket.

Reports have shown that the AFIs of twin pregnancies follow a pattern similar to those of singleton gestations. The AFI increases significantly during the second trimester, stabilizes during the early third trimester, and begins to decline between 33 and 36 weeks (40–42). In their series of 91 twin gestations, Chau et al. (42) were able to determine the fifth and ninety-fifth percentiles of AFI. Although the values varied throughout pregnancy, the percentiles approximated the norms established for singleton pregnancies. In regard to each twin's maximum vertical pocket depth, the ninetieth percentile confidence intervals were also approximately the same as the values seen in singleton gestations (3 to 8 cm) (39,42).

Porter et al. (41) established normative AFI measurements for twin pregnancies after 27 weeks' gestation. Their results were similar to those reported by Chau et al. (42). When the data collected by Porter et al. were compared with AFI data reported for singletons (37), the fifth and fiftieth percentile values for twins were found to be slightly higher at each gestational age than comparable values for singletons. This was not the case for the ninety-fifth percentile values, which were slightly lower for the twin pregnancies.

The amniotic fluid volume in uncomplicated diamniotic twin gestations has been found to increase independently in each sac as the gestational age progresses (43). Magann et al. (43) established that the average amniotic fluid volume for each twin was similar to the volume reported for singleton gestations. Because this value was independent of both fetal weight and position, the authors suggested that a single AFI was appropriate for evaluation of diamniotic twin pregnancies.

Although Watson et al. (40) found the amniotic fluid volume of twin gestations to be substantially greater than that of singleton pregnancies at all gestational ages, they noted that the AFI correlated closely with the DVP from either gestational sac ($r = 0.71$; $p < .0001$). At 20, 27, and 36 weeks of pregnancy, the mean AFI was 16.7 ± 4.8 cm, 21.1 ± 3.1 cm, and 14.6 ± 3.4 cm, respectively. This is in contrast to AFI values of 14.1 cm, 14.6 cm, and 13.8 cm for a singleton pregnancy at similar gestational ages (37). Therefore, Watson et al. suggested that either method of sonographic amniotic fluid assessment is appropriate for twin gestations.

The major deficiency in the literature is that no one method has been validated for predicting perinatal outcome for multiple gestations. Until those data are available, it is recommended that the same values be used to define oligohydramnios and polyhydramnios as are currently used for singleton gestation. Oligohydramnios is a concern if the DVP in either gestational sac is less than 2 cm or if the overall AFI is less than 5 cm. Polyhydramnios is suggested by a DVP greater than 8 cm in either sac or an overall AFI greater than 25 cm. In both of these circumstances, a subjective evaluation of amniotic fluid volume may also contribute to clinical decision making.

THIRD-TRIMESTER ULTRASONOGRAPHY

Intrauterine Growth Restriction

Abnormal fetal growth is one of the most common complications encountered in multifetal pregnancies. Although some studies have shown no difference in fetal growth between singletons and twins (44), the majority have shown decreased fetal growth in the third trimester among normal twin gestations (45–47). It appears that twins grow with the same velocity as singletons until the third trimester, when twin growth slows, even in healthy gestations. The slowing of growth velocity of normal twin gestations appears to occur at approximately 30 to 32 weeks' gestation. When plotted on a typical singleton growth chart, the mean estimated weight for twins is at approximately the fiftieth percentile for singletons until these gestational ages. Between 32 and 36 weeks, the estimated weight for twins typically decreases to between the tenth and the fiftieth percentile for singletons. After 36 weeks, twin weights often are below the tenth percentile compared with the weights of singletons of the same gestational age (46,48).

Growth velocity of triplets begins to show the same slowing as seen in twin gestations but with an onset at approximately 28 weeks (48,49). When the components of fetal growth are analyzed, it appears most likely that the biparietal diameter of normal twins does not differ greatly from that of matched singletons that are appropriate for gestational age throughout pregnancy (44). Other reports have suggested a reduction in the biparietal diameter of twins compared to singletons (45,46). It is important to remember, however, that biparietal diameter measurements in twins may be difficult due to both intrauterine crowding and a higher rate of malpresentation resulting in a greater frequency of dolichocephalic breech presentations. Socol et al. (46) found that birth length and head circumferences of twins usually are comparable with those of singletons matched for gestational age. The slowing of growth of twins approaching term is primarily accounted for by reductions in the measurement of the abdominal circumference (47). These findings suggest that the reduction in twin growth velocity in multiple gestations near term is most consistent with asymmetric intrauterine growth retardation (IUGR).

The reason for this asymmetric intrauterine growth restriction in multiple gestations likely involves the same etiology that results in asymmetric growth abnormalities in singleton pregnancies—placental insufficiency magnified by the inherent competition for nutrients presented by multiple fetuses and a greater frequency of abnormal placental implantations. Other causes of IUGR may occur, such as early placental infection, chromosomal and structural abnormalities, or chronic intertwin transfusion syndrome, but these are the less likely explanations. By 36 weeks' gestation, a large percentage of undelivered twins have IUGR according to singleton growth norms. IUGR also is a clinically significant contributor to intertwin growth discordance (see Chapter 8).

Many investigators have suggested that although the incremental growth of twin fetuses is less than that of singletons, the clinical difference is too small to warrant generation of separate nomograms for the evaluation of fetal growth in twin pregnancies. We prefer to use established singleton growth curves but understand the anticipated deviations that multiple gestations take from these singleton norms. The limitations of the current nomographic data available for twins make adoption of universal twin growth standards unfeasible. It is clear that without a baseline for growth established with early diagnosis and accurate dating of the multiple gestation, interpretation of individual twin growth rates will be hampered by the normally occurring variation in fetal growth. IUGR among multiples is best predicted with an estimated fetal weight calculated from multiple values, including abdominal circumference. Chitkara et al. (50) determined that a combined estimated fetal weight and femur length measurement had a sensitivity of 92% for IUGR, which was superior to that of any individual measurement.

Although a great deal of data have been generated describing intrauterine growth in multiple gestations, curiously few studies have specifically addressed either the clinical value of serial ultrasound assessment of fetal growth or the appropriate interval for screening in the setting of a multiple gestation. It can be easily inferred, however, that ultrasound examination has an important role in the antepartum assessment of the fetal well-being of twins: (a) The percentage of newborns experiencing IUGR is significantly higher in multiple gestations than in singleton pregnancies; (b) At every gestational age, perinatal mortality is increased in multiple gestations relative to singletons, and much of this excess is related to growth restriction; (c) Identification of multiple gestations with growth restriction involving one or more fetuses could lead to antenatal surveillance or delivery in an effort to decrease the incidence of perinatal morbidity and mortality; (d) Fundal height measurements are of minimal usefulness in the identification of abnormal fetal growth in a multiple gestation; ultrasound still is the only modality that allows accurate assessment of fetal growth; (e) Ultrasound is the only modality that can be used to identify twin–twin transfusion syndrome, for which intervention can lead to improved outcomes.

To assess the ideal interval between serial ultrasonography, Grobman and Parilla (51) identified 31 twin gestations over a 6-year period with normal fetal growth and no anomalies identified between 20 and 24 weeks that subsequently developed ultrasound evidence of fetal growth aberrations. These aberrations included abdominal circumference measurement less than fifth percentile, estimated fetal weight less than tenth percentile, or greater than 20% difference in the estimated fetal weights. The mean interval between scans was 4.4 ± 2 weeks with 10.3 ± 3.9 weeks elapsing before a growth abnormality was first suspected. If no growth abnormalities were identified between 28 and 32 weeks, the mean elapsed time until the subsequent development of abnormal growth identified by ultrasound was 6.3 ± 1.6 weeks. The positive predictive value was 47.7% if abnormal growth was observed at any ultrasound examination. The authors concluded that with the relatively poor predictive value and the long interval after a normal scan for an abnormality to become apparent, that ultrasound every 2 to 3 weeks is unnecessary when normal growth had been previously observed. No appropriate interval was suggested by these authors.

In conclusion, it is clear that ultrasound plays an important role in the management of multiple gestations and is essential for the diagnosis of intrauterine growth abnormalities. In the second half of gestation in multiple pregnancies, fetal growth should be assessed periodically with serial ultrasound examinations. In general, the scans can be scheduled on a monthly basis, but the interval between scans should be based on the clinical situation. The interval can be extended if results of previous examinations suggest appropriate growth, particularly in dichorionic gestations. Shorter intervals may be needed for complicated pregnancies. The identification of abnormal fetal growth in a multiple gestation provides the foundation for initiation of fetal surveillance or for the consideration of delivery just as it would in a singleton pregnancy.

Antepartum Fetal Surveillance

Doppler velocimetry has been advocated for use in high-risk pregnancies, such as multiple gestations affected with growth restriction or discordance. Previous studies have shown the umbilical artery systolic to diastolic (S/D) ratio measured throughout gestation to be similar in singleton and twin pregnancies (52,53). It also is known that the higher the resistance index, the more frequent the evidence of fetal compromise. In a retrospective study of 94 twins and 7 triplets by Gaziano et al. (54), 17 fetuses were found to have abnormal results of Doppler flow studies. Fifteen of the 17 fetuses had serious morbidity. Seven were small for gestational age, and 8 of the other 10 were admitted to a neonatal intensive care unit (NICU).

In a retrospective study of 52 twins and four triplets by Gerson et al. (55), 44 pregnancies were judged to be normal by Doppler velocimetry. Concordant, appropriate for gestational age infants were delivered in each case. One abnormal Doppler velocimetry result occurred in a pregnancy that was concordant, while 9 abnormal Doppler findings were associated with discordant birth weights. In this small study, the sensitivity of Doppler velocimetry for birth-weight discordance was 81.8%. The specificity was 97.9%, and the positive and negative predictive values were 90% and 95.6% respectively. In a single small study investigating umbilical artery waveform analysis of higher-order gestations, Giles et al. (56) studied 20 triplet and 1 quadruplet pregnancies throughout the latter part of pregnancy. Nine of the triplet pregnancies produced one or more small for gestational age babies which highly correlated with abnormal results of Doppler flow studies. The two stillbirths in the series both had absent end diastolic flow for several weeks prior to their deaths. When there is a persistent absence of diastolic flow, the risk of adverse fetal outcome becomes substantial. Results of prospective, but small, studies of Doppler ultrasonography in the management of twin pregnancies have suggested a reduction in fetal death (combined odds ratio, 0.14; 95% CI, 0.03–0.77) when Doppler velocimetry was used in the evaluation of fetal well-being (57,58).

Studies have suggested that twin discordance may be associated with abnormal findings at Doppler velocimetry. Umbilical artery blood flow velocimetry has been advocated for prediction of this condition. In a study of 58 consecutive twin pregnancies, of which 18 were growth discordant, Divon et al. (59) found that the diagnostic accuracy of ultrasound was not significantly different from that of Doppler velocimetry. The investigators compared biparietal diameter, abdominal circumference, femur length, and estimated fetal weight measurements with Doppler results for fetuses of each twin pair. Overall, the best predictor seemed to be the presence of either a difference in the S/D ratio of more than 15% or a difference in estimated fetal weight of more than 15%. On the basis of these differences, investigators correctly identified 14 of 18 discordant twin pairs and misclassified 5 of 40 concordant gestations (59).

Other investigators have found a combination of results of umbilical artery Doppler velocimetry and sonographic estimation of fetal weight to have a sensitivity for detection of growth restriction higher than either individual study alone. For example, Berkowitz et al. (60) showed that the combination of these tests has a sensitivity of 85% for IUGR, which was better than the individual sensitivities of either Doppler velocimetry (55%) or estimated fetal weight (76%). These observations were confirmed by both Gaziano et al. (61) and Degani et al. (62). Interestingly some authors have found that Doppler velocimetry can help detect intrauterine growth restriction anywhere from 3 to 7 weeks earlier than does sonographic biometry (53,62,63).

The role of Doppler ultrasound in the detection and evaluation of chronic intertwin transfusion syndrome is not well defined. Investigative results are not consistent. Most studies suggest that an S/D ratio difference greater than 15% is associated with intrauterine growth restriction, whereas twin–twin transfusion syndrome is rarely associated with a substantial difference in the S/D ratio until late in gestation, when one or both of the fetuses are significantly compromised. Rizzo et al. (60) compared the S/D ratio differences for 15 sets of discordant twins who exhibited no evidence of chronic intertwin transfusion syndrome with the S/D ratio differences for 10 sets of discordant twins with chronic intertwin transfusion syndrome. In the group without chronic intertwin transfusion, substantial differences in the S/D ratios were detected at the time of the initial Doppler ultrasound screening. In the group with chronic intertwin transfusion syndrome, the S/D ratio differences were not apparent until very close to the time of delivery (64). It is likely that abnormal results of Doppler studies reflect the placental pathology associated with uteroplacental insufficiency and fetal growth restriction. In most instances of chronic intertwin transfusion syndrome, the pathological process producing a small twin is typically not placental but rather hematological.

Another form of antepartum fetal surveillance useful in multiple gestations besides Doppler velocimetry is fetal biophysical profile (BPP) testing. Biophysical testing includes sonographic evaluation of fetal movement, tone, and breathing, in addition to the previously mentioned assessment of amniotic fluid. Ultrasound and biophysical assessment allow noninvasive evaluation of fetal status, especially for an immature fetus. The appropriate use of ultrasound assessment allows for conservative management of selected pregnancies and appropriately timed intervention and delivery of other gestations.

There are two retrospective studies devoted exclusively to the BPP in twin and triplet gestations. Lodeiro et al. (65) performed a full BPP study with a nonstress test (NST) on 49 consecutive twin pairs, of which 40 had additional high-risk factors including IUGR, maternal hypertension, diabetes, or bleeding. Testing was repeated on a weekly basis as long as scores were 8 or 10. When the BPP score was 8 or 10, 62 of 64 fetuses had a good outcome (2 died of extreme prematurity). When the BPP score was 7 or less, all fetuses experienced distress, but no deaths occurred. Lodeiro et al. (65) found that the final BPP was normal for all fetuses with a reactive NST and for more than 80% of fetuses with a nonreactive NST. The full BPP had a sensitivity of 83% for adverse perinatal outcomes, suggesting that the BPP is a fairly reliable way to observe twins in the antepartum period.

Alcalay et al. (66) reviewed the outcomes of 35 triplet pregnancies delivered between 1984 and 1989. The last BPP (excluding the NST) preceding delivery was analyzed if it was within 1 week of delivery. A BPP of 8/8 was obtained for 99 fetuses, and the 5-minute Apgar score was 7 or more for 93 of the 99. The BPP was 6/8 in six fetuses of which 5 had an Apgar score of 7 or more at 5 minutes. There were two stillbirths, both of which had a normal BPP within 1 week of the demise. The failure of the BPP to help identify these two stillbirths is obviously concerning. Firm conclusions regarding the reliability of the BPP in multiple gestations are limited by the paucity of available evidence and represent another area awaiting additional investigation.

Intrapartum Use

Ultrasound is also of vital importance to the management of multiple gestations during labor and delivery. It allows for determination of fetal lie, and therefore appropriate counseling of the pre-labor or laboring patient regarding mode of delivery. In addition, ultrasound is used during the second stage of labor to aid the physician in delivery of the second or third infant, who may benefit from external cephalic version, internal podalic version, or complete breech extraction, all of which can be guided by the information provided by ultrasound.

SUMMARY

The importance of ultrasound in the management of multiple gestations cannot be understated. As mentioned at the outset, the use of ultrasound in multiple pregnancy has enormous potential to decrease the morbidity and mortality associated with fetal anomalies, growth disturbances, and preterm delivery. In addition, the outcomes of multiple pregnancies have been greatly affected by the contribution ultrasound makes toward fetal surveillance and management of labor.

REFERENCES

1. Luke B, Bryan E, Sweetland C, et al. Prenatal weight gain and the birth weight of triplets. *Acta Genet Med Gemellol (Roma)* 1995;44:93–101.
2. Chasen ST, Chervenak FA. What is the relationship between the universal use of ultrasound, the rate of detection of twins, and outcome differences? *Clin Obstet Gynecol* 1998;41:67–77.
3. Doubilet PM, Benson CB. "Appearing twin": undercounting of multiple gestations on early first trimester sonograms. *J Ultrasound Med* 1998;17:199–203.
4. Landy HJ, Weiner S, Corson S, et al. The "vanishing twin": ultrasonographic assessment of fetal disappearance in the first trimester. *Am J Obstet Gynecol* 1986;155:14–18.
5. LeFevre ML, Bain RP, Ewigman BG, et al. A randomized trial of prenatal ultrasonographic screening: impact on maternal management and outcome. *Am J Obstet Gynecol* 1993;169:483–489.
6. Saari-Kemppainen A, Karjalainen O, Ylostalo P, et al. Ultrasound screening and perinatal mortality: controlled trial of systematic one-stage screening in pregnancy. *Lancet* 1990;336:387–391.
7. Waldenstrom U, Axelsson O, Nilsson S, et al. Effects of routine one-stage ultrasound screening in pregnancy: a randomized controlled trial. *Lancet* 1988;2:585–588.
8. Hughey MJ, Olive DL. Routine ultrasound scanning for the detection and management of twin pregnancies. *J Reprod Med* 1985; 30:427–430.
9. Persson PH, Grennart RL, Gennser G, et al. Improved outcome of twin pregnancies. *Acta Obstet Gynecol Scand* 1979;58:3–7.
10. Grennart L, Persson PH, Gennser G. Benefits of ultrasonic screening of a pregnant population. *Acta Obstet Gynecol Scand Suppl* 1978;78:5–10.
11. Ewigman BG, Crane JP, Frigoletto FD, et al. Effect of prenatal ultrasound screening on perinatal outcome. *N Engl J Med* 1993; 329:821–827.

12. Divon MY, Weiner Z. Ultrasound in twin pregnancy. *Semin Perinatol* 1995;19:404–412.
13. Sebire NJ, Snijders RJM, Hughes K, et al. The hidden mortality of monochorionic twin pregnancies. *Br J Obstet Gynaecol* 1997; 104:1207–1209.
14. D'Alton ME, Dudley DK. The ultrasonic prediction of chorionicity in twin gestation. *Am J Obstet Gynecol* 1989;160:557–561.
15. Vayssiere CF, Neim N, Camus EP, et al. Determination of chorionicity in twin gestations by high-frequency abdominal ultrasonography: counting the layers of the dividing membrane. *Am J Obstet Gynecol* 1996;175:1529–1533.
16. Townsend RR, Simpson GF, Filly RA. Membrane thickness in ultrasound prediction of chorionicity of twin gestations. *J Ultrasound Med* 1988;7:326–332.
17. Winn HN, Gabrielli S, Reece EA, et al. Diagnosis of placental chorionicity in twin gestations. *Am J Obstet Gynecol* 1989;161: 1540–1542.
18. Stagiannis KD, Sepulveda W, Southwell D, et al. Ultrasonographic measurement of the dividing membrane in twin pregnancy during the second and third trimesters: a reproducibility study. *Am J Obstet Gynecol* 1995;173:1546–1550.
19. Sepulveda W, Sebire NJ, Hughes K, et al. Evolution of the lambda or twin-chorionic peak sign in dichorionic twin pregnancies. *Obstet Gynecol* 1997;89:439–441.
20. Wood SL, St Onge R, Connors G, et al. Evaluation of the twin peak or lambda sign in determining chorionicity in multiple pregnancy. *Obstet Gynecol* 1996;88:6–9.
21. Babinski A, Mukherjee T, Kerenyi T, et al. Diagnosing amnionicity at 6 weeks of pregnancy with transvaginal three-dimensional ultrasonography: case report. *Fertil Steril* 1999;71:1161–1164.
22. Norton ME, D'Alton ME, Bianchi DW. Molecular zygosity studies aid in the management of discordant multiple gestations. *J Perinatol* 1997;17:202–207.
23. Scardo JA, Ellings JM, Newman RB. Prospective determination of chorionicity, amnionicity and zygosity in twin gestations. *Am J Obstet Gynecol* 1995;173:1376–1380.
24. Derom C, Vlietinick R, Derom R, et al. Increased monozygotic twinning rate after ovulation induction. *Lancet* 1982;1:1236–1238.
25. Sepulveda W, Sebire NJ, Odibo A, et al. Prenatal determination of chorionicity in triplet pregnancy by ultrasonographic examination of the ipsilon zone. *Obstet Gynecol* 1996;88:855–858.
26. Snijders RJM, Sebire NJ, Nicolaides KH. Maternal age and gestational age specific risk for chromosomal defects. *Fetal Diagn Ther* 1995;10:356–367.
27. Baldwin VJ. Anomalous development of twins. In: Baldwin VJ, ed. *Pathology of multiple pregnancy*. New York: Springer-Verlag, 1994:169–197.
28. Spellacy WN, Handler A, Ferre CD. A case controlled study of 1253 twin pregnancies from a 1982–1987 perinatal database. *Obstet Gynecol* 1990;75:168–171.
29. Edwards MS, Ellings JM, Newman RB, et al. Predictive value of antepartum ultrasound examination for anomalies in twin gestations. *Ultrasound Obstet Gynecol* 1995;6:43–49.
30. D'Alton ME, Mercer BM. Antepartum management of twin gestation: ultrasound. *Clin Obstet Gynecol* 1990;33:42–51.

31. Sebire NJ, Nicolaides KH. Screening for fetal abnormalities in multiple pregnancies. *Baillieres Clin Obstet Gynecol* 1998;12:19–36.
32. Goldenberg RL, Iams JD, Miodovnik M, et al. The preterm prediction study: risk factors in twin gestations. *Am J Obstet Gynecol* 1996;175:1047–1053.
33. Souka AP, Heath V, Flint S, et al. Cervical length at 23 weeks in twins in predicting spontaneous preterm delivery. *Obstet Gynecol* 1999;94:450–454.
34. Imseis HM, Albert TA, Iams JD. Identifying twin gestations at low risk for preterm birth with a transvaginal ultrasonographic cervical measurement at 24–26 weeks gestation. *Am J Obstet Gynecol* 1997;177:1149–1155.
35. Chamberlain PF, Manning FA, Morrison I, et al. Ultrasound evaluation of amniotic fluid volume, I: the relationship of marginal and decreased amniotic fluid volume to perinatal outcome. *Am J Obstet Gynecol* 1984;150:245–249.
36. Chamberlain PF, Manning FA, Morrison I, et al. Ultrasound evaluation of amniotic fluid volume, II: the relationship of increased fluid volumes to perinatal outcome. *Am J Obstet Gynecol* 1984; 150:250–244.
37. Moore TR, Cayle JE. The amniotic fluid index in normal human pregnancy. *Am J Obstet Gynecol* 1990;162:1168–1173.
38. Rutherford SE, Smith CV, Phelan JP, et al. Four-quadrant assessment of amniotic fluid volume: interobserver and intraobserver variation. *J Reprod Med* 1987;32:587–589.
39. Moore TR. Superiority of the four-quadrant sum over the single deepest pocket technique in ultrasonographic identification of abnormal amniotic fluid volumes. *Am J Obstet Gynecol* 1990; 163:762–767.
40. Watson WJ, Harlass FE, Menard MK, et al. Sonographic assessment of amniotic fluid in normal twin pregnancy. *Am J Perinatol* 1995;12:122–124.
41. Porter TF, Dildy GA, Blanchard JR, et al. Normal values for amniotic fluid index during uncomplicated twin pregnancy. *Obstet Gynecol* 1996;87: 699–702.
42. Chau AC, Kjos SL, Kovacs BW. Ultrasonographic measurement of amniotic fluid volume in normal diamniotic twin pregnancies. *Am J Obstet Gynecol* 1996;174:1003–1007.
43. Magann EF, Whitworth NS, Bass JD, et al. Amniotic fluid volume of third trimester diamniotic twin pregnancies. *Obstet Gynecol* 1995;85:957–960.
44. Crane JP, Tomich PG, Kopta M. Ultrasonic growth patterns in normal and discordant twins. *Obstet Gynecol* 1980;55:678–683.
45. Leveno K, Santos-Roamos R, Duen Hoelter J, et al. Sonar cephalometry in twins: a table of biparietal diameters for normal twin fetuses and a comparison with singletons. *Am J Obstet Gynecol* 1979;135:727–736.
46. Socol ML, Tamura RK, Sabbagha RE, et al. Diminished biparietal diameter and abdominal circumference growth in twins. *Obstet Gynecol* 1984;64:235–238.
47. Grumbach K, Coleman B, Arger PH, et al. Twin and singleton growth patterns compared during ultrasound. *Radiology* 1986; 158:237–242.
48. McKeown T, Record RG. Observation on foetal growth in multiple pregnancy in man. *J Endocrinol* 1952;8:386–400.

49. Jones JS, Newman RB, Miller MC. Cross-sectional analysis of triplet birth weight. *Am J Obstet Gynecol* 1991;168:135–140.
50. Chitkara U, Berkowitz GS, Levine R, et al. Twin pregnancy: routine use of ultrasound examinations in the prenatal diagnosis of intrauterine growth retardation and discordant growth. *Am J Perinatol* 1985;2:483–486.
51. Grobman WA, Parilla BV. The positive predictive value of suspected growth aberration in twin gestations. *Am J Obstet Gynecol* 1999;181:1139–1141.
52. Giles WB, Trudinger BJ, Cook CM. Fetal umbilical artery flow velocity–time waveforms in twin pregnancies. *Br J Obstet Gynaecol* 1985;92:490–497.
53. Farmakides G, Schulman H, Saldama LR, et al. Surveillance of twins with umbilical artery velocimetry. *Am J Obstet Gynecol* 1985;153:789–792.
54. Gaziano EP, Knox GE, Bendel RP, et al. Is pulsed Doppler velocimetry useful in the management of multiple gestation pregnancies? *Am J Obstet Gynecol* 1991;164:1426–1433.
55. Gerson AG, Wallace DM, Bridgens NK, et al. Duplex Doppler ultrasound in the evaluation of growth in twin pregnancies. *Obstet Gynecol* 1987;70:419–423.
56. Giles WB, Trudinger BJ, Cook CM, et al. Umbilical artery waveforms in triplet pregnancy. *Obstet Gynecol* 1990;75:813.
57. Omtzigt AWJ. *Clinical value of umbilical Doppler velocimetry: a randomized controlled trial* [doctoral thesis]. Utrecht, The Netherlands: University of Utrecht, 1990.
58. Johnstone FD, Prescott R, Hoskins P, et al. The effect of introduction of umbilical Doppler recordings to obstetric practice. *Br J Obstet Gynaecol* 1993;100:733–741.
59. Divon MY, Guidetti DA, Braverman JJ, et al. Intrauterine growth retardation: a prospective study of the diagnostic value of real-time sonography combined with umbilical artery flow velocimetry. *Obstet Gynecol* 1988;72:611–614.
60. Berkowitz GS, Chitkara U, Rosenberg J, et al. Sonographic estimation of fetal weight and Doppler analysis of umbilical artery velocimetry in the prediction of intrauterine growth retardation: a prospective study. *Am J Obstet Gynecol* 1988;158:1149–1153.
61. Gaziano E, Knox E, Wager GP, et al. The predictability of the small-for-gestational-age infant by real-time ultrasound derived measurements combined with pulsed Doppler umbilical artery velocimetry. *Am J Obstet Gynecol* 1988;158:1431–1439.
62. Degani S, Gonen R, Shapiro I, et al. Doppler flow velocity waveforms in fetal surveillance of twins. *J Ultrasound Med* 1992;11:537–541.
63. Devoe LD, Ware DJ. Antenatal assessment of twin gestation. *Semin Perinatol* 1995;19:413–423.
64. Rizzo G, Arduini D, Romanini C. Cardiac and extracardiac flows in discordant twins. *Am J Obstet Gynecol* 1994;170:1321–1327.
65. Lodeiro JG, Vintzelous AM, Feinstein SJ, et al. Fetal biophysical profile in twin gestation. *Obstet Gynecol* 1986;67:824–827.
66. Alcalay M, Lipitz S, Ben Rapael Z, et al. Fetal biophysical profile score in triplet pregnancies. *J Reprod Med* 1994;39:436–440.

Maternal Nutrition

In the United States, the rates of low birth weight and preterm birth have remained essentially unchanged for the past 20 years. Part of this stagnation of previous progress stems from the rise in the number of multiple births, masking disparate patterns by plurality (1,2). Although many investigators have focused on the clinical pathways of these outcomes, no consistent mechanism has emerged. Although numerous nonmodifiable factors that may contribute to both low birth weight and prematurity, including maternal age, ethnicity, parity, and obstetric history, the most promise may lie in the nutritional factors that can be modified during pregnancy (3–5).

Multiple pregnancy is a state of magnified nutritional requirements, resulting in a greater nutrient drain on maternal resources and an accelerated depletion of nutritional reserves. Most studies to date have evaluated the effects of nutritional factors on the course and outcome of singleton pregnancies. The body of literature on multiple gestations is growing, but there are still many gaps in our knowledge of normal and abnormal physiologic changes and effective interventions. This chapter summarizes current research on the effect of maternal pregravid weight, gestational weight gain, carbohydrate metabolism, iron status, and vitamin and mineral intake on fetal growth and length of gestation of singletons, and when known, in twin and triplet gestations.

Guidelines for Perinatal Care (6) acknowledges that nutrition counseling is an integral component of perinatal care and that it is most effectively accomplished by referral to a nutritionist or registered dietitian. The recommendations, issued jointly by the American Academy of Pediatrics and the American College of Obstetricians and Gynecologists and which are for singleton pregnancies only, cover preconception care, nutrition in pregnancy, postpartum guidelines, and neonatal nutrition. In reality, nutrition counseling and interventions often are overlooked in the prenatal care of multiples, with few studies citing specific nutrition interventions (7–11). This is unfortunate because nutrition may provide a powerful mechanism by which to improve intrauterine growth and length of gestation in these high-risk pregnancies.

MATERNAL PREGRAVID WEIGHT AND GESTATIONAL WEIGHT GAIN

Singletons

The factors most strongly correlated with both length of gestation and birth weight are maternal height, pregravid or early pregnancy body weight, maternal fat deposition, and gestational weight gain. Although each factor independently influences birth weight and length of gestation, the effects are neither equal nor additive. The landmark studies in this area have been from the Collaborative Perinatal Project, which was conducted between 1959 and 1964 (12–15). Based on term singleton pregnancies, these studies demonstrated that: (a) a progressive increase in weight gain is paralleled by an increase in mean birth weight and a decline in the incidence of low birth weight (LBW); (b) increasing pregravid weight diminishes the effect of weight gain on birth weight; (c) there is an inverse relation between weight gain and perinatal mortality, with gains up to 30 pounds (13.6 kg); and (d) higher gestational weight gains are related to higher birth weights and better growth and development during the first postnatal year. As a result of these and subsequent studies, in 1990 the Institute of Medicine issued pregravid body mass index (BMI)–specific weight gain guidelines for singleton pregnancies (16). Table 6-1 provides estimates of BMI for height and pregravid weight status. Many investigators have subsequently confirmed these associations, including the link between low prepregnancy weight and both prematurity and intrauterine growth retardation (IUGR). The reported increased risk ranges from 1.7 to 3.0, depending on the study population (17). The population-attributable risk for early preterm birth (before 32 weeks) with low prepregnancy weight is as much as 31% to 43%, depending on race and ethnicity (18). Low maternal weight gain also has been significantly associated with both IUGR and preterm birth, with reported risks in the range of 2.1 to 4.3 (16,19–23). Significant interaction also has been documented between the effect of low pregravid weight and low weight gain on the risk of preterm birth (adjusted odds ratio [AOR], 5.63; 95% confidence interval [CI], 2.35–13.8) (24).

Pattern of Weight Gain

Although cumulative or total weight gain is an important predictor of birth weight, the pattern of weight gain and rate of gain also play significant roles in modifying birth weight and predicting preterm delivery (25,26). Hediger et al. (25,26) demonstrated that both early weight gain (before 24 weeks' gestation) and later weight gain (after 24 weeks) have independent effects on the outcome of singleton births. In a multiracial sample of 1,790 teenagers from Camden County, New Jersey, early inadequate weight gain (less than 4.3 kg by 24 weeks) was associated with an increased risk of small-for-gestational-age outcomes (SGA) (less than tenth percentile for gestation) (AOR, 2.08; 95% CI, 1.31–3.30) (25). Even if there were compensatory gains after 24 weeks to bring the cumulative total gain up to a level deemed adequate, the risk of an SGA birth still was increased (AOR, 1.88; 95% CI, 1.08–3.27). This finding strongly suggests that early weight gain, which presumably reflects gains in maternal nutrient stores, is important in enhancing fetal growth by serving as a nutrient reserve later in pregnancy or as a marker for adequate placental growth and development. In these studies, the rate of preterm delivery (before 37 weeks) was relatively unaffected by early inadequate weight gain but increased with late inadequate weight gain (less than 400 g/week). This occurred even when the total pregnancy weight gain never fell below the targets set in clinical standards (AOR, 1.69; 95% CI, 1.12–2.55) (25).

Weight Gain in Twin Pregnancies

In its 1990 report, the Institute of Medicine suggested a range of maternal weight gain of 35 to 45 pounds (16 to 20 kg) for term (38 to 41 weeks) twin pregnancies (16). The general consensus among researchers who have evaluated these guidelines for twins is that total gain should be at least 40 to 45 pounds (18 to 20 kg) with

Table 6-1. Prepregnancy weight for height by body frame size

Height (inches)	Small Frame			Medium Frame			Large Frame		
	Underweight	Normal Weight	Overweight	Underweight	Normal Weight	Overweight	Underweight	Normal Weight	Overweight
57	94	104	125	100	112	134	109	122	146
58	95	105	126	102	114	137	112	124	149
59	96	107	128	105	117	140	114	127	152
60	98	109	131	107	119	143	116	129	155
61	101	112	134	110	122	146	118	132	158
62	104	115	138	113	125	150	122	136	163
63	106	118	142	115	128	154	126	140	168
64	109	121	145	118	131	157	128	143	172
65	112	124	149	120	134	161	132	147	176
66	114	127	152	123	137	164	135	150	180
67	117	130	156	126	140	168	138	154	185
68	120	133	160	129	143	172	141	157	188
69	122	136	163	131	146	175	144	160	192
70	125	139	167	134	149	179	146	163	196
71	128	142	170	137	152	182	149	166	199
72	131	145	174	140	155	186	152	169	203

Note: Weight is in pounds. Underweight is 10% or more less than normal weight for height and frame size. Overweight is 20% or more above normal weight for height and frame size.

From Luke B, Eberlein T. When you're expecting twins, triplets, or quads. New York: Harper Collins, 1999; 54.

an emphasis on adequate weight gain before 24 weeks' gestation (27–37) (Table 6-2). Recent research has demonstrated a "ripple" effect of maternal weight gain on twin fetal growth, with gains before 20 weeks and between 20 and 28 weeks both affecting fetal growth from 20 to 28 weeks and 28 weeks to delivery (Table 6-3) (36). Prior to 20 weeks, the only factors affecting fetal growth are monozygosity and smoking; both are negative factors.

For twins, an average birth weight of 2,500 g or more is associated with maternal weight gains of 40 to 45 pounds (18.1 to 20.4 kg), as 24 pounds (11 kg) by 24 weeks (31,32). A low rate of gain before 24 weeks (less than 0.85 lb/week), regardless of rate of gain after 24 weeks, is significantly associated with poor intrauterine growth and higher morbidity (32). Luke and Leurgans (33) reported that advised weight gain for twin gestations averaged 30 pounds (13.6 kg), whereas actual gains averaged 40 to 45 pounds (18.1 to 20.4 kg). This study also evaluated the Institute of Medicine recommendations of 35 to 45 pounds (16 to 20 kg) for twin pregnancies and concluded that weight gains above this range were associated with twin birth weights of 2,500 to 2,800 g at 36 to 38 weeks, the optimal birth weight for gestational age for these pregnancies.

Several studies on twin gestations have clearly established the importance of maternal weight gain before 20 weeks' gestation on twin birth weight (29,34,36). The first, based on 646 twin pregnancies at three study sites, demonstrated that twin birth weight was significantly associated with weight gain before 20 weeks among underweight women, before 20 weeks and after 28 weeks among overweight women, and during all three gestational periods among normal-weight women (34). The second study, based on 1,564 twin pregnancies, confirmed and expanded the earlier findings and showed that both early maternal weight gain (before 20 weeks) and midpregnancy weight gain (between 20 to 28 weeks) significantly affected the rate of fetal growth between 20 to 28 weeks and 28 weeks to birth (36). It is clear, then, that by improving weight gain early in pregnancy fetal growth can be enhanced, and, by extension, lengthen gestation.

Based on these studies, Luke et al. (38) proposed BMI-specific weight gain guidelines for twin pregnancies. These guidelines were modeled using multiple regression for the gestational periods of 0 to 20 weeks (early), 20 to 28 weeks (middle), and 28 weeks to delivery (late). The guidelines were based on achieving optimal rates of fetal growth (between the twin and singleton fiftieth percentiles at 20 to 28 weeks, and between the twin seventy-fifth to ninetieth percentiles at 28 to 38 weeks) and average birth weights between the singleton fiftieth percentile and the twin ninetieth percentile at 38 weeks (2,700 to 2,800 g). Optimal rates of fetal growth and optimal birth weights were associated with rates of maternal weight gain (lb/week) as follows:

BMI Group	Early	Middle	Late	Total Gain (lb)
Underweight	1.25–1.75	1.50–2.0	1.25	47–61
Normal weight	1.00–1.50	1.25–2.0	1.00	38–54
Overweight	1.00–1.25	1.00–1.5	1.00	36–45
Obese	0.75–1.25	1.00	0.75	29–39

Weight Gain in Triplet Pregnancies

In their analysis of 1,138 triplet pregnancies, Elster et al. (9) reported several factors to be predictive of higher average fetal weight for a given gestational age, including male gender, older maternal age, maternal height, pregravid weight and weight gain, and parity. These investigators also reported that length of gestation correlated with maternal age, parity, and weight gain. Maternal weight gain was even more strongly associated with outcomes for triplets than for twins. Gains in different periods of gestation affected birth weight, birth weight for gestation (birth weight z score), and length of gestation were demonstrated in a study of 144 triplets by Luke et al. (38). Regression analyses indicated that the most significant periods of maternal weight gain for average triplet birth weight were from conception to 20 weeks and between 20 to 28 weeks (158 g per pound per week, $p = .001$, and 111 g per pound per week, $p = .001$, respectively). For average triplet birth weight, the z score between 20 and 28 weeks was 0.53 SD units per pound per week, $p < .0001$). For length of gestation from 28 weeks to delivery the z score was 4.6 days per pound per week, $p < .0001$). A summary of the distribution of low birth weight and very low birth weight infants, maternal weight gain recommendations, and average birth weights by plurality are given in Table 6-4.

The effect of higher weight gain before 20 or 24 weeks on twin and triplet birth weight is most pronounced among infants of underweight gravidas (29,32). This early weight gain may reflect the acquisition of maternal nutrient stores, particularly the deposition of body fat (39). In addition, levels of fat-mobilizing hormones, such as follicle-stimulating hormone (FSH) and human placental lactogen (hPL), may be higher among normal-weight and overweight women as well as among women with dizygotic twin pregnancies (40). Therefore, underweight women with low early weight gain may lack appropriate nutrient reserves, including maternal stored fat, and adequate levels of hormones to mobilize the nutrient stores that are available. The result is a higher incidence of birth weights in the tenth percentile or lower among their infants.

High early weight gain may be particularly important in multiple pregnancies for two distinct reasons. First, pregnancy is usually much shorter for multiple gestations, as much as 4 to 12 weeks, thereby shortening the period for intrauterine growth. As shown by Williams et al. (41), the peak rate of increase in weight for multiples occurs at about 31 weeks compared with 33 weeks for singletons. Second, higher weight gains during early gestation may influence the structural and functional development of the placenta (42). In multiple pregnancies the placenta ages more quickly, shortening the gestational period during which the placenta can most effectively transfer nutrients to the developing fetuses. Higher gains during early gestation therefore may initially benefit placental structure and function, and subsequently augment fetal growth through more effective placental function and the transfer of a higher level of nutrients.

CHANGES IN MATERNAL BODY FAT

Singletons

A substantial portion of gestational weight gain is maternal body fat. Measured as triceps skinfold thickness or mid-upper arm

Table 6-2. Comparison of maternal weight gain by plurality

Reference	Twins		Triplets		Quadruplets	
	No. of Women	Gain (lb)	No. of Women	Gain (lb)	No. of Women	Gain (lb)
Fenton and Thirsk, 1994 (125)[a]	100	31.0 ± 9.0				
Lantz et al., 1996 (29)	189	35.2 ± 15.2				
Luke et al., 1993 (32)	163	36.4 ± 15				
Luke et al., 1998 (36,37)	1,564	38.4 ± 15.1				
Luke et al., 1991 (30)	275	43.3 ± 17.1				
Seoud et al., 1992 (11)	94	45.3 ± 1.8				
Pederson et al., 1989 (22)[b]						
<90% ideal body weight	37	42 ± 10				
90%–120% ideal body weight	22	48 ± 12				
>120% ideal body weight	2	33 ± 4				
Lantz et al., 1996 (29)[c]						
BMI <19.8	7	52.6 ± 4.3				
BMI 19.8–26.0	17	43.1 ± 2.6				
BMI >26.0	11	40.3 ± 5.8				
Luke et al., 1992 (31)[c]						
BMI <19.8	14	43.6				
BMI 19.8–26.0	36	41.9				
BMI >26.0	8	43.5				

Study			
Levene, 1991 (126)			
Spontaneous	35	24.4 ± 12.5	
Assisted reproduction	64	28.4 ± 13.0	
Pons et al., 1988 (7)	21	31.9	
Syrop and Varner, 1985 (127)	20	34.1	
Luke et al., 1998 (36,37)	78	41.8 ± 12	
Luke et al., 2000 (38)	78	42 ± 17	
Luke et al., 1995 (128)	38	43.9 ± 15.5	
Elster et al., 1991 (9)	1,138	45.1	
Seoud et al., 1992 (11)	13	50.6 ± 16.9	
Pons et al., 1996 (118)	65		39.2
Collins and Bleyl, 1990 (129)	71		45.8
Elliott and Radin, 1992 (8)	10		57.4 ± 19.6
Seoud et al., 1992 (11)	4		68.2 ± 9.0

[a] Maternal weight gain to 34 weeks only.
[b] Maternal gain associated with optimal outcomes: both twins ≥2,500 g, Apgar score at 5 minutes ≥7, and Dubowitz scores >37 wk.
[c] Maternal weight gains associated with both twin birth weights ≥2,500 g.
BMI, body mass index.

Table 6-3.   The ripple effect of maternal weight gain on fetal growth and birth weight in twin pregnancies

Variable	Rate of Sum of Twin Fetal Growth (g/wk)			Sum of Twin Pair Birth Weight (g)
	0–20 wk	20–28 wk	28 wk–Delivery	
Maternal age (per yr)		0.7	1.0	
Maternal pregravid weight (per lb)		0.2	0.3	4.0
Maternal height (per in)				28.1
Multiparity		8.1	11.7	231
Dichorionic placenta	2.6			
Male twins (per twin)				116
Smoking	−4.3	−14.9	−26.2	−353
Preeclampsia		−7.1	−11.5	
Early rate of gain (per lb/wk, 0–20 wk)		10.9	16.9	283
Mid rate of gain (per lb/wk, 20–28 wk)		15.9	23.9	164
Late rate of gain (per lb/wk, 28–36 wk)				69.8

Adapted from Luke B, Min SJ, Gillespie B, et al. The importance of early weight gain on the intrauterine growth and birth weight of twins. *Am J Obstet Gynecol* 1998;179:1155–1161, with permission.

circumference (MUAC), the amount of maternal body increases in the first two trimesters and decreases in the third, reflecting the early accretion of maternal body fat and the subsequent utilization in late gestation to meet increasing energy needs. The components of maternal weight gain, particularly changes in body fat, may be more important determinants of pregnancy outcome than is absolute weight gain. Prior studies involving well-nourished women, based on deuterium oxide and underwater weighing (43–46) or anthropometric measures (47–49) have shown a pattern of small gains in maternal body fat early in pregnancy, rapid accumulation between 20 and 30 weeks' gestation, and a leveling off between 30 weeks and delivery. A consistent finding in studies with diverse ethnic and racial groups is the correlation between triceps skinfold or MUAC measures during the second trimester and birth weight. Loss of upper arm fat or the failure to accrue

Table 6-4. Comparison of low-birth-weight (LBW), very-low-birth-weight (VLBW), and weight gain recommendations by plurality

| Plurality | No. of Infants | Percentage | | Maternal Weight Gain (lb) | | Range of Gestation (wk) | Average Birth Weight (g) |
		LBW	VLBW	To 24 wk	Total		
Singletons	3,770,020	6	1	12	25–35	39–41	3,700–4,000
Twins	104,137	50	10	24	40–45	36–38	2,500–2,800
Triplets	6,148	90	32	36	50–60	34–35	1,900–2,200
Quadruplets	589	98	75	50	65–80	31–33	1,500–1,800

From 1997 U.S. live births.

maternal fat during the second trimester is associated with poor fetal growth and lower birth weights (47–51).

Examining the components of weight gain in pregnancy, Hediger et al. (52) demonstrated that for teenagers and adults whose pregravid weights were above the twenty-fifth percentile for age, the loss of subcutaneous fat (more than 6.4 cm^2) from 28 weeks through 4 to 6 weeks post partum (measured at the mid-upper arm) was associated with a higher birth weight ($+144$ g, $p < .01$). At the same time there appeared to be a mobilization of fat stores, there was an increase in arm muscle area. However, when pregravid weight was below the twenty-fifth percentile for age, a loss of upper arm fat was associated instead with a lower birth weight (-339 g, $p < .01$). This finding suggested that the nutrient stores of these women may have been relatively depleted. Continued weight gain, increases in upper arm fat area (more than 5 cm^2), and loss of upper arm muscle also were associated with lower birth weight (-123 g, $p < .02$). Thus, a change in amount of upper arm fat is a significant predictor of variation in infant birth weight. Serial monitoring by arm anthropometry, as well as maternal weight, may help determine risk of IUGR.

Multiples

Changes in arm anthropometry have also been used to determine the risk of IUGR in twin pregnancies (53). Serial data on MUAC and maternal weight gain were collected for 72 women pregnant with twins. MUAC changes were determined from 20 to 34 weeks, that is, subsequent to the early gestational weight gains strongly associated with fetal growth of twins (less than 20 weeks), but before the onset of edema. Over this period, MUAC should increase, reflecting early increases in maternal fat and lean body mass (LBM) and after 28 to 30 weeks, increases in LBM alone. The baseline MUAC measured at 20 weeks averaged 29.7 ± 3.8 cm. From 20 to 34 weeks, there was no net change in MUAC (-0.002 ± 0.16 cm/week), but a highly significant correlation between weight gain at 20 weeks and subsequent change in MUAC ($r = 0.41, p < .001$). The cutoff for change in MUAC most closely associated with twin birth weight was determined to be -0.2 cm/week (-2 mm/week). Women with a change in MUAC less than -0.2 cm/week differed in that they were significantly shorter and heavier, and had less weight gain. In models adjusted for gestation, race, number of males per sibship, chorionicity, and baseline MUAC at 20 weeks, the decrement in total twin birth weight attributable to a change in MUAC of less than -0.2 cm/week was -446 ± 97 g ($p < .03$) and decrement in average birth weight z score of -0.53 ± 0.23 SD unit ($p < .03$). Changes in MUAC from 20 to 34 weeks thus were significantly associated with fetal growth in twin pregnancies. Serial measurements of MUAC that indicate a loss of more than -0.2 cm/week from 20 to 34 weeks are significantly associated with lower twin birth weight and reduced fetal growth. Such a loss of MUAC may indicate that dietary intake or nutrient stores are inadequate. These findings also raise the possibility that serial measurements of MUAC, a simple but relatively precise measure of change in maternal body composition, for obese women, for whom weight gain guidelines are not clear, could be used as a proxy for weight gain to determine risk of poor fetal growth.

Effect of Parity

It is well known that there are changes in body composition with pregnancy, with parous women generally being heavier and having a higher proportion of body fat compared with nulliparous women. This difference is particularly important in multiple pregnancies. Luke et al. (34–37) reported multiparity significantly increased sum of twin pair birth weight by 231 to 368 g and significantly increased the rate of the sum of twin pair fetal growth between 20 and 28 weeks by 8.13 g and between 28 and 36 weeks by 11.72 g. In their study of 144 triplet pregnancies, Luke et al. (38) reported primiparity to be significantly associated with lower average birth weight (–124 g, $p = .005$) and lower average birth weight z score (–.615 SD units, $p = .001$). Crowther and Hamilton (54) reported that triplet perinatal mortality was significantly higher among primigravidas compared with grand multigravidas ($p < .001$) (mean gestation 31.1 ± 5.2 versus 34.0 ± 3.4, or about 20.3 days). Gonen et al. (55) reported that multiparous women with triplet and higher-order pregnancies delivered their infants about 1 week later than nulliparous women. Among triplet pregnancies, Ron-El et al. (56) reported mean gestations about 10 days longer for multiparous than for nulliparous women (240 days versus 230 days).

NUTRIENT REQUIREMENTS

Maternal and nutritional factors contribute to fetal growth and birth weight to a larger degree in multiple than in singleton pregnancies. Maternal diet and nutritional status have a more important role in multiple pregnancy, with increases in all nutrient requirements. Because of the greater expansion in blood volume, increase in maternal tissues (body fat and muscle, breast, uterine) and fetal mass, caloric requirements are estimated to increase by about 40% for twin pregnancies and by about 80% for triplet and higher-order pregnancies. Although there are no national guidelines for individual nutrient requirements, based on physiologic changes in multiple pregnancy, an estimate of nutrient needs is given in Table 6-5.

Carbohydrate Metabolism in Multifetal Pregnancy

During pregnancy alteration of carbohydrate metabolism results in lower fasting glucose levels and an exaggeration of the insulin response to eating (Figs. 6-1 and 6-2). In both diabetic and twin gestations, these changes are magnified, particularly during the second half of pregnancy, resulting in accelerated starvation (57). Women pregnant with multiples have significantly lower blood glucose and insulin levels, and higher plasma levels of β-hydroxybutyrate than do women pregnant with singletons (57). This finding indicates more rapid depletion of glycogen stores and resultant metabolism of fat between meals and during an overnight fast. Both fasting and ketonuria have been linked to an increase in preterm labor and preterm delivery (58,59). In animal studies, fasting during pregnancy results in higher plasma levels of prostaglandin metabolites, which cause uterine contractions and preterm birth (60–62). An exaggeration of this effect may be partially responsible for the increased incidence of early preterm births of multiple pregnancies.

Table 6-5. Recommended dietary allowances (RDAs) for nonpregnant women and women pregnant with singletons and estimated dietary requirements for women pregnant with twins, triplets, and quadruplets

Nutrient	Nonpregnant[a]	Singleton Pregnancy[a]	Twin Pregnancy[b]	Triplet or Quadruplet Pregnancy[b]	Dietary Sources
Calories	2,200 kcal	2,500 kcal	3,500 kcal	4,500 kcal	Proteins, fats, and carbohydrates
Protein (20%)	110 g	126 g	176 g	225 g	Meats, seafood, poultry, dairy products
Carbohydrate (40%)	220 g	248 g	350 g	450 g	Breads, cereals, pasta, dairy, fruits
Fat (40%)	98 g	112 g	155 g	200 g	Dairy products, nuts, oils
Folic acid	180 µg	400 µg	800 µg	1,200 µg	Dark green vegetables, citrus fruits
Niacin	15 mg	17 mg	25 mg	35 mg	Meats, nuts, beans
Riboflavin	1.3 mg	1.6 mg	3.0 mg	4.0 mg	Meats, liver, breads, cereals, pasta
Thiamin	1.1 mg	1.5 mg	3.0 mg	4.0 mg	Pork, meats, breads, cereals, pasta
Vitamin A	800 µg RE	800 µg RE	1,000 µg RE	1,200 µg RE	Dark green, orange, or yellow produce, liver
Vitamin B$_6$	1.6 mg	2.2 mg	4.4 mg	6.0 mg	Meats, liver, breads, cereals, pasta

					Sources
Vitamin B$_{12}$	2.0 μg	2.2 μg	3.0 μg	4.0 mg	Meats, poultry
Vitamin C	60 mg	70 mg	150 mg	200 mg	Citrus fruits
Vitamin D	5 μg	10 μg	15 μg	20 μg	Fortified dairy products
Vitamin E	8 mg	10 mg	14 mg	16 mg	Nuts, oils, enriched grains
Calcium	800 mg	1,200 mg	2,000 mg	3,000 mg	Milk, cheese, ice cream
Iodine	150 μg	175 μg	300 μg	400 μg	Iodized salt, seafood
Iron	15 mg	30 mg	60 mg	90 mg	Meats, eggs, breads, cereals, pasta
Magnesium	280 mg	320 mg	500 mg	750 mg	Seafood, beans, breads, cereals, pasta
Phosphorus	800 mg	1,200 mg	2,000 mg	3,000 mg	Meats
Selenium	55 μg	65 μg	75 μg	90 μg	Breads, cereals
Zinc	12 mg	15 mg	30 mg	45 mg	Meats, seafood, eggs

[a] Adapted from the National Research Council, Food and Nutrition Board. *Recommended dietary allowances*, 10th ed. Washington, DC: National Academy Press, 1989, with permission.

[b] Estimated dietary requirements for multiple pregnancies, based on the RDAs for singleton pregnancies.

RE, retinol equivalents.

From Luke B. Maternal nutrition. In: Reece EA, Hobbins JC, eds. *Medicine of the fetus and mother.* Philadelphia: Lippincott Williams & Wilkins, 1999: 935–950.

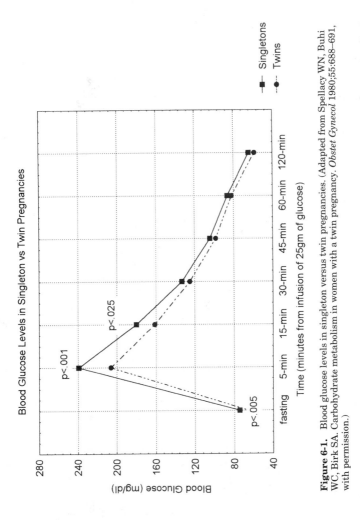

Figure 6-1. Blood glucose levels in singleton versus twin pregnancies. (Adapted from Spellacy WN, Buhi WC, Birk SA. Carbohydrate metabolism in women with a twin pregnancy. *Obstet Gynecol* 1980;55:688–691, with permission.)

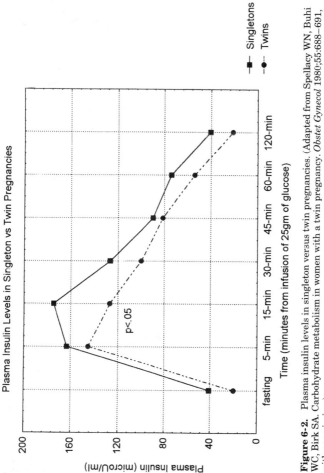

Figure 6-2. Plasma insulin levels in singleton versus twin pregnancies. (Adapted from Spellacy WN, Buhi WC, Birk SA. Carbohydrate metabolism in women with a twin pregnancy. *Obstet Gynecol* 1980;55:688–691, with permission.)

The adverse effects of maternal ketonemia extend beyond premature birth. Studies involving women with diabetes during pregnancy have shown significant correlations between second- and third-trimester glycemic regulation and neurobehavioral deficits in the neonates (63). These alterations in neurodevelopment have been demonstrated in the children of diabetic women through 9 years of age (63–65). Although similar studies have not been conducted with women pregnant with multiples, the alterations are similar to those seen in diabetic pregnancies and may therefore explain a component of the excess disability among children of multiple pregnancies.

Mineral Intake and Supplementation

In addition to being the nutrients most often lacking in women's diets, calcium, magnesium, and zinc have been identified as having the most potential for reducing pregnancy complications and improving outcomes (66–69). A recent review by the World Health Organization concluded that these nutrients "be rigorously evaluated as these interventions may have effects on both impaired fetal growth and preterm delivery" (67).

Iron

Iron deficiency anemia is significantly associated with LBW, preterm delivery, and inadequate maternal weight gain. In a study involving adolescent and young gravidas, iron deficiency anemia (based on the Centers for Disease Control and Prevention criteria of hemoglobin values less than 11.0 g/dL in the first and third trimester, and less than 10.5 g/dL in the second trimester) was significantly associated with inadequate maternal weight gain (AOR, 2.67; 95% CI, 1.13–6.30), preterm delivery (AOR 2.66; 95% CI, 1.15–6.17), and low birth weight (AOR, 3.10; 95% CI, 1.16–4.39) (70). Iron deficiency anemia during the second trimester of pregnancy also has been significantly associated with preterm delivery (AOR 4.3; 95% CI, 1.2–15.5), particularly among black women (AOR, 1.9; 95% CI, 1.5–2.3) (71).

Iron deficiency anemia, as measured at 16 to 18 weeks (second trimester) and at 25 to 32 weeks (third trimester), is significantly associated with preterm delivery. The increase in risk ranges from 2.7 to 4.3 and 1.8 to 3.5, respectively, depending on the age and racial composition of the study population (70–73). Serum ferritin levels, which are elevated in the presence of infection and decreased with iron deficiency, also have been linked to prematurity. Extreme levels of maternal serum ferritin, measured early in the second trimester (15 to 17 weeks), as well as elevated levels at 24, 26, or 28 weeks have been associated with preterm birth (74–78). It has been shown that elevated third-trimester serum ferritin levels that reflect a failure to decline from the beginning of care are significantly associated with preterm and very preterm birth (AOR, 8.77; 95% CI, 3.9–19.7 and AOR, 3.81; 95% CI, 1.93-7.52, respectively). Iron deficiency anemia and poor maternal nutrition underlie the relationship (78).

The few studies that have evaluated iron status in multiple pregnancies have reported lower hemoglobin levels in the first and second trimesters, higher rates of iron deficiency anemia, and even residual iron deficiency anemia among the infants up to 6 months of age (79–81). Hediger and Luke (82) evaluated hemodynamics during twin pregnancy and the association of hemoglobin (Hgb) and hematocrit (Hct) levels with maternal nutritional status and twin outcome. Serial measures of iron status (Hgb, Hct) and measures of maternal nutritional status, including weight gain, were collected for 293 twin pregnancies. As in singleton pregnancies, levels of Hgb and Hct declined through the first trimester to a nadir at 20 to 24 weeks. As with greater volume expansion in twin pregnancies, the levels were even lower in the second trimester than for singleton pregnancies. By the third trimester, lower levels of serum ferritin (indicating better volume expansion) were associated with pregravid BMI (-0.50 ± 0.21 µg/L per kg gain, $p =$ .02) and rate of weight gain to 20 weeks (-11.6 ± 5.0 µg/L per kg weight gain, $p =$ .02). As shown in prior studies, both maternal pregravid BMI and rate of weight gain before 20 weeks' gestation are consistently strong predictors of twin birth weight outcomes. Mean levels by trimester were as follows:

	First Trimester	Second Trimester	Third Trimester
Hemoglobin (g/dL)	12.8	11.3	11.0
Hematocrit (%)	37.3	32.8	32.0
Ferritin (µg/L)	56.6	34.3	12.2

Iron status during pregnancy also has been linked to fetal programming and the development of chronic disease. A low maternal hemoglobin level is strongly related to the development of a large placenta and high placental weight to birth weight ratio, which is seen as predictive of long-term programming of hypertension and cardiovascular disease. Because the iron demands of pregnancy can exceed 1 g, with nearly half this amount in the red cell mass increase in blood volume, the maternal preconceptional and early pregnancy iron status are extremely important. Severe maternal iron deficiency anemia leads to placental adaptive hypertrophy, a decrease in the cortisol metabolizing system, and increased susceptibility to hypertension in later life.

Zinc

During pregnancy plasma zinc concentrations decline 20% to 30% compared with nonpregnant values, reflecting the transfer of zinc from mother to fetus and the normal expansion of the maternal plasma volume (83,84). Plasma zinc concentrations and available zinc intakes are significantly correlated, with zinc supplementation increasing maternal plasma levels (85,86). Using plasma zinc as an indicator of zinc status, Neggers et al. (85) found a positive correlation between duration of gestation and zinc concentration at entry to prenatal care. A recent randomized trial of zinc supplementation among women with plasma zinc levels below the median showed that zinc supplementation resulted in an increase in gestation duration by approximately 0.5 weeks and an increase in birth weight (76). Plasma zinc levels in the lowest quartiles are associated with significantly greater frequency of maternal complications, including infection (87,88). Maternal zinc nutriture, as a composite index of zinc measured from maternal whole blood, hair, and colostrum, has been shown to be related to the risk of premature rupture of membranes (PROM) (88). Women with PROM were found to have significantly lower levels of zinc than were women who gave birth at term.

Scholl et al. (89) evaluated the association between dietary zinc intake and pregnancy outcome for a cohort of 818 low-income, mostly minority women in Camden, New Jersey. Low zinc intake during pregnancy (less than 6 mg/day or less than 40% of the recommended daily allowance for pregnancy) was associated with an increased incidence of iron deficiency anemia at entrance to care, lower use of prenatal supplements during pregnancy, and a higher incidence of inadequate weight gain during pregnancy. Even after adjusting for other confounding variables, such as energy intake, maternal age, ethnicity, and cigarette smoking, a low dietary intake of zinc was associated with a twofold increase in the risk of LBW (AOR, 2.10; 95% CI, 1.19–3.67), a nearly twofold increase in preterm delivery (AOR, 1.86; 95% CI, 1.11–3.09), and a threefold increase in risk of early preterm birth (before 33 weeks' gestation) (AOR, 3.46; 95% CI, 1.04–11.47). In addition, there was a joint effect of iron deficiency anemia at entrance to care and a low zinc intake during pregnancy. When both were present, there was a fivefold increase in risk of preterm delivery (AOR, 5.44; 95% CI, 1.58–18.79).

Although maternal zinc nutriture has been significantly related to length of gestation, infection, and risk of premature rupture of membranes (85,87,88), clinical trials of zinc supplementation have yielded equivocal results (90,91). In a trial in which only randomly selected women with plasma zinc levels below the median received supplementation, investigators found an increase in length of gestation of approximately 0.5 week ($p = .06$) and an increase in birth weight about half of which was explained by the longer duration of gestation (92). Consistent with prior results, effects were increased for nonobese women (pregravid BMI less than 26.0). Studies of prenatal zinc supplementation have found an improvement in fetal neurobehavioral development (93).

Calcium

During pregnancy, there is an increased physiologic demand for calcium such that a full-term infant accretes about 30 g, primarily in the third trimester, when there is active ossification of the fetal skeleton. Prenatal diets low in calcium have been associated with increased blood pressure because of heightened smooth-muscle reactivity, resulting in an increased risk of pregnancy-induced hypertension and preterm delivery. Nearly all calcium supplementation trials have been shown to lower blood pressure levels (94–99).

Results of calcium supplementation trials among high-risk women have been promising. There have been significant reductions in the number of preterm deliveries among teenagers (7.4% versus 21.1%, $p < .007$) and significantly longer mean gestations among women with very low dietary calcium intakes (37.4 versus 39.2 weeks, $p < .01$) (95–97). Other studies have shown inconsistent results in lowering the rates of pregnancy-induced hypertension, or no effect on preterm delivery and small-for-gestational-age births (98,99).

Calcium supplementation trials among high-risk women (teenagers in Baltimore and women with very low calcium intakes in Quito, Ecuador) have had promising results in decreasing the rate of preterm delivery. Among teenagers (16 years of age) in Baltimore with similar overall dietary calcium intakes, the group that received calcium supplementation had a lower incidence of preterm delivery than did the placebo group (7.4% versus 21.1%, $p < .007$) (95). Life-table analysis demonstrated an overall shift to a higher gestational age among the calcium supplementation group. In Ecuador, length of gestation increased from 37.4 to 39.2 weeks for the calcium supplementation group versus the placebo group (96,97). On the other hand, a large calcium supplementation trial involving more than 1,000 women from Argentina showed a decrease in pregnancy-induced hypertension but no effect on preterm delivery (98). A multicenter trial of calcium supplementation in the United States with more than 4,500 adult women showed no difference in the incidence of pregnancy-induced hypertension, preterm delivery, or small-for-gestational-age birth (99). The ability of supplemental calcium to decrease the risk of preterm delivery may be confined to high-risk populations where there is either a severe dietary restriction of calcium, or where, as in the case of adolescents and multiple pregnancy, there is an increased demand for this nutrient.

Prenatal calcium supplementation may have far-reaching effects beyond pregnancy. Belizàn et al. (100) evaluated blood pressure among 7-year-old children whose mothers had received calcium supplementation during pregnancy. They reported significantly lower systolic blood pressure and lower risk of high systolic blood pressure (relative risk [RR], 0.59; 95% CI, 0.39–0.90), particularly among children in the highest quartile of BMI (RR, 0.43; 95% CI, 0.26–0.71).

Magnesium

Magnesium supplementation trials have shown inconsistent results (101–103). These inconsistencies may have been due to differences in study design, study populations, and the concurrent use of other medications such as β-sympathomimetic agents (103). More recent studies, however, have demonstrated that magnesium is not only effective as therapy for and prophylaxis against eclampsia, but is safe and potentially beneficial for neonates (104, 105). In a case–control study examining the risk of cerebral palsy among premature infants exposed to magnesium *in utero,* Nelson and Grether (106) found a protective effect (odds ratio [OR], 0.14; 95% CI, 0.05–0.51), whether or not the magnesium had been given for preeclampsia or as treatment for preterm labor. In a population-based cohort study of prenatal magnesium exposure among children who had very low birth weights, Schendel et al. (107) found a protective effect against cerebral palsy (OR, 0.11; 95% CI, 0.02–0.81) and possibly against mental retardation (OR, 0.30; 95% CI, 0.07–1.29). Recent analyses indicate that reduced long-term morbidity with prenatal magnesium exposure is unlikely due to selective mortality of vulnerable infants (108). Magnesium therapy, as prenatal supplementation or as therapy for preeclampsia or preterm labor, may play a neuroprotective role.

ROLE OF THE PLACENTA IN FETAL GROWTH

As a factor in the causal pathway between maternal nutritional status and fetal growth, placentation plays a pivotal role (see Chapter 2). The placenta influences fetal growth with its size, capacity to transport oxygen and nutrients, and its own metabolism. It is known that placental weight and levels of placental hormones are affected by maternal nutritional status. Human placental lactogen (hPL) is a placental hormone that has structural, immunological, and biologic similarities to both pituitary growth hormone and human prolactin. Maternal serum levels parallel placental weight, increasing throughout gestation to maximum levels in the third trimester. The increase in hPL levels during the second half of pregnancy also stimulates lipolysis, which allows for the availability and transfer of increased amounts of glucose and amino acids to the fetus during the critical period of maximal fetal growth. Levels of hPL are known to be higher in multiple gestations.

There is a positive correlation between placental and fetal weights, specifically related to placental villous surface area, indicating that the functional component of the placenta is of prime importance in the support of fetal growth. In addition, uteroplacental blood flow is a recognized factor influencing fetal growth. In animal models, experimentally induced reductions in uterine blood flow have been shown to decrease fetal growth (109). Experimental embolization of the placenta results in significantly decreased DNA synthesis in the cotyledons (trophoblasts), left fetal ventricular wall, and fetal quadriceps (109). These growth consequences of decreased uteroplacental perfusion are compatible with the clinical findings among fetuses with growth retardation, who display abnormal Doppler waveforms that show high resistance to flow in the umbilical circulation.

Research findings suggest that maternal weight gain before 20 weeks' gestation and parity are related to placental weight at term (110). Other researchers have linked the composition of the maternal diet to both placental weight and birth weight. They found that a high carbohydrate intake in early pregnancy (before 17 weeks) suppresses placental growth, particularly if combined with a low dairy and meat protein intake later in pregnancy (111). Hediger et al. (112) demonstrated that by 32 weeks' gestation, fetuses subsequently delivered preterm were already significantly smaller than those later delivered at term. These investigators reported that infants delivered preterm after PROM or failed tocolysis were proportionately smaller, indicating an overall slowing of growth originating in early pregnancy and persisting throughout gestation. Recent work on first-trimester crown–rump length supports these findings (113). These investigators concluded that a suboptimal intrauterine environment during the first trimester, secondary to altered placentation resulting in reduced nutrient transfer or inadequate maternal nutritional status, may adversely influence fetal growth throughout pregnancy, as well as length of gestation. Smaller-than-expected crown–rump length was significantly associated with LBW at term (RR, 2.1; 95% CI, 1.2–3.5) and early preterm birth (24 to 32 weeks) (RR, 2.2; 95% CI, 1.2–4.1), but not late preterm birth (33 to 36 weeks) (RR, 1.0; 95% CI, 0.7–1.5). These findings are consistent with the hypothesis that the pathophysiology of early versus late preterm birth may be different (114).

SPECIALIZED PRENATAL PROGRAMS FOR MULTIPLES

Several researchers have attempted to improve outcomes in multiple pregnancies with programs of specialized prenatal care, all of which have included a maternal nutrition component. These studies demonstrated fewer antenatal hospitalizations, early preterm births, and delivery of fewer very low birth weight infants (7,8,115–119).

There have been only two specific prenatal nutrition programs for multiples (38,68,120). The Higgins Nutrition Intervention Program in Montreal, Canada, which recommends an additional 1,000 calories and 50 g of protein to baseline singleton dietary recommendations, has demonstrated an 80 g improvement in twin birth weight and a 15% reduction in preterm births (before 37 weeks) (from 47% to 40%) in their analysis of 177 program twin pregnancies versus 343 non-program twin pregnancies (120).

The other prenatal nutrition program for multiples is at the University of Michigan (38,68). This program includes patient education, risk monitoring, and nutrition recommendations of 3,500 calories per day with an emphasis on heme-rich sources of iron and protein. Results of preliminary analyses based on the first three years of the program indicated that program participants had higher weight gains to 24 weeks (27.4 lb [12.4 kg] versus 25.2 lb [11.4 kg]) and higher total gains (45.0 lb [20.4 kg] versus 38.8 lb [17.6 kg], $p < .05$) than women who did not participate in the program. The program participants also had better birth weights (2,488 g versus 2,051 g, $p < .001$) and lengths of gestation (35.9 weeks versus 34.0 weeks, $p < .001$). Program mothers were less likely to give birth preterm (before 37 weeks, 61% versus 72%) or early preterm (before 33 weeks, 11% versus 37%, $p < .01$; AOR, 0.24; 95% CI, 0.10–0.57), or to have preterm premature rupture of membranes (7% versus 23%; AOR, 0.29; 95% CI, 0.10–0.82), preterm labor (24% versus 48%, $p < .01$, AOR, 0.45; 95% CI, 0.23–0.90), or low birth weight infants (<2,500 g, 37% versus 71%, AOR 0.27; 95% CI, 0.14–0.53). Program mothers were more likely to meet all of the target goals of the program, including gestation of 36 to 38 weeks (AOR, 3.16; 95% CI, 1.62–6.18), birth weight between 2,500 and 2,800 g (AOR, 3.69; 95% CI, 1.68–8.12), and birth weights greater than seventy-fifth percentile for twins (AOR, 2.01; 95% CI, 1.03–3.89).

In addition to averaging higher birth weights and longer gestations, infants of program mothers also had significantly shorter birth hospitalizations, including shorter stays in the NICU. Based on regression analysis, infants of program mothers averaged 435 g higher birth weights ($p < .001$), 13.1 days' longer gestation ($p < .001$), and 7.4 fewer hospital days ($p < .001$). Infants of program mothers also required fewer medical interventions and had lower odds of having respiratory distress syndrome (AOR, 0.53; 95% CI, 0.31–0.90), bronchopulmonary dysplasia (AOR, 0.11; 95% CI, 0.01–0.55), apnea of prematurity (AOR, 0.52; 95% CI, 0.30–0.87), anemia (AOR, 0.32; 95% CI, 0.16–0.61), retinopathy (AOR, 0.20; 95% CI, 0.05–0.59), or patent ductus arteriosus

(AOR, 0.15; 95% CI, 0.02–0.54). These infants also had lower odds of requiring NICU admission (AOR, 0.44; 95% CI, 0.28–0.68), mechanical ventilation (AOR, 0.39; 95% CI, 0.22–0.66), total parenteral nutrition (AOR, 0.25; 95% CI, 0.13–0.45), or blood transfusions (AOR, 0.09; 95% CI, 0.02–0.27). The reduction in morbidity greatly decreased hospital charges ($31,594 versus $79,428 per twin pair, $p = .001$) and charges per day ($2,348 versus $3,618 per twin pair, $p < .0001$). Newborn savings due to program participation averaged $52,553 per twin pair.

PRENATAL ANTECEDENT OF CHILDHOOD AND ADULT HEALTH

In recent years there has been growing interest in the possible link between prenatal growth and childhood and adult health and disease, termed *metabolic imprinting* or *programming* (121). Barker et al. (122) provided the first direct evidence that some adult-onset diseases can originate from IUGR. These authors showed an association between essential hypertension and low birth weight. Data from the British National Study of Children born in 1946 have provided additional evidence for the link between low birth weight and the development of hypertension, as well as insulin resistance (123). Fetal adaptation to uteroplacental insufficiency, particularly the decreased DNA synthesis in the myocardium (109), may be the basis for the association between IUGR and subsequent risk of cardiovascular disease in adult life. Poor maternal nutritional status, determined by means of triceps skinfold measurement at 18 and 28 weeks' gestation, has been correlated with the subsequent development of higher blood pressure among the children at 11 years of age (124). Conversely, prenatal interventions to improve prenatal nutrition may have far-reaching positive effects on health beyond the perinatal period. For example, Belizàn et al. (100) demonstrated that 7-year-old children whose mothers had received calcium supplementation prenatally had significantly lower systolic blood pressures and lower risk of high systolic blood pressure (RR, 0.59; 95% CI, 0.39–0.90). This effect was particularly evident among children in the highest quartile of BMI (RR, 0.43; 95% CI, 0.26–0.71).

CLINICAL CONSIDERATIONS AND KEY POINTS

- Multiple pregnancy represents a state of magnified nutritional requirements, resulting in a greater nutrient drain on maternal resources, and an accelerated depletion of nutritional reserves.
- The factors most strongly correlated with both length of gestation and birth weight are maternal height, pregravid or early pregnancy body weight, maternal fat deposition, and weight gain.
- Maternal weight gain to 20 weeks and between 20 and 28 weeks has the greatest effect on birth weight in twin and triplet pregnancies, particularly among underweight women.
- Parity, which most likely represents a higher proportion of body fat, has a positive effect on pregnancy outcome, averaging 7 to 10 days longer gestation for multiparous versus nulliparous women.
- In addition to being the nutrients most often lacking in women's diets, calcium, magnesium, and zinc have been identified as hav-

ing the most potential for reducing pregnancy complications and improving outcomes.

REFERENCES

1. Impact of multiple births on low birthweight—Massachusetts, 1989–1996. *Morb Mortal Wkly Rep* 1999;48:289–292.
2. Martin JA, Taffel SM. Current and future impact of rising multiple birth ratios on low birthweight. *Stat Bull* 1995;76:10–18.
3. Brown JE. Improving pregnancy outcomes in the United States: the importance of preventive nutrition services. *J Am Diet Assoc* 1989;89:631–633.
4. Brown JE. Prenatal nutrition counseling: two caveats. *J Am Diet Assoc* 1996;96:448–449.
5. Alexander GR, Weiss J, Hulsey TC, et al. Preterm birth prevention: an evaluation of programs in the United States. *Birth* 1991; 18:160–169.
6. American Academy of Pediatrics and American College of Obstetricians and Gynecologists. *Guidelines for perinatal care,* 4th ed. Washington, DC. AAP/ACOG, 1997.
7. Pons JC, Mayenga JM, Plu G, et al. Management of triplet pregnancy. *Acta Genet Med Gemellol (Roma)* 1988;37:99–103.
8. Elliot JP, Radin TG. Quadruplet pregnancy: contemporary management and outcome. *Obstet Gynecol* 1992;80:421–424.
9. Elster AD, Bleyl JL, Craven TE. Birth weight standards for triplets under modern obstetric care in the United States, 1984–1989. *Obstet Gynecol* 1991:77:387–393.
10. Levene MI, Wild J, Steer P. Higher multiple births and the modern management of infertility in Britain. *Br J Obstet Gynaecol* 1992;99:607–613.
11. Seoud MAF, Toner JP, Kruithoff C, et al. Outcome of twin, triplet, and quadruplet in vitro fertilization pregnancies: the Norfolk experience. *Fertil Steril* 1992;57:825–834.
12. Eastman NJ, Jackson E. Weight relationships in pregnancy: the bearing of maternal weight gain and prepregnancy weight on birthweight in full term pregnancies. *Obstet Gynecol Surv* 1968; 23:1003–1025.
13. Niswander KR, Singer J, Westphal M, et al. Weight gain during pregnancy and prepregnancy weight: association with birth weight of term gestations. *Obstet Gynecol* 1969;33:482–491.
14. Niswander K, Jackson E. Physical characteristics of the gravida and their association with birth weight and perinatal death. *Am J Obstet Gynecol* 1974;119:306–313.
15. Singer JE, Westphal M, Niswander K. Relationship of weight gain during pregnancy to birth weight and infant growth and development in the first year of life. *Obstet Gynecol* 1968;31:417–423.
16. Institute of Medicine. *Nutrition during pregnancy.* Washington, DC: National Academy Press, 1990.
17. World Health Organization. Physical status: the use and interpretation of anthropometry. WHO Technical Report Series 854. Geneva, Switzerland: World Health Organization, 1995.
18. Goldenberg RL, Iams JD, Mercer BM, et al. The preterm prediction study: the value of new versus standard risk factors in predicting early and spontaneous preterm births. *Am J Public Health* 1998;88:233–238.

19. Abrams B, Newman V, Key T, et al. Maternal weight gain and preterm delivery. *Obstet Gynecol* 1989;74:577–583.
20. Abrams B, Newman V. Small-for-gestational-age birth: maternal predictors and comparison with risk factors of spontaneous preterm delivery in the same cohort. *Am J Obstet Gynecol* 1991; 164:785–790.
21. Spinillo A, Capuzzo E, Piazzi G, et al. Risk for spontaneous preterm delivery by combined body mass index and gestational weight gain patterns. *Acta Obstet Gynecol Scand* 1998;77:32–36.
22. Virji SK, Cottington E. Risk factors associated with preterm deliveries among racial groups in a national sample of married mothers. *Am J Perinatol* 1991;8:347–353.
23. Berkowitz GS. Clinical and obstetric risk factors for preterm delivery. *Mt Sinai J Med* 1985;52:239–247.
24. Spinillo A, Stronati M, Ometto A, et al. The influence of presentation and method of delivery on neonatal mortality and infant neurodevelopmental outcome in nondiscordant low-birthweight (<2500 g) twin gestations. *Eur J Obstet Gynecol Reprod Biol* 1992;47:189–194.
25. Hediger ML, Scholl TO, Belsky DH, et al. Patterns of weight gain in adolescent pregnancy: effects on birth weight and preterm delivery. *Obstet Gynecol* 1989;74:6–12.
26. Hediger ML, Scholl TO, Salmon RW. Early weight gain in pregnant adolescents and fetal outcome. *Am J Hum Biol* 1989;1: 665–672.
27. Pederson AL, Worthington-Roberts B, Hickok DE. Weight gain patterns during twin gestation. *J Am Diet Assoc* 1989;89:642–646.
28. Brown JE, Schloesser PT. Prepregnancy weight status, prenatal weight gain, and the outcome of term twin gestations. *Am J Obstet Gynecol* 1990;162:182–186.
29. Lantz ME, Chez RA, Rodriguez A, et al. Maternal weight gain patterns and birth weight outcome in twin gestations. *Obstet Gynecol* 1996;87:551–556.
30. Luke B, Keith L, Johnson TRB, et al. Pregravid weight, gestational weight gain and current weight of women delivered of twins. *J Perinat Med* 1991;19:333–340.
31. Luke B, Minogue J, Abbey H, et al. The association between maternal weight gain and the birthweight of twins. *J Matern Fetal Med* 1992;1:267–276.
32. Luke B, Minogue J, Witter FR, et al. The ideal twin pregnancy: patterns of weight gain, discordancy, and length of gestation. *Am J Obstet Gynecol* 1993;169:588–597.
33. Luke B, Leurgans S. Maternal weight gains in ideal twin outcomes. *J Am Diet Assoc* 1996;96:178–181.
34. Luke B, Gillespie B, Min SJ, et al. Critical periods of maternal weight gain: effect on twin birthweight. *Am J Obstet Gynecol* 1997;177:1055–1062.
35. Luke B, Keith L, Keith D. Maternal nutrition in twin gestations: weight gain, cravings and aversions, and sources of nutrition advice. *Acta Genet Med Gemellol (Roma)* 1997;46:157–166.
36. Luke B, Min SJ, Gillespie B, et al. The importance of early weight gain on the intrauterine growth and birthweight of twins. *Am J Obstet Gynecol* 1998;179:1155–1161.
37. Luke B. What is the influence of maternal weight gain on the fetal growth of twins? *Clin Obstet Gynecol* 1998;41:57–64.

38. Luke B, Min L, Newman RB, et al. BMI–specific weight gain guidelines for twin pregnancies. *Am J Obstet Gynecol* 2000; 182(2):S141 (abst).

39. Taggart NR, Holiday RM, Billewicz WZ. Changes in skinfolds during pregnancy. *Br J Nutr* 1967;21:439–451.

40. MacGillivray I, Campbell DM. The physical characteristics and adaptations of women with twin pregnancies. In: *Twin research: clinical studies.* New York: Alan R. Liss, 1978:81–86.

41. Williams RL, Creasy RK, Cunningham GC, et al. Fetal growth and perinatal viability in California. *Obstet Gynecol* 1982;59:624–632.

42. Young M. Placental factors and fetal nutrition. *Am J Clin Nutr* 1981;34:738–743.

43. Pipe NGG, Smith T, Halliday D, et al. Changes in fat, fat-free mass and body water in human normal pregnancy. *Br J Obstet Gynaecol* 1979;86:929–940.

44. Hytten FE, Thomson AM, Taggart N. Total body water in normal pregnancy. *J Obstet Gynaecol Br Commonw* 1966;73:553–561.

45. Seitchik J, Alper C, Szutka A. Changes in body composition during pregnancy. *Ann NY Acad Sci* 1963;110:821 829.

46. Van Raaji JMA, Schonk CM, Vermaat-Miedema SH, et al. Body fat mass and basal metabolic rate in Dutch women before, during, and after pregnancy: a reappraisal of energy cost of pregnancy. *Am J Clin Nutr* 1989;49:765–772.

47. Villar J, Cogswell M, Kestler E, et al. Effect of fat and fat-free mass deposition during pregnancy on birthweight. *Am J Obstet Gynecol* 1992;167:1344–1352.

48. Viegas OAC, Cole TJ, Wharton BA. Impaired fat deposition in pregnancy: an indicator for nutritional intervention. *Am J Clin Nutr* 1987;45:23–28.

49. Neggers Y, Goldenberg RL, Cliver SP, et al. Usefulness of various maternal skinfold measurements for predicting newborn birth weight. *J Am Diet Assoc* 1992;92:1393–1394.

50. Bissenden JG, Scott PH, King J, et al. Anthropometric and biochemical changes during pregnancy in Asian and European mothers having well grown babies. *Br J Obstet Gynaecol* 1981; 88:992–998.

51. Bissenden JG, Scott PH, King J, et al. Anthropometric and biochemical changes during pregnancy in Asian and European mothers having light for gestational age babies. *Br J Obstet Gynaecol* 1981;88:999–1008.

52. Hediger ML, Scholl TO, Schall JI, et al. Changes in maternal upper arm fat stores are predictors of variation in infant birth weight. *J Nutr* 1994;124:24–30.

53. Luke B, Hediger ML, Wanty S. Mid–upper arm circumference (MUAC) changes in late pregnancy predict fetal growth in twins. Presented at the 24th Annual Meeting of the Human Biology Association, Columbus, OH, April 26–28, 1999.

54. Crowther CA, Hamilton RA. Triplet pregnancy: a 10–year review of 105 cases at Harare Maternity Hospital, Zimbabwe. *Acta Genet Med Gemellol (Roma)* 1989;38:271–278.

55. Gonen R, Heyman E, Asztalos EV, et al. The outcome of triplet, quadruplet, and quintuplet pregnancies managed in a perinatal unit: obstetric, neonatal, and follow-up data. *Am J Obstet Gynecol* 1990;162:454–459.

56. Ron-El R, Mor Z, Weinraub Z, et al. Triplet, quadruplet and quintuplet pregnancies. *Acta Obstet Gynecol Scand* 1992;71:347–350.
57. Casele HL, Dooley SL, Metzger BE. Metabolic response to meal eating and extended overnight fast in twin gestation. *Am J Obstet Gynecol* 1996;175:917–921.
58. Frentzen BH, Johnson JWC, Simpson S. Nutrition and hydration: relation to preterm myometrial contractility. *Obstet Gynecol* 1987;70:887–891.
59. Kaplan M, Eidelman AI, Aboulafia Y. Fasting and the precipitation of labor: the Yom Kippur effect. *JAMA* 1983;250:1317–1318.
60. Binienda Z, Massmann A, Mitchell MD, et al. Effect of food withdrawal on arterial blood glucose and plasma 13,14-dihydro-15-keto-prostaglandin $F_{2\alpha}$ concentrations and nocturnal myometrial electromyographic activity in the pregnant rhesus monkey in the last third of gestation: a model for preterm labor? *Am J Obstet Gynecol* 1989;160:746–750.
61. Silver M, Fowden AL. Uterine prostaglandin F metabolite production in relation to glucose availability in late pregnancy and a possible influence of diet on time of delivery in the mare. *J Reprod Fertil Suppl* 1982;32:511–519.
62. Fowden AL, Silver M. The effect of the nutritional state on uterine prostaglandin F metabolite concentrations in the pregnant ewe during late gestation. *Q J Exp Physiol* 1983;68:337–349.
63. Rizzo T, Frienkel N, Metzger BE, et al. Correlations between antepartum maternal metabolism and newborn behavior. *Am J Obstet Gynecol* 1990;163:1458–1464.
64. Rizzo T, Metzger BE, Burns K. Correlations between antepartum maternal metabolism and intelligence of offspring. *N Engl J Med* 1991;325:911–916.
65. Rizzo TA, Dooley SL, Metzger BE, et al. Prenatal and perinatal influences on long-term psychomotor development in offspring of diabetic mothers. *Am J Obstet Gynecol* 1995;173:1753–1758.
66. Enns CW, Goldman JD, Cook A. Trends in food and nutrient intakes by adults: NFCS 1977–78, CSFII 1989–91, and CSFII 1994–95. *Fam Econ Nutr Rev* 1997;10:2–15.
67. Gülmezoglu M, de Onis M, Villar J. Effectiveness of interventions to prevent or treat impaired fetal growth. *Obstet Gynecol Surv* 1997;6:139–149.
68. Luke B. Nutrition and prematurity. *Prenat Neonat Med* 1998; 3:32–34.
69. Ramakrishnan U, Manjrekar R, Rivera J, et al. Micronutrients and pregnancy outcome: a review of the literature. *Nutr Res* 1998;19:103–159.
70. Scholl TO, Hediger ML, Fischer RL, et al. Anemia versus iron deficiency: increased risk of preterm delivery. *Am J Obstet Gynecol* 1992;55:985–988.
71. Klebanoff MA, Shiono PH, Selby JV, et al. Anemia and spontaneous preterm birth. *Am J Obstet Gynecol* 1991;164:59–63.
72. Siega-Riz A, Adair LS, Hobel CJ. Maternal hematologic changes during pregnancy and the effect of iron status on preterm delivery in a West Los Angeles population. *Am J Perinatol* 1998;15: 515–522.
73. Mitchell MC, Lerner E. Maternal hematologic measures and pregnancy outcome. *J Am Diet Assoc* 1992;92:484–486.

74. Holzman C, Katnik R, Jetton J, et al. Do maternal serum ferritin levels have a role in predicting preterm delivery? *Am J Epidemiol* 1996;143:S73(abst).

75. Tamura T, Goldenberg RL, Johnston KE, et al. Serum ferritin: a predictor of early spontaneous preterm delivery. *Obstet Gynecol* 1996;87:360–365.

76. Goldenberg RL, Tamura T, DuBard M, et al. Plasma ferritin and pregnancy outcome. *Am J Obstet Gynecol* 1996;175:1356–1359.

77. Goldenberg RL, Mercer BM, Miodovnik M, et al. Plasma ferritin, premature rupture of membranes, and pregnancy outcome. *Am J Obstet Gynecol* 1998;179:1599–1604.

78. Scholl TO. High third-trimester ferritin concentration: associations with very preterm delivery, infection, and maternal nutritional status. *Obstet Gynecol* 1998;92:161–166.

79. Spellacy WN, Handler A, Ferre CD. A case–control study of 1,253 twin pregnancies from a 1982–1987 prenatal data base. *Obstet Gynecol* 1990;75:168–171.

80. Blickstein I, Goldschmit R, Lurie S. Hemoglobin levels during twin versus singleton pregnancies. *J Reprod Med* 1995;40:47–50.

81. Ben Miled S, Bibi D, Khalfi N, et al. Iron stocks and risk of anemia in twins. *Arch Inst Pasteur Tunis* 1989;66:221–241.

82. Hediger ML, Luke B. Hemodynamics and maternal weight gain in twin pregnancies. Presented at the 127th Annual Meeting of the American Public Health Association, Chicago, IL, November 9–11, 1999.

83. Swanson CA, King JC. Zinc and pregnancy outcome. *Am J Clin Nutr* 1987;46:763–771.

84. Hambridge KM, Krebs NF, Jacobs MA, et al. Zinc nutritional status during pregnancy: a longitudinal study. *Am J Clin Nutr* 1983;37:429–442.

85. Neggers YH, Cutter GR, Acton RT, et al. A positive association between maternal serum zinc concentration and birth weight. *Am J Clin Nutr* 1990;51:678–684.

86. Neggers YH, Goldenberg RL, Tamura T, et al. Plasma and erythrocyte zinc concentrations and their relationship to dietary zinc intake and zinc supplementation during pregnancy in low-income African-American women. *J Am Diet Assoc* 1997;97: 1269–1274.

87. Mukherjee MD, Sandstead HH, Ratnaparkhi MV, et al. Maternal zinc, iron, folic acid, and protein nutriture and outcome of human pregnancy. *Am J Clin Nutr* 1984;40:496–507.

88. Sikorski R, Juszkiewicz T, Paszkowski T. Zinc status in women with premature rupture of membranes at term. *Obstet Gynecol* 1990;76:675–677.

89. Scholl TO, Hediger ML, Schall JI, et al. Low zinc intake during pregnancy: its association with preterm and very preterm delivery. *Am J Epidemiol* 1993;137:1115–1124.

90. Hunt IF, Murphy NJ, Lleaver AE, et al. Zinc supplementation during pregnancy: effects on selected blood constituents and on progress and outcome in low-income women of Mexican descent. *Am J Clin Nutr* 1984;40:508–521.

91. Cherry FF, Sandstead HH, Rojas P, et al. Adolescent pregnancy: associations among body weight, zinc nutriture, and pregnancy outcome. *Am J Clin Nutr* 1989;50:945–954.

92. Goldenberg RL, Tamura T, Neggers Y, et al. The effect of zinc supplementation on pregnancy outcome. *JAMA* 1995;274:463–468.
93. Merialdi M, Caufield LE, Zavaleta N, et al. Adding zinc to prenatal iron and folate tablets improves fetal neurobehavioral development. *Am J Obstet Gynecol* 1998;180:483–490.
94. Repke JT, Villar J. Pregnancy-induced hypertension and low birth weight: the role of calcium. *Am J Clin Nutr* 1991;272:237–241S.
95. Villar J, Repke JT. Calcium supplementation during pregnancy may reduce preterm delivery in high-risk populations. *Am J Obstet Gynecol* 1990;163:1124–1131.
96. Belizàn JM, Villar J, Gonzalez L, et al. Calcium supplementation to prevent hypertensive disorders of pregnancy. *N Engl J Med* 1991;325:1399–1405.
97. Lòpez-Jaramillo P, Narvàez M, Weigel RM, et al. Calcium supplementation reduces the risk of pregnancy-induced hypertension in an Andes population. *Br J Obstet Gynecol* 1989;96:648–655.
98. Lòpez-Jaramillo P, Narvàez M,, Felix C, et al. Dietary calcium supplementation and prevention of pregnancy hypertension. *Lancet* 1990;335:293.
99. Levine RJ, Hauth JC, Curet LB, et al. Trial of calcium to prevent preeclampsia. *N Engl J Med* 1997;337:69–76.
100. Belizàn JM, Villar J, Bergel E, et al. Long term effect of calcium supplementation during pregnancy on the blood pressure of offspring: follow-up of a randomized controlled trial. *BMJ* 1997; 315:281–285.
101. Sibai BM, Villar MA, Bray E. Magnesium supplementation during pregnancy: a double–blind randomized controlled clinical trial. *Am J Obstet Gynecol* 1989;161:115–119.
102. Conradt A, Weidinger H, Algayer H. On the role of magnesium in fetal hypotrophy, pregnancy-induced hypertension and preeclampsia. *Magnes Bull* 1984;6:68–76.
103. Spätling L, Spätling G. Magnesium supplementation in pregnancy: a double-blind study. *Br J Obstet Gynaecol* 1988;95: 120–125.
104. Lucas MJ, Leveno KJ, Cunningham FG. A comparison of magnesium sulfate with phenytoin for the prevention of eclampsia. *N Engl J Med* 1995;333:201–205.
105. Eclampsia Trial Collaborative Group. Which anticonvulsant for women with eclampsia? Evidence from the Collaborative Eclampsia Trial. *Lancet* 1995;345:1455–1463.
106. Nelson KB, Grether JK. Can magnesium sulfate reduce the risk of cerebral palsy in very low birthweight infants? *Pediatrics* 1995;95:263–269.
107. Schendel DE, Berg CJ, Yeargin-Allsopp M, et al. Prenatal magnesium sulfate exposure and the risk of cerebral palsy or mental retardation among very low-birth-weight children aged 3 to 5 years. *JAMA* 1996;276:1805–1810.
108. Grether JK, Hoogstrate J, Selvin S, et al. Magnesium sulfate tocolysis and risk of neonatal death. *Am J Obstet Gynecol* 1998;178:1–6.
109. Gagnon R, Rundle H, Johnston L, et al. Alterations in fetal and placental deoxyribonucleic acid synthesis rates after chronic fetal placental embolization. *Am J Obstet Gynecol* 1995;172:1451–1458.
110. Hindmarsh PC, Geary M, Rodeck CH, et al. Placental weight is influenced by early maternal nutritional status. *J Soc Gynecol Investig* 1999;6 (Suppl):187A(abst).

111. Godfrey K, Robinson S, Barker DJP, et al. Maternal nutrition in early and late pregnancy in relation to placental and fetal growth. *BMJ* 1996;312:410–414.
112. Hediger ML, Scholl TO, Schall JI, et al. Fetal growth and the etiology of preterm delivery. *Obstet Gynecol* 1995;85:175–182.
113. Smith GCS, Smith MFS, McNay MB, et al. First-trimester growth and the risk of low birth weight. *N Engl J Med* 1998;339: 1817–1822.
114. Novy MJ, McGregor JA, Iams JD. New perspectives on the prevention of extreme prematurity. *Clin Obstet Gynecol* 1995;38: 790–808.
115. O'Connor MC, Arias E, Royston JP, et al. The merits of special antenatal care for twin pregnancies. *Br J Obstet Gynaecol* 1981; 88:222–230.
116. Vergani P, Ghidini A, Bozzo G, et al. Prenatal management of twin gestation: experience with a new protocol. *J Reprod Med* 1991;36:667–671.
117. Gardner MO, Amaya MA, Sakakini J. Effects of prenatal care on twin gestations. *J Reprod Med* 1990;35:519–521.
118. Pons JC, Nekhlyudov L, Dephot N, et al. Management and outcomes of 65 quadruplet pregnancies: sixteen years' experience in France. *Acta Genet Med Gemellol (Roma)* 1996;45:367–375.
119. Newman RB, Ellings JM. Antepartum management of the multiple gestation: the case for specialized care. *Semin Perinatol* 1995;19:387–403.
120. Dubois S, Doughtery C, Duquette MP, et al. Twin pregnancy: the impact of the Higgins Nutrition Intervention Program on maternal and neonatal outcomes. *Am J Clin Nutr* 1991;53:1397–1403.
121. Waterland RA, Garza C. Potential mechanisms of metabolic imprinting that lead to chronic disease. *Am J Clin Nutr* 1999; 69:179–197.
122. Barker DJ, Bull AR, Osmond C, et al. Fetal and placental size and risk of hypertension in adult life. *Br Med J* 1990;301:259–262.
123. Fall CHD, Osmond C, Barker DJP, et al. Fetal and infant growth and cardiovascular risk factors in women. *BMJ* 1995; 310:428–432.
124. Clark PM, Atton C, Law CM, et al. Weight gain in pregnancy, triceps skinfold thickness, and blood pressure of offspring. *Obstet Gynecol* 1998;91:103–107.
125. Fenton TR, Thirsk JE. Twin pregnancy: the distribution of maternal weight gain of non-smoking normal weight women. *Can J Public Health* 1994;85:37–40.
126. Levene MI. Assisted reproduction and its implications for paediatrics. *Arch Dis Child* 1991;66:1–3.
127. Syrop CH, Varner MW. Triplet gestation: maternal and neonatal implications. *Acta Genet Med Gemellol (Roma)* 1985;34:81–88.
128. Luke B, Leurgans S, Keith LG, et al. The childhood growth of twin children. *Acta Genet Med Gemellol (Roma)* 1995;44:169–178.
129. Collins M, Bleyl J. Seventy-one quadruplet pregnancies. *Am J Obstet Gynecol* 1990;162:1384–1392.
130. Spellacy WN, Buhi WC, Birk SA. Carbohydrate metabolism in women with a twin pregnancy. *Obstet Gynecol* 1980;55:688–691.

Preterm Birth Prediction and Prevention

It has long been appreciated that there is an inverse relation between number of fetuses and length of gestation. Approximately one-half of twin gestations and more than 80% of triplet gestations are delivered prematurely. Premature delivery is the single most important contributor to the high rates of adverse perinatal outcomes among these pregnancies. Published perinatal mortality rates for twins in developed countries range from 47 to 120 per 1,000 twin births (1). Population-based data in the United States reveal that rates of neonatal death are five- to sevenfold higher among twin than among singleton gestations regardless of race (2). The majority of this perinatal mortality is a consequence of early preterm delivery of very low birth weight infants.

As a result of these high rates of premature birth, multiple gestations contribute disproportionately to the overall burden of prematurity and its perinatal consequences. In Europe, multiple gestations account for 17% of births between 20 and 27 weeks; 21% of births between 28 and 31 weeks; and 17% of births between 32 and 36 weeks (3). In New Zealand, more than one-fourth of all deliveries at less than 32 weeks' gestation are multiple (4). In the United States, twins represent fewer than 2% of the live births but account for more than 15% of all very low birth weight infants, almost 14% of low birth weight infants, 11% of all neonatal deaths, 3.4% of postneonatal deaths, and 8.4% of infant deaths (2).

Appropriately therefore, the prediction and prevention of preterm birth among twins are important obstetrical issues. In general, prenatal care has been as poorly studied and is as highly individualized as any aspect of medicine. Fortunately however, prediction and prevention of preterm birth in multiple gestations has generated considerable attention in the obstetrical literature. Much of this attention is in the form of randomized clinical trials, which provide the highest quality of evidence on which to base obstetrical management.

Although techniques to predict and prevent premature birth are considered separately herein, it is important to remember that these two issues are intertwined. The ability to ascertain which women are at greater risk for preterm birth is of limited value without effective intervention to prevent premature birth. Alternatively, prevention strategies that appear to have little or no efficacy among the general population of twins may prove effective for a more selective, higher-risk subgroup. Identifying characteristics predictive of preterm birth allows us to focus the expenditure of resources and provides insights that help generate hypothesis testing of interventions to prevent early delivery.

Ascertaining which women are at greatest risk of preterm birth and establishing effective means to prevent preterm delivery or at least to postpone it until sufficient fetal growth and development have occurred represents the most important advance possible in the prenatal care of women with multiple pregnancies.

PREDICTION OF PRETERM BIRTH

Risk Scoring

Risk-scoring systems have been developed in an effort to identify which women are at increased risk of giving birth preterm. These risk-scoring systems have applied primarily to singleton gestations because multiple pregnancy is such an independently powerful risk factor for preterm birth (5). In fact, in the most well known of all the proposed risk-scoring systems, twin gestation confers a score of 10, which by itself identifies that pregnancy as being high risk in the Creasy scoring system (6). Even for singleton gestations, most risk-scoring systems have not proved efficient in identifying who is likely to deliver prematurely. At best these scoring systems have a sensitivity of less than 50% and positive predictive values that are even lower. They also have proved to be poorly reproducible among different populations (7).

Other well-described risk factors for preterm birth, such as the extremes of maternal age, black race, low socioeconomic status, substance abuse, small stature, poor maternal weight gain, occupational fatigue, assisted reproduction, or coincidental obstetric and medical complications may place a woman with a multiple gestation at increased risk of prematurity. However, these other risk factors have little overall effect because of the overwhelming influence of fetal number.

In an analysis of traditional historical and medical risk factors associated with preterm birth among 147 twin gestations, Goldenberg et al. (8) could not identify any factors that were significantly associated with delivery at less than 32 weeks. Although smoking, prior spontaneous preterm birth, and various medical complications were more common among women delivering twins at less than 35 weeks' gestation, only urinary tract infection (odds ratio [OR], 3.2; 95% confidence interval [CI], 1.3–7.9) was significantly associated with this outcome. For delivery at less than 37 weeks, only a prior spontaneous preterm birth (OR, 4.0; 95% CI, 1.1–18.2) was significantly associated with this outcome. This same association between spontaneous preterm birth of twins and prior spontaneous preterm birth of a singleton has been described by other investigators (9).

Ultrasonic Cervical Length Measurements

Transvaginal ultrasonography for cervical length measurement was originally described by Anderson et al. (10). They found a relation between a shortened cervical length at 30 weeks' gestation and an increased risk of preterm delivery among asymptomatic singleton pregnancies. In a large prevention study of preterm birth that was sponsored by the National Institutes of Health, Iams et al. (11) used endovaginal sonography to measure cervical length at 24 weeks' gestation for 2,915 randomly enrolled women with singleton pregnancies and again at 28 weeks' gestation for 2,531 women from the original cohort. A cervical length of 25 mm or less had sensitivities for preterm delivery prior to 35 weeks' gestation of 37.3% and 49.4% at 24 and 28 weeks' gestation, respectively. The positive predictive values of a cervical length of 25 mm or less at 24 or 28 weeks' gestation were 17.8% and 11.3%, respectively. With continuous evaluation, there was a strong association between decreasing cervical length and increasing risk of preterm birth (11).

The use of endovaginal sonography to measure cervical length has also been studied to determine its predictive value for preterm delivery in twin gestations. Kushnir et al. (12) found no difference in cervical length between singleton and twin gestations up to 19 weeks of gestation. Thereafter however, the cervix was significantly shorter in twin pregnancies than in singletons even though all the twins delivered at term. In a large multicenter study sponsored by the National Institute of Child Health and Human Development (NICHD) Maternal-Fetal Medicine Unit Network, predictors of preterm delivery were evaluated in twin gestations (8). A shortened cervical length of 25 mm or less was significantly more common in twin pregnancies than in singletons at both 24 (17.7% versus 9.1%) and 28 (32.8% versus 14.5%) weeks' gestation. Of all the potential predictors of preterm delivery considered, a cervical length of 25 mm or less at 24 weeks' gestation had the strongest association with preterm delivery before 32 weeks' (OR, 6.9; 95% CI, 2.0–24.2), 35 weeks' (OR, 3.2; 95% CI, 1.3–8.0), and 37 weeks' gestation (OR, 2.8; 95% CI, 1.1–7.7) for twin pregnancies (8). At 28 weeks, the presence of a shortened cervix (25 mm or less) was significantly associated with preterm birth at less than 35 weeks' ($p = .047$) but not at less than 32 or less than 37 weeks' gestation (8).

In a similar observational study in England, Souka et al. (13) performed endovaginal ultrasound cervical length measurements at 23 weeks' gestation for 215 twin pregnancies. For this cohort, the investigators reported a median cervical length at 22 to 24 weeks of 38 mm. The fifth percentile was 19 mm, and the first percentile was 7 mm. The cervical length measurements were the same for both monochorionic and dichorionic gestations. The sensitivity of a cervical length less than 20 mm at 24 weeks' gestation to predict spontaneous preterm delivery was 100% for deliveries occurring at 28 weeks' gestation or before; 80% for deliveries at 30 weeks' gestation or before; and 47% for deliveries 32 weeks' gestation or before (13).

The negative predictive value of endovaginal cervical length measurements also is important. In the previously cited study by Iams et al. (11) regarding an unselected singleton population, the negative predictive value of an endovaginal cervical length measurement of more than 25 mm for preterm delivery prior to 35 weeks' gestation was 97% at 24 weeks' and 98% at 28 weeks' gestation. Imseis et al. (14) performed a retrospective analysis of 85 twins who had undergone second-trimester endovaginal ultrasound for cervical length measurement. These investigators determined that a transvaginal cervical length of more than 35 mm between 24 and 26 weeks' gestation identified twin gestations at low risk (less than 3%) for spontaneous delivery prior to 34 weeks. Similar to the other investigations, Imseis et al. were able to demonstrate significant shortening of cervical length among twins destined to be born prematurely.

Whether cervical shortening is a preexisting condition that predisposes women to premature delivery or whether it is a consequence of pathological processes associated with prematurity identifiable in midgestation is not clear. The higher frequency of cervical shortening in multiple gestations than in singletons would seem to suggest that a short cervix most likely develops during the pregnancy rather than before pregnancy. Regardless, short cervical measurements at transvaginal ultrasound correlate with preterm delivery for both singleton and twin gestations. Normal second-trimester cervical lengths, however, have been associated with low rates of delivery prior to 34 weeks' gestation. Unfortunately, there have not been any intervention trials testing innovative management strategies predicated on endovaginal cervical length measurements. Specifically, there is insufficient evidence to conclude that cerclage of an abnormally short cervix will improve outcome, although this is clearly an area for further investigation. However, cervical measurements that are normally long identify a twin gestation at relatively low risk of spontaneous preterm delivery and a pregnancy for which there is little need for prophylactic obstetrical intervention.

Digital Cervical Assessment

The value of antepartum digital cervical examination of women with twin gestations lies in its ability to provide ongoing risk assessment. Most of the available information regarding prediction of preterm delivery with antepartum cervical examination derives from studies of high- and low-risk singleton pregnancies. In a prospective study of serial changes in cervical status in more than 8,000 singleton pregnancies, Bouyer et al. (15) showed that term labor and preterm labor were preceded by cervical changes that could be detected by means of digital cervical examination. Early dilatation of the internal cervical os 1 cm or more was predictive of the highest risk of premature delivery, while a cervical length 1 cm or less was of secondary importance.

Because of the higher risk of preterm delivery, antepartum management of twin gestation has frequently included serial digital cervical examination. In a study involving an observational cohort, O'Connor et al. (16) performed routine cervical examination as part of a special antepartum twin clinic. In their study, cervical dilatation of 2 cm or more before 30 weeks' gestation was predictive of preterm birth with a sensitivity of only 20%. This low sensitivity might not have been unexpected, given the early gestational age at which the examinations were performed. Of the 28 primigravid patients in O'Connor's study, only 2 had cervical dilatation before 30 weeks and 1 of these delivered her infant before term. Of the 72 multigravid patients, only 14 had cervical dilatation of 2 cm or more on or before 30 weeks' gestation, and 6 of these women delivered their infants prematurely. Houlton et al. (17), in Durbin, South Africa, followed 128 twin pregnancies with weekly cervical examinations. Women were seen in a special clinic for purposes of calculating a cervical score.

Cervical score is calculated as follows: cervical length (cm) minus cervical dilatation at the internal os (cm). For example, a cervix that is 2 cm long with a closed internal os has a score of +2. A cervix that is 1 cm long and dilated 1 cm at the internal os gives a cervical score of 0. A cervix that is 1 cm long with an internal os dilated 3 cm gives a cervical score of –2. Cervical examinations continued until the spontaneous onset of labor without benefit of tocolytics or bed rest. Houlton et al. (17) found that a cervical score of 0 or less during any single examination was predictive of preterm labor within 14 days for 69% of the women with such changes. When only multiparous women were considered, the predictive value rose to 80%, suggesting the predictive value of the cervical score may be marginally less for nulliparous women. In the study by Houlton et al., the false-positive rate for a low cervical score and labor within 2 weeks was only 3% (1 of 34) (17).

Neilson et al. (18) followed 223 twin pairs in a specialty clinic in Zimbabwe. They performed frequent cervical examinations for calculation of a cervical score. No attempt was made to inhibit preterm labor with tocolytic drugs. The investigators focused on the prognostic importance of a cervical score of 0 or less on or before 34 weeks' gestation. The positive predictive value of such a score was 66%. As the score became more negative, the predictive value rose. A cervical score of −2 or less identified a subgroup of women at 76% risk of preterm delivery. In the entire series of 223 twin pregnancies, no woman delivered within 1 week of having a cervical score more than 0 (18). Because this study was composed entirely of parous women in Zimbabwe, the results may not apply to other populations.

Newman et al. (19) performed weekly digital cervical examinations on 86 twin and 7 triplet gestations at a specialized twin clinic in Charleston, South Carolina. At each prenatal visit, a cervical score was calculated in the manner described by Houlton et al. (17). Weekly cervical assessment revealed a progressive decrease in cervical score throughout the latter half of gestation most notable after 30 weeks' gestation. As the cervical score decreases, the mean time until delivery shortens. A cervical score of 0 or less on or before 34 weeks' gestation had a sensitivity of 88% for spontaneous preterm delivery in multiple pregnancies. The same cervical score of 0 or less prior to 34 weeks also had a positive predictive value of 75% and a fourfold increased relative risk of delivery prior to 37 weeks' gestation. The earlier in gestation that a cervical score of 0 or less is detected, the greater is the positive predictive value that can be ascribed to it (Table 7-1). As the cervical score becomes more negative at earlier gestational ages, the positive predictive value for preterm delivery approaches 100%. Unfortunately, the sensitivity remains low because of the relative rarity of such abnormal antepartum cervical examinations so early in pregnancy. Parous women tend to have lower mean cervical scores than nulliparous women; however, this does not significantly alter either the positive predictive value or the relative risk of preterm birth that can be ascribed to a given score. As in the study by Neilson et al. (18), only 2 of 78 (2.6%) women experienced spontaneous preterm labor or preterm premature rupture of the membranes (PROM) within 1 week of being found to have a cervical score greater than 0 (19).

A final consideration is the safety of antepartum cervical examination, particularly one that endeavors to assess the internal cervical os. In a prospective, nonrandomized, nonconcurrent, cohort trial by Bivins et al. (20), outcomes for 86 patients observed in the specialized twin clinic between 1988 and 1991 who underwent routine cervical examination at each visit were compared with outcomes for 288 other women with twin gestations observed in a high-risk obstetrical clinic between 1981 and 1991 who under-

Table 7-1. Predictive validity of a cervical score of zero or less on or before 34 weeks' gestation for spontaneous preterm delivery in multiple gestations

Value	Entire Cohort	Nulliparous Patients	Parous Patients	Cervical Score ≤0	
				20–28 wk	29–34 wk
Sensitivity (%)	88	83	91	33	87
Specificity (%)	62	75	58	96	81
Positive predictive value (%)	75	83	72	92	73
Negative predictive value (%)	81	75	83	61	81
Relative risk	3.9	3.3	4.3	2.0	3.8
95% Confidence limit	1.8–8.7	1.0–11.4	1.5–12.4	1.4–2.9	1.7–8.5

From Newman RB, Godsey RK, Ellings JM, et al. Quantification of cervical change: relationship to preterm delivery in multifetal gestation. *Am J Obstet Gynecol* 1991;165:264–269.

went cervical examinations for obstetrical indications only. Comparison of these two groups revealed no significant differences in patient demographics or pregnancy complications, including preterm delivery, bleeding, intraamniotic infection, or neonatal sepsis. Importantly, premature rupture of the membranes was significantly less frequent in the group that underwent routine cervical examination (12.4%) than among the women bearing twins who were examined less frequently (23.6%).

Antepartum digital cervical examination for assessment of preterm delivery risk appears to be both safe and efficacious. The cervical score is recommended because of its simplicity, capability to be quantified and reproduced, and focus on cervical dilatation and effacement. It appears reasonable to use a cervical score of 0 or less as a marker of abnormal cervical status and increased risk of preterm delivery. Women who maintain a cervical score greater than 0 appear to be good candidates for continued observation without specific obstetrical intervention. Antepartum digital cervical examination should be performed on a 1 or 2 week basis between 20 and 36 weeks' gestation. Ideally, the examinations should be performed by one examiner for consistency, and any changes in the findings or a reduction in the cervical score should be warning signs for the clinician.

Better identification of patients at risk of preterm labor may allow more specific application of interventions capable of reducing the likelihood of preterm delivery. Unfortunately, there are no prospective, randomized trials demonstrating that antepartum digital cervical examination is associated with an improvement in perinatal outcome. In a prospective, nonrandomized, cohort study, patients treated in a specialized twin clinic that emphasized education for prevention of preterm birth, frequent digital cervical examination for calculation of a cervical score, activity reduction, and limited care providers were compared to a contemporary cohort of patients with twin gestations treated in private obstetricians' offices or a high-risk obstetrical clinic under the supervision of housestaff and attending physicians. There were no differences in the demographic characteristics of the groups, the adequacy of prenatal care, or antepartum complications. However, patients attending the twin clinic had fewer early preterm deliveries due to spontaneous preterm labor or preterm PROM. As a consequence, they had lower numbers of very low birth weight infants, admissions to a neonatal intensive care unit, and perinatal mortality (21). Papiernik et al. (22), in France, developed a special program for multifetal gestations that emphasized frequent patient visits, early work leave, antepartum digital cervical assessment, and home visits by midwives. In this retrospective observational study, the program was able to reduce the numbers of very low birth weight infants and perinatal deaths in relation to multifetal pregnancy outcomes prior to development of the program. Although the results of neither study (21,22) can define the relation between antepartum cervical examination and improvement in pregnancy outcome, they do support the inclusion of digital cervical examination as part of a comprehensive program for multifetal pregnancy care. They also support the conclusion of Bivins et al. (20) that there is no evidence that antepartum digital cervical examination of women with multiple gestations increases the frequency of adverse pregnancy outcome.

Fetal Fibronectin

Fetal fibronectin is a high-molecular-weight, extracellular matrix glycoprotein that is normally found in amniotic fluid, fetal membranes, and placental tissue. Results of a number of observational trials involving singleton gestations have demonstrated that the presence of fetal fibronectin in cervical vaginal secretions at concentrations greater than 50 ng/mL between 21 and 37 weeks' gestation is abnormal and predictive of impending preterm labor (23,24). This finding has led to the hypothesis that disruption of the chorionic–decidual interface by either inflammatory or infectious processes may precede the onset of preterm labor in some pregnancies and be heralded by the release of fetal fibronectin into the cervical vaginal secretions. Studies have analyzed the predictive capabilities of fetal fibronectin in both symptomatic and asymptomatic singleton pregnancies. Several of these trials included small numbers of multiple gestations; however, multiple gestations typically are not analyzed separately or in sufficient number for meaningful interpretation. Four trials specifically had findings related to fetal fibronectin testing in multiple gestations. All of the studies were observational without mention of the frequency of tocolytic use.

In the previously described NICHD Maternal-Fetal Medicine Unit Network preterm prediction study, Goldenberg et al. (8) reported on 147 women with twin gestations who underwent assessment in the second and third trimesters for cervical-vaginal fetal fibronectin, bacterial vaginosis, and cervical length. Positive fetal fibronectin results at 28 weeks' ($p = .047$) and 30 weeks' ($p = .002$) gestation were significantly associated with increased risk of deliv-

ery before 32 weeks but not at other gestational age intervals or of
delivery prior to 35 or 37 weeks. The association of fetal fibronectin
with preterm delivery was no longer significant after control for
cervical length with logistic regression analysis (8).

Wennerholm et al. (25) observed 121 asymptomatic women carrying twins who underwent repeated screening for fetal fibronectin,
bacterial vaginosis, and endotoxin and underwent endovaginal cervical length measurements between 24 and 34 weeks' gestation. A
positive fetal fibronectin result in at least one sample was associated with a relative risk of 2.0 for birth before 35 weeks' gestation
and a relative risk of 18.0 for birth before 35 weeks if all fetal
fibronectin samples were positive. A positive fetal fibronectin test
at 24 weeks had a sensitivity of 37% for delivery prior to 35 weeks'
gestation, a specificity of 91%, a positive predictive value of 54%,
and a negative predictive value of 84%. The corresponding rates for
a positive result at 28 weeks' gestation were 50%, 92%, 62%, and
87%. A positive fetal fibronectin result at 28 weeks also was associated with neonatal morbidity (relative risk [RR], 5.1) and intensive care nursery admission more than 7 days (RR, 5.4) (25). In this
study, testing for bacterial vaginosis, endotoxin, and cervical length
had no predictive value for preterm birth (25).

Oliveira et al. (26) analyzed the outcomes for 52 women who had
twin gestations and underwent cervical-vaginal secretion testing
every 2 weeks between 24 and 34 weeks' gestation. The occurrence
of at least one positive test result for fetal fibronectin was associated with a significantly increased risk of birth prior to 37 weeks
(RR, 3.4) but not before 34 weeks. Tolino et al. (27) also explored
the usefulness of fetal fibronectin as a predictor of preterm labor
in 62 twin and 6 triplet pregnancies. Cervical-vaginal secretions
were assayed for fetal fibronectin on a weekly basis from 24 weeks
onward. Fifteen women delivered prior to 34 weeks' gestation. A
single positive test result was predictive of preterm labor at less
than 34 weeks with a sensitivity of 93.3%, a specificity of 66%, a
positive predictive value of 37.8%, and a negative predictive value
of 96.7%. If two consecutive samples had positive results, the sensitivity decreased to 90.9% but the specificity increased to 77.1%.
The positive and negative predictive values remained similar at
38.4% and 97.6%, respectively (27).

Based on the results of the foregoing studies, it is reasonable
to conclude that fetal fibronectin in cervical-vaginal secretions in
the late second and early third trimesters is associated with an
increased risk of preterm birth among asymptomatic women carrying multiple fetuses. There are conflicting data about whether
fetal fibronectin testing has predictive value that is additive to that
of endovaginal ultrasound cervical length measurements or even
digital cervical examination. Although serial testing of cervical-
vaginal secretions for fetal fibronectin may identify a patient with
multiple gestations at increased risk of preterm birth, alterations
in clinical management based on fetal fibronectin testing have not
yet been evaluated for multifetal gestations. As such, improved
pregnancy outcomes from fetal fibronectin testing have not yet
been demonstrated.

Bacterial Vaginosis

Emerging clinical evidence suggests an association between the
presence of cervical vaginal infections, such as bacterial vaginosis,

and subsequent spontaneous preterm labor or preterm premature rupture of the membranes (28,29). Women with positive fetal fibronectin assays also are significantly more likely to harbor bacterial vaginosis than are women negative for fetal fibronectin in cervical-vaginal secretions (30). Most of these studies, however, have involved singleton gestations. There are many reasons to be suspicious that the causes of preterm delivery in singletons may be significantly different from those in multiple gestations. In the NICHD preterm prediction study (8), in twin pregnancies, the presence of bacterial vaginosis at either 24 or 28 weeks' gestation was not associated with spontaneous preterm birth. A similar lack of association between bacterial vaginosis and spontaneous preterm birth of twins also was reported by Wennerholm et al. (25). Consistent with the lack of association between bacterial vaginosis and preterm birth of multiple gestations is the fact that prospective treatment trials for bacterial vaginosis have not shown modification of pregnancy outcome (31,32).

Other mediators of infection such as inflammatory cytokines also have been linked to premature labor. Increased local production of inflammatory cytokines associated with infection can increase the production of prostaglandins within the genital tract; the increased production may achieve both cervical ripening and initiation of uterine contractility (33). The presence of cytokines in both the amniotic fluid and the cervical-vaginal secretions during singleton pregnancies has been associated with the occurrence of premature labor; however, the contribution of these cytokines to premature labor in multiple gestations has not been established. The role of cytokines as predictors of preterm delivery in multiple gestations awaits further, appropriately designed investigations.

Combined Markers

Prediction of spontaneous preterm delivery of multiple gestations continues to be a clinical challenge. As we learn more about the pathophysiology of premature labor, identification of more efficient predictors will likely be possible. In the meantime, describing the predictive capability of factors such as cervical shortening by either digital or ultrasonic examination or the presence of fetal fibronectin in cervical-vaginal secretions contributes in small ways to our understanding of the phenomenon of preterm birth.

Another approach to the prediction of preterm delivery is the use of combined markers. Because of the individual strength of the markers, many clinicians have looked at the combination of cervical length measurement and fetal fibronectin. In the study of 147 twin gestations conducted by Goldenberg et al. (8), the investigators found that at 24 weeks' gestation, 21 patients had a short cervix only, 3 had a positive fetal fibronectin result only, and 4 had positive results of both tests (8). At 28 weeks, 30 women had a short cervix only, 2 had a positive fetal fibronectin result only, and 5 had positive results of both tests. The likelihood of spontaneous preterm birth at any gestational age was substantially higher if both tests results were positive than when only one test result was positive or both results were negative (Tables 7-2 and 7-3) (8).

In contradistinction to singleton gestation, in multiple gestation, the shortened cervix appears to be a more powerful predictor of prematurity than is the presence of fetal fibronectin and appears to be predictive of preterm delivery risk earlier (24 weeks) than does fetal fibronectin (28 to 30 weeks). The pattern in which these markers appear suggests that for twins shortening of the cervix likely precedes disruption of the choriodecidual interface, which is believed to be origin of the cervical-vaginal fetal fibronectin. For singletons, early identification of fetal fibronectin and later development of cervical shortening suggest a different pathway to prematurity, possibly intrauterine inflammation or infection.

As we become more efficient at identifying women at increased risk of preterm delivery, even those with multiple gestations, treatment options will have to be devised and the effectiveness of these interventions proven. Interventions that have been explored to date are discussed in the next section.

Table 7-2. **Comparison of the predictive value of endovaginal cervical length measurement, cervical and vaginal fetal fibronectin, and a combination of the two tests for spontaneous preterm birth of twins when tested at 24 weeks' gestation**

Risk Factor	Occurrence (%)	Preterm Birth Rate (%)		
		<32 wk	<35 wk	<37 wk
Number	147	13	47	80
Cervical length (mm)				
≤25	17.7	26.9	53.9	73.1
>25	82.3	5.0	26.5	48.8
		$p = .002$	$p = .01$	$p = .03$
Fetal fibronectin				
Positive	4.8	28.6	42.9	85.7
Negative	95.2	6.5	29.7	50.7
		NS	NS	NS
Combined				
Both negative	80.7	4.3	26.5	47.9
One positive	16.6	16.7	41.7	66.7
Both positive	2.7	50.0	75.0	100
		$p = .003$	$p = .043$	$p = .031$

NS, not significant.
From Goldenberg RL, Iams JD, Miodovnik M, et al. The preterm prediction study: risk factors in twin gestations. *Am J Obstet Gynecol* 1996;175:1047–1053.

Table 7-3. Comparison of the predictive value of endovaginal cervical length measurement, cervical and vaginal fetal fibronectin, and a combination of the two tests for spontaneous preterm birth of twins when tested at 28 weeks' gestation

Risk Factor	Occurrence (%)	Preterm Birth Rate (%)		
		<32 wk	<35 wk	<37 wk
Number	147	13	47	80
Cervical length (mm)				
≤25	32.5	13.2	42.1	65.8
>25	67.5	3.8	24.1	46.8
		NS	$p = .047$	NS
Fetal fibronectin				
Positive	6.4	28.6	57.1	71.4
Negative	93.6	3.9	26.5	50.0
		$p = .047$	NS	NS
Combined				
Both negative	65.1	1.5	21.7	44.9
One positive	30.2	9.4	40.6	62.5
Both positive	4.7	40.0	60.0	80.0
		$p = .004$	$p = .042$	NS

NS, not significant.
From Goldenberg RL, Iams JD, Miodovnik M, et al. The preterm prediction study: risk factors in twin gestations. *Am J Obstet Gynecol* 1996;175:1047–1053.

PREVENTION OF PRETERM BIRTH

Early Diagnosis

The Routine Antenatal Diagnostic Imaging with Ultrasound (RADIUS) trial was a practice-based multicenter study involving women at low risk of adverse pregnancy outcome. The RADIUS trial was unable to prove its primary hypothesis that routine screening with standardized ultrasonography would reduce perinatal morbidity and mortality (34). A significant secondary finding, however, was the improved diagnosis of multiple gestations among the group undergoing routine ultrasound screening. Multiple pregnancies were detected in 68 patients in the screened group and in 61 patients in the control group. All but one noncompliant patient in the screened group received the diagnosis of multiple pregnancy before 26 weeks' gestation. In contrast, and despite the liberal use of ultrasound in the control group, 23 multiple gestations (37%) were not identified until after 26 weeks' gestation, and 8 were undetected until the delivery admission (35). After a systematic review of randomized clinical trials of routine ultrasound examinations in early pregnancy, Neilson (36), using the Cochrane database, concluded that routine use of ultrasound increases the early diagnosis of multiple gestation and reduces the possibility that a multiple gestation would remain undetected at 26 weeks' gestation.

Although making the diagnosis of multiple gestation is a prerequisite to any effective intervention to prolong pregnancy, it is unclear from the available evidence that making an early diagnosis improves pregnancy outcome for multiples. Persson et al. (37) performed routine early ultrasound screening, which allowed them to detect 98% of 254 twin gestations presenting at Malmo General Hospital in Sweden for obstetric care. Among this prospective cohort, the investigators found a reduction in risk of perinatal loss that they believed was related to early diagnosis. In the RADIUS trial (34), the rate of adverse perinatal outcomes among the multiple pregnancies was 25% for the routine ultrasound screening group and 37.7% for the control group. This represents a 50% increase in the frequency of adverse perinatal outcome among the twins in the control group. This difference was not significant ($p = .13$) because of the small sample size for this secondary analysis. However, with a larger sample size, a difference of this degree in the frequency of moderate and severe neonatal morbidities would be clinically significant.

Prophylactic Cervical Cerclage

Two prospective, randomized trials have been performed to assess the value of prophylactic cervical cerclage in twin pregnancies. Neither revealed any difference in the risk of preterm birth or in perinatal mortality (38,39). Dor et al. (38) prospectively randomized 50 twin gestations diagnosed ultrasonographically in the first trimester and found no differences with respect to late miscarriage (up to 26 weeks' gestation), severe prematurity, or perinatal death (182 per 1,000 with cerclage versus 152 per 1,000 without cerclage). The Medical Research Council/Royal College of Obstetricians and Gynecologists Working Party on Cervical Cerclage prospectively randomized 905 patients in nine countries if the provider was uncertain whether cerclage was indicated (39). Included among those 905 patients were 60 pregnant with twins who underwent cerclage and 14 who did not. There were no significant differences in the number who delivered their infants before 33 weeks (10% cerclage versus 29% no cerclage) or in the percentage of patients delivering their infants before 37 weeks (60% cerclage versus 50% no cerclage). Although neither study demonstrated a benefit of prophylactic cerclage, both studies lacked substantial statistical power because of the small sample sizes.

The two prospective trials also demonstrated that cervical cerclage imparts risk to the pregnancy, specifically increased risk of maternal infection and preterm premature rupture of the membranes. The findings of these prospective randomized trials were supported by results of several retrospective studies, none of which revealed any difference in mean gestational age at delivery or proportion of preterm deliveries (40–42).

For triplet pregnancies, the literature is dominated by retrospective, nonrandomized studies. The most provocative was conducted by Goldman et al. (43). The results revealed significant prolongation of pregnancy among 12 women carrying triplets to underwent elective cerclage at 13 to 14 weeks compared to 10 women with triplets who did not undergo cerclage (35.0 versus 30.7 weeks). This prolongation of pregnancy was associated with a concomitant reduction in perinatal morbidity and mortality. However, there was a confounding effect of parity, which would tend to shift the mean gestational age at delivery in favor of the cerclage group. In addition, the gestational age at delivery of the 10 sets of triplets whose mothers did not undergo cerclage was significantly less than that anticipated from other large clinical experiences.

In two other small, retrospective, nonrandomized studies, investigators specifically studied the value of elective cervical suture in triplet pregnancies. Neither study found a difference in mean gestational age at delivery (44,45). These findings were consistent with those of several relatively large clinical experiences, none of which demonstrated any benefit of elective cervical cerclage in triplet pregnancy (46–48). Unpublished data from the Triplet Connection (a nonprofit support group for mothers with high-order multiples) reveals a mean gestational age at delivery of 32.7 weeks among 3,140 triplet gestations without cerclage and 32.8 weeks for 58 triplet pregnancies with cerclage before 16 weeks' gestation. The quality of these data is limited by the biases inherent in postpartum retrospective data collection with questionnaires.

The two prospective, randomized trials involving twins and the preponderance of retrospective studies do not appear to provide sufficient evidence to support elective cervical cerclage for twin or triplet pregnancy. Cervical cerclage should be reserved for patients likely to have cervical incompetence on the basis of reproductive history and clinical findings.

Prophylactic Tocolytic Therapy

Prescription of prophylactic oral β-mimetic agents to women with twin pregnancies to reduce the risk of premature birth has been evaluated in seven prospective, randomized, controlled trials (49–55). Evaluation of these trials is difficult because of their heterogenicity. Although oral β-mimetic agents were used in all the studies, a variety of drugs and various dosages were used, and administration of medication was begun at different gestational ages. Despite this heterogenicity, a metaanalysis of these trials failed to show any consistent beneficial effect on the risk of preterm birth, birth weight, or neonatal mortality (56). There was a reduction in the risk of respiratory distress syndrome in four of the seven trials but not in the metaanalysis. Other tocolytic agents, such as prostaglandin synthetase inhibitors, calcium channel antagonists, intramuscular progesterone, and oral magnesium sulfate, have not been studied for use as prophylactic tocolytic therapy during multifetal pregnancy. It is also worthy of emphasis that the potential risk of prolonged fetal exposure to β-mimetic agents or other tocolytics is not completely known (57).

There is little evidence of efficacy of prophylactic tocolysis in triplet gestations, although the data are obtained solely from retrospective review of clinical experience. Of 198 women with triplet pregnancies treated in the United States from 1985 to 1988, 115 (58.1%) received prophylactic tocolytics, primarily oral terbutaline sulfate (58). There was no difference in either gestational age (33.8 weeks) or birth weight (1,894 g) for the 115 women receiving prophylactic tocolysis compared to the 83 who did not

(33.2 weeks and 1,869 g). Ron-el et al. (47) reported no improvement in gestational length with use of prophylactic β-adrenergic agents. The lack of identifiable efficacy of prophylactic tocolysis for triplet gestation might have been biased if the prophylactic tocolysis was used more often by patients perceived to be at greater risk than as a routine intervention.

Despite the aforementioned recognized limitations of retrospective data, the prophylactic use of oral β-mimetic agents is not associated with improved outcomes or a meaningful prolongation of pregnancy and therefore cannot be recommended for routine use.

Routine Hospitalization

There have been four prospective randomized trials of hospitalized bed rest for women with uncomplicated twin pregnancy (59–62). The Cochrane systematic review of these four trials showed that the risk of preterm birth was not reduced by a policy of elective hospitalization (63). Significantly more women delivered low birth weight infants and infants before 34 weeks' gestation in the hospitalized cohort. There also were no differences in perinatal mortality or neonatal outcome (63). In another relatively large study, Andrews et al. (64), using a prospective sequential study design, evaluated the effects of elective hospitalization on the management of twin pregnancies (64). In this study, a policy of elective hospitalization until 34 weeks' gestation was used between 1983 and 1985 and encompassed 134 twin deliveries. This was followed by a policy, enforced between 1985 and 1987, of outpatient management in the absence of complications. This policy encompassed 177 twin deliveries. There were no differences in prematurity rates or perinatal morbidity between the two groups. The twins of women electively admitted to the hospital had a higher mortality rate and incurred significantly higher costs (64).

It should be noted that in the all the aforementioned studies, the randomized twin pregnancies were uncomplicated, representing a general twin population. Women with twins who may be at increased risk of preterm delivery because of an abnormally short endovaginal cervical length measurement or a cervical score of 0 or less may benefit from an intervention such as hospitalized bed rest. In one trial in which hospitalized bed rest was offered to women with twin gestations and a low cervical score, no differences occurred in rate of preterm birth, perinatal mortality, or fetal growth (65). Unfortunately, the conclusions that can be drawn from this trial are limited by its small sample size.

There has been only one small, prospective, randomized trial of hospitalization of women carrying triplets (66). At 29 weeks of gestation, 10 women carrying triplets were randomized to undertake hospitalized bed rest while 9 remained at home as a control group. Six of the control patients ultimately required hospital admission for obstetrical complications. The hospitalized group had a longer duration of pregnancy, decreased incidence of delivering very low birth weight infants, increased fetal weights, and a decrease in neonatal morbidity (66). However, due to the small sample size, the wide confidence limits around these treatment effects made the observed differences between the groups compatible with chance variation.

Adams et al. (67) reported provocative results of a retrospective, sequential cohort study in which they compared two time periods in which differing management strategies were used. Between 1985 and 1993, 34 triplet pregnancies were managed with elective hospitalization at 24 weeks as the primary management strategy. The outcomes of these pregnancies were compared with those for 32 other triplet pregnancies managed between 1993 and 1996, when bed rest at home was prescribed beginning at 24 weeks' gestation. Routine hospitalization increased the gestational age at delivery 1 week (33.5 versus 32.5 weeks' gestation; $p = .16$), but this difference did not achieve statistical significance. The outpatient management group experienced a significant increase in the frequency of pregnancy-induced hypertension compared to those electively hospitalized (31.3% versus 8.8%; $p = .02$) (67). Evaluating the role of elective hospitalization of women pregnant with triplets will continue to be difficult due to the high rate of hospital admission for higher-order multiple pregnancy. In the review of triplet management by Newman et al. (58), 88 (44.4%) of the women carrying triplets required hospitalization for reasons other than preterm labor.

In twin gestations, routine hospitalization does not appear to reduce the frequency of premature birth, improve mean gestational age at delivery, reduce perinatal mortality, or improve neonatal outcome. For triplet gestations, only one small, prospective, randomized trial (66) showed a trend toward improved outcome with routine hospitalization. However, the authors acknowledged that there were too few patients to draw definitive conclusions. They urged further research to help clarify whether there are any benefits to routine hospitalization of women pregnant with triplets that will outweigh the social and financial costs associated with such a policy. A second retrospective sequential cohort study (67) found an insignificant 1-week improvement in gestational age at delivery and a significantly lower incidence of pregnancy-induced hypertension among the routinely hospitalized triplets. This study was limited by its nonrandomized nature and the changes in management inherent in studies using historical cohorts. As a consequence, it appears that for triplet gestations the data supporting routine hospitalization are at present inconclusive.

Restricted Activity and Maternal Rest

Although there does not appear to be any benefit to routine hospitalization for multifetal gestation, activity restriction and increased maternal rest at home are recommended during most twin and triplet pregnancies. There are probably few clinical practices that are as widely used with so little supportive scientific evidence. There are no prospective, randomized trials that have been conducted to evaluate the benefit of this intervention. In a retrospective study Jeffrey and Bowes (68) considered three historical cohorts of women delivering twins between 1966 and 1971 at the University of Colorado Medical Center. These cohorts included 42 women who were not diagnosed as having twins until they were in labor or until delivery, 31 women diagnosed as having twins during the antepartum period but who were not advised to undertake bed rest, and 41 women diagnosed as having twins during the antepartum period and for whom bed rest was recommended.

There was no significant difference in the length of gestation among any of the three groups. The perinatal mortality rate was significantly lower among the group who rested compared to either the intrapartum diagnosis and no bed rest groups (6.1% versus 21.7% versus 22.9%; $p < .05$). This difference in perinatal mortality disappeared if deliveries at less than 30 weeks' gestation were excluded.

Fetal weight was significantly increased among the rested group. When weight and gestational age were considered, the incidence of small-for-gestational-age infants also was significantly reduced among the rested group (23.4% versus 40.5% versus 37.3%; $p < .05$) (68). These differences in fetal weight and the incidence of small-for-gestational-age infants persisted even when deliveries at less than 30 weeks were excluded. The infants of rested mothers were consistently larger than infants of unrested mothers at every gestational week. The authors concluded that bed rest for multiple gestation promotes intrauterine growth and lowers the incidence of small-for-gestational-age infants.

Activity restriction also may influence the length of gestation. Studies of antepartum uterine contractile activity performed with a 24-hour home tocodynamometer identified a reduction in frequency of uterine contractions associated with maternal rest and an increase in contractility after intercourse (69). Further study is needed to more clearly define the influence of activity restriction and maternal rest on both fetal growth and uterine contractility in multiple gestation and to identify those patients for whom this intervention may be most beneficial.

In a prospective but nonrandomized trial, Vergani et al. (70) developed a specific protocol for management of twin pregnancy. The protocol emphasized frequent prenatal visits along with work leave from 28 weeks' gestation onward and home bed rest for at least 2 hours a day. Patients enrolled into the protocol had a lower incidence of delivery before 34 weeks' gestation and of very low birth weight delivery compared to a cohort of women with multiples who did not participate in the management protocol. In another retrospective review, Tafforeau et al. (71) reported the results of a preterm birth prevention program for twins that emphasized early diagnosis, education to prevent preterm birth, reduced activity, and work leave. Twins enrolled in the intervention had a lower frequency of very low birth weight delivery, NICU admission, and perinatal mortality.

Syrop and Varner (72) performed a retrospective analysis of obstetrical outcome among triplets whose mothers were prescribed unrestricted activity compared with those whose mothers were prescribed restricted activity. Division of mothers into a restricted activity category was based on chart documentation of patient instruction that included restrictions such as modified home bed rest two or three times a day, bed rest with use of the bathroom, strict bed rest, or unspecified bed rest. Absence of documented maternal activity restriction resulted in a classification of unrestricted activity. The authors reported that mothers with restricted activity levels had an average first prenatal visit at 20.4 weeks with triplets detected at an average gestation of 29.8 weeks. The mean gestational age at delivery was 34.3 weeks. Three of the 39 infants died, 1 of which was small for gestational age. Mothers with unrestricted activity levels had their first prenatal visit at 24.6 weeks, and their triplets were detected at an average gestation of 31.2 weeks. The mean gestational age at delivery for this group was 31.3 weeks. Ten of the 18 infants died, and 67% of these were small for gestational age (72). The improvements in outcome for mothers with restricted activity may have been due to the marked differences in the early registration for prenatal care and the earlier diagnosis of triplet gestation. In a series of triplets described by Ron-El et al. (47), there were no differences in fetal outcome with or without maternal bed rest.

Although restriction of activity and maternal rest are widely used, there is little evidence to demonstrate a beneficial effect of these practices in twin or triplet gestations. Further research is needed to define the effect of restriction of activity and maternal rest on duration of pregnancy, fetal growth, and risk of pregnancy-induced hypertension. Research should explore the role of restriction of activity and maternal rest when women carrying multiples are found to be at increased risk of preterm delivery. Questions about when restriction of activity and rest should be initiated and for how long they should be continued have not been answered. The majority of perinatal morbidity and mortality for multiple gestations occurs before 30 weeks' gestation; therefore, any intervention to reduce maternal activity and increase rest would have to be instituted in the midgestational period if benefit is to be anticipated. Despite the limited data available to support it, use of this intervention suggests that it is considered to be reasonable and probably beneficial by most obstetricians caring for women with twin gestations and by almost all those caring for women with triplet and higher-order gestations.

Home Uterine Activity Monitoring

Few issues are as controversial as home uterine activity monitoring (HUAM). Some obstetricians have advocated HUAM for multiple gestations because of the increased risk of premature labor and because observational data indicate a higher frequency of contractions in multiple than in singleton pregnancies (73–75). Other observational data suggest that women with multiple gestations may be less accurate than women with singleton pregnancies in self-detection of prelabor uterine activity (76). HUAM has been advocated in an attempt to increase maternal awareness of the frequency of uterine contractions and potentially allow earlier diagnosis of preterm labor among these women.

Prospective, randomized trials evaluating the efficacy of HUAM in multiple pregnancies have provided conflicting results (Table 7-4). Knuppel et al. (77) performed a prospective, randomized intervention whereby 45 women with twin gestations were assigned to either daily HUAM and perinatal nursing support or to a program of patient education of preterm labor symptomatology and self-palpation of uterine activity. Equal numbers of patients in both groups (62% and 74%) had preterm labor. Among the patients practicing HUAM, all 14 who had preterm labor were dilated 3 cm or less at the time of presentation compared to 10 of 16 in the education group. The mean cervical dilatation was significantly lower among the HUAM group (1.6 cm) than that among the education group (2.9 cm; $p = .01$) at the time that preterm labor was diagnosed.

Table 7-4. Outcomes of prospective, randomized clinical trials of home uterine activity monitoring (HUAM) in twin gestations

Procedure	n	Preterm Labor (%)	Cervical Diameter at Diagnosis (cm)	Dilation ≤2 cm (%)	Tocolytic Candidate	Mean No. of Days Gravid	Preterm Birth	Neonatal Outcomes
Knuppel et al., 1990 (77)		(<37 wk)					(<37 wk)	
Education	26	62	2.9	38	62	—	50%	Not described
PNS + HUAM	19	74	1.6[a]	79[a]	100[a]	—	81%	
Dyson et al., 1991 (78)		(<36 wk)					(<36 wk)	
Standard care	80	45	—	—	27	6	46	
Education and palpation	57	42	—	—	67[a]	27[b]	30[a]	Improved
Education and palpation with HUAM	52	48	—	—	96[a]	35[b]	23[a]	
Dyson et al., 1998 (79)		(<35 wk)					(<35 wk)	
Weekly PNS	280	35	1.8	75	—	22	22%	
Daily PNS	277	34	1.7	76	—	23	24%	Unchanged
Daily PNS + HUAM	287	40	1.4	80	—	29	24%	

[a] $p < .05$.
[b] $p < .01$.
PNS, perinatal nursing services.

Of the 14 patients using HUAM who had preterm labor, only 1 (7%) delivered her infants prematurely because of failed tocolysis. Seven of 16 in the education group delivered their infants prematurely after failed tocolysis (44%; $p = .03$). Overall, more patients in the education group delivered prior to 37 weeks' gestation than in the HUAM group (81% versus 50%) (77).

In 1991, Dyson et al. (78) published a prospective, randomized trial in which 394 women with high-risk pregnancies were allocated to undergo one of three interventions. The first group was a standard care population instructed in the signs and symptoms of preterm labor. This cohort was taught the technique of self-palpation of uterine activity and underwent weekly cervical examinations. The second group was called the education and palpation group. Patients in this group performed daily HUAM and transmitted the data in such a way that the uterine activity data could not be analyzed. The members of the education and palpation group were contacted at least 5 days a week by a study nurse to elicit any symptoms of preterm labor and record the number of contractions detected by means of the patient's self-palpation. All patients were instructed to report to the hospital for evaluation if they had more than five contractions per hour that persisted for more than 1 hour despite bed rest and oral hydration. The third group received the same education and palpation instruction as the second group but also underwent daily HUAM, the data from which were interpreted by a study nurse. Asymptomatic patients who had more than five contractions per hour with routine monitoring were asked to lie down, drink fluids, and be monitored for a second hour. If they persisted with more than five contractions, they were referred to the hospital for evaluation. In the entire study group, 189 women had twin gestations and participated in a separate analysis.

Among the twin gestations, the incidence of preterm labor was similar for all three groups. The incidence of preterm birth at less than 36 weeks' gestation was significantly lower among the education and palpation group (29.8%; $p < .05$) and markedly lower among the HUAM group (23.1%; $p < .01$) than among the standard care group (46.3%) (78). There were no significant differences in the frequency of preterm birth between the HUAM and the education and palpation groups. A significant reduction also occurred in the incidence of delivery as a result of failed tocolysis at less than 34 weeks' gestation in both the education and palpation and the HUAM groups. When neonatal outcomes were considered, the education and palpation group tended to have better outcomes than the standard care group, while the infants in the HUAM group had significant improvements in all measures compared with the standard care group. The HUAM twins also were less likely to weigh less than 1,500 g, to be admitted to the NICU, and had shorter hospital stays than were infants in the education and palpation group. It is important to note that the addition of HUAM to the education and palpation program was not found to significantly improve outcomes for singleton gestations.

Following their initial publication, Dyson et al. embarked on a second prospective, randomized, multicenter trial of HUAM that involved 2,422 pregnant women in the Kaiser health system (79). Included were 844 women pregnant with twins, all of whom participated in the standard education program for prevention of preterm birth. This education program was then combined by means of random assignment with three subsequent levels of surveillance: 1) weekly contact with a perinatal nurse; 2) daily contact with a perinatal nurse; or 3) daily contact with a perinatal nurse and HUAM. The primary end point was the incidence of preterm birth at less than 35 weeks' gestation.

Among the women with twin pregnancies, there were no differences in the frequency of preterm birth at less than 35 weeks between women receiving weekly nursing contact (22%), daily nursing contact (24%), or HUAM (24%). There also were no differences in mean cervical dilatation at the diagnosis of preterm labor between the weekly contact (1.8 ± 1.7 cm), daily contact (1.7 ± 1.3 cm), or HUAM (1.4 ± 1.2 cm) groups. Ninety percent or more of the patients in all three groups had 3 cm or less dilatation when preterm labor was diagnosed, whereas 75% of the weekly contact, 76% of the daily contact, and 80% of the HUAM patients had 2 cm or less dilatation at the diagnosis of preterm labor. None of the three groups had any significant differences in frequency of low birth weight or very low birth weight, mean number of days gained with tocolysis, or number of unscheduled office visits. A higher percentage (16%) of patients in the HUAM group received prophylactic tocolytic therapy than did in the weekly contact group (8%). In contradistinction to their previous findings (78), Dyson et al. (79) found that neither daily contact with a perinatal nurse or HUAM provided additional benefits in twin gestations compared with more intensive patient education, daily uterine self-palpation, and weekly contact with a perinatal nurse.

HUAM for twin gestations is associated with better outcomes than is standard care; however, less obvious benefit can be ascribed when the comparison group is intensively educated and provided with frequent if not daily perinatal nursing contact. In situations in which frequent or daily contact with the provider's office is not practical, HUAM may be a reasonable alternative. Although twins are at high risk of preterm delivery, further ability to stratify risk within the population with multiple gestations may increase the efficacy and cost-effectiveness of HUAM. At present, the benefits of HUAM in the care of women pregnant with twins is controversial, and its use should be highly selective.

SUMMARY

In order to have a significant beneficial impact on the outcome of multiple pregnancy, we must continue to identify markers of increased risk of preterm delivery and design intervention trials that improve pregnancy outcome. Reduction in the frequency of delivery at less than 37 weeks' gestation and of low birth weight may not be achievable given the inherent limitations of the human uterus to maintain multiple fetuses beyond certain limits. However, rates of early preterm delivery (before 32 weeks' gestation) and delivery of very low birth weight infants (less than 1,500 g) do appear to be outcomes that can be reduced. Continuing studies should focus on identifying which women are at risk of these outcomes and enrolling them in better designed or novel clinical interventions to improve perinatal outcome.

REFERENCES

1. Botting BJ, MacDonald-Davies I, MacFarland AJ. Recent trends in the incidence of multiple births and associated mortality. *Arch Dis Child* 1987;62:941–948.
2. Powers WF, Kiely JL. The risk confronting twins: a national perspective. *Am J Obstet Gynecol* 1994;170:456–461.
3. Lumley J. The epidemiology of preterm birth. *Baillieres Clin Obstet Gynecol* 1993;7:477–498.
4. Donoghue D, Lancaster P, Henderson-Smart D, et al. Australian and New Zealand Neonatal Network 1995. Sydney: National Perinatal Statistics Unit, Australian Institute of Health and Welfare, 1997.
5. Gardner MO, Goldenberg RL, Cliver SP, et al. The origin and outcome of preterm twin pregnancies. *Obstet Gynecol* 1995;85:553–557.
6. Creasy RK, Gummer BA, Liggins GC. System for predicting spontaneous preterm birth. *Obstet Gynecol* 1980;55:692–695.
7. Keirse MJNC. An evaluation of formal risk scoring for preterm birth. *Am J Perinatol* 1989;6:226–233.
8. Goldenberg RL, Iams JD, Miodovnik M, et al. The preterm prediction study: risk factors in twin gestations. *Am J Obstet Gynecol* 1996;175:1047–1053.
9. Menard MK, Newman RB, Keenan A, et al. Prognostic significance of prior preterm twin delivery on subsequent singleton pregnancy. *Am J Obstet Gynecol* 1996;174:1429–1432.
10. Anderson HF, Nugent CE, Wanty SD, et al. Prediction of risk for preterm delivery by ultrasonographic measurement of cervical length. *Am J Obstet Gynecol* 1990;163:859–867.
11. Iams JD, Goldenberg RL, Meis PJ, et al. The length of the cervix and the risk of spontaneous premature delivery. *N Engl J Med* 1996;334:567–572.
12. Kushnir O, Izquierdo LA, Smith JF, et al. Transvaginal sonographic measurement of cervical length: evaluation of twin pregnancies. *J Reprod Med* 1995;40:380–382.
13. Souka AP, Heath V, Flint S, et al. Cervical length at 23 weeks in twins in predicting spontaneous preterm delivery. *Obstet Gynecol* 1999;94:450–454.
14. Imseis HM, Albert TA, Iams JD. Identifying twin gestations at low risk for preterm birth with a transvaginal ultrasonographic cervical measurement at 24–26 weeks gestation. *Am J Obstet Gynecol* 1997;177:1149–1155.
15. Bouyer J, Papiernik E, Dreyfus J, et al. Maturation signs of the cervix and prediction of preterm birth. *Obstet Gynecol* 1986;78:209–214.
16. O'Connor MC, Arias E, Royston JP, et al. The merits of special antenatal care for twin pregnancies. *Br J Obstet Gynaecol* 1981;88:222–228.
17. Houlton MCC, Marivate M, Philpott RH. Factors associated with preterm labour and changes in the cervix before labour in twin pregnancy. *Br J Obstet Gynaecol* 1982;89:190–194.
18. Neilson JP, Verkuyl DAA, Crowther CA, et al. Preterm labor in twin pregnancies: prediction by cervical assessment. *Obstet Gynecol* 1988;72:719–723.
19. Newman RB, Godsey RK, Ellings JM, et al. Quantification of cervical change: Relationship to preterm delivery in the multifetal gestation. *Am J Obstet Gynecol* 1991;165:264–269.

20. Bivins HA, Newman RB, Ellings JM, et al. Risk of antepartum cervical examination in multifetal gestations. *Am J Obstet Gynecol* 1993;169:22–25.
21. Ellings JM, Newman RB, Hulsey TC, et al. Reduction in very low birth weight deliveries and perinatal mortality in a specialized, multi-disciplinary twin clinic. *Obstet Gynecol* 1993;81:387–391.
22. Papiernik E, Mussy MA, Vial M, et al. A low rate of perinatal deaths for twin births. *Acta Genet Med Gemellol (Roma)* 1985; 34:201–206.
23. Lockwood CJ, Senyei AE, Dische MR, et al. Fetal fibronectin in cervical and vaginal secretions as a predictor of preterm delivery. *N Engl J Med* 1991;325:669–674.
24. Goldenberg RL, Mercer BM, Meis PJ et al. The preterm prediction study: fetal fibronectin testing and spontaneous preterm birth. *Obstet Gynecol* 1996;87:643–648.
25. Wennerholm UB, Holm B, Mattsby-Baltzer I, et al. Fetal fibronectin, endotoxin, bacterial vaginosis, and cervical length as predictors of preterm birth and neonatal morbidity in twin pregnancies. *Br J Obstet Gynaecol* 1997;104:1398–1404.
26. Oliveira T, de Souza E, Mariani-Neto C, Camano L. Fetal fibronectin as a predictor of preterm delivery in twin gestations. *Int J Gynaecol Obstet* 1998;62:135–139.
27. Tolino A, Ronsini S, Zullo F, et al. Fetal fibronectin as a screening test for premature delivery in multiple pregnancies. *Int J Gynaecol Obstet* 1996;52:3–7.
28. McGregor JA, French JI, Parker R, et al. Prevention of premature birth by screening and treatment for common genital tract infections: results of a prospective controlled evaluation. *Am J Obstet Gynecol* 1995;173:157–167.
29. Meis PJ, Goldenberg RL, Mercer B, et al. The preterm prediction study: significance of vaginal infections. *Am J Obstet Gynecol* 1995;173:1231–1235.
30. Goldenberg RL, Thom E, Moawad AH, et al. The preterm prediction study: fetal fibronectin, bacterial vaginosis, and peripartum infection. *Obstet Gynecol* 1996;87:656–660.
31. Chaim W, Mazor M, Leiberman JR. The relationship between bacterial vaginosis and preterm birth: a review. *Arch Gynecol Obstet* 1997;259:51–58.
32. Carey JC, Klebanoff MA, Hauth JC, et al. Metronidazole to prevent preterm delivery in pregnant women with asymptomatic bacterial vaginosis. *N Engl J Med* 2000;342:534–540.
33. Mitchell MD, Trautman MS, Dudley DJ. Immuno-endocrinology of preterm labour and delivery. *Baillieres Clin Obstet Gynecol* 1993;7:553–575.
34. Ewigman BG, Crane JP, Frigoletto FD, et al. Effect of prenatal ultrasound screening on perinatal outcome. *N Engl J Med* 1993; 329:821–837.
35. LeFevre ML, Bain RP, Ewigman BG, et al. A randomized trial of prenatal ultrasonographic screening: Impact on maternal management and outcome. *Am J Obstet Gynecol* 1993;169:483–489.
36. Neilson JP. Routine ultrasound in early pregnancy. In: Neilson JP, Crowther CA, Hodnett ED, et al., eds. Pregnancy and childbirth module, Cochrane Database of Systematic Reviews. Issue 3. Oxford, UK: Cochrane Collaboration, 1997 [updated June 3, 1997].

37. Persson PH, Grennert RL, Gennser G, et al. Improved outcome of twin pregnancies. *Acta Obstet Gynecol Scand* 1979;58:3–7.
38. Dor J, Shalev J, Mashiach J, et al. Elective cervical suture of twin pregnancies diagnosed ultrasonically in the first trimester following ovulation induction. *Gynecol Obstet Invest* 1982;13:55–59.
39. Medical Research Council/Royal College of Obstetrician and Gynaecologists Working Party on Cervical Cerclage. Interim report of the Medical Research Council/Royal College of Obstetrician and Gynaecologists Multicenter Trial of Cervical Cerclage. *Br J Obstet Gynaecol* 1988;95:437–445.
40. Weekes ARL, Mengies DN, DeBoer CH. The relative efficacy of bed rest, cervical suture, and no treatment in the management of twin pregnancy. *Br J Obstet Gynaecol* 1977;84:161–164.
41. Plank K, Mikulaj V, Stencl J, et al. Prevention and treatment of prematurity in twin gestation. *J Perinat Med* 1993;21:309–313.
42. Sinha DP, Nandakumar VC, Brough AK, et al. Relative cervical incompetence in twin pregnancy: assessment and efficacy of cervical suture. *Acta Genet Med Gemellol (Roma)* 1979;28:327–331.
43. Goldman GA, Dicker D, Peleg D, et al. Is elective cerclage justified in the management of triplet and quadruplet pregnancy? *Aust N Z J Obstet Gynecol* 1989;29:9–12.
44. Mordel N, Zajicek G, Benshushan A, et al. Elective suture of the uterine cervix in triplets. *Am J Perinatol* 1993;10:14–16.
45. Zakut H, Insher V, Serr DM. Elective cervical suture in preventing premature delivery in multiple pregnancies. *Isr J Med Sci* 1977;13:488–492.
46. Itzkowic DV. A survey of 59 triplet pregnancies. *Br J Obstet Gynaecol* 1979;86:23–28.
47. Ron-El R, Caspi E, Schreyer P, et al. Triplet and quadruplet pregnancies and management. *Obstet Gynecol* 1981;57:458–463.
48. Lipitz S, Reichman BN, Paret G, et al. The improving outcome of triplet pregnancies. *Am J Obstet Gynecol* 1989;161:1279–1284.
49. O'Connor MC, Murphy H, Dalrymple IJ. Double blind trial of ritodrine and placebo in twin pregnancy. *Br J Obstet Gynaecol* 1979; 86:706–709.
50. Marivate M, DeVilliera KQ, Fairbrother P. The effect of prophylactic outpatient administration of fenoterol on the time of onset of spontaneous labor and fetal growth rate in twin pregnancy. *Am J Obstet Gynecol* 1977;128:707–708.
51. Skjaerris J, Aberg A. Prevention of prematurity in twin pregnancy by orally administered terbutaline. *Acta Obstet Gynecol Scand* 1982;108[suppl]:39–40.
52. O'Leary JA. Prophylactic tocolysis of twins. *Am J Obstet Gynecol* 1986;154:904–905.
53. Mathews DD, Friend JB, Michael CA. A double-blind trial of oral isoxuprine in the prevention of premature labour. *J Obstet Gynaecol Br Commonw* 1967;74:68–70.
54. Cetrulo CL, Freeman RK. Ritodrine HCl for the prevention of premature labor in twin pregnancies. *Acta Genet Med Gemellol (Roma)* 1976;25:321–324.
55. Ashworth MF, Spooner SF, Verkuyl DAA, et al. Failure to prevent preterm labor and delivery in twin pregnancy using prophylactic oral salbutamol. *Br J Obstet Gynaecol* 1990;97:878–882.
56. Keirse MJNC. Prophylactic oral betamimetics in twin pregnancies. In: Keirse MJNC, Renfrew MJ, Neilson JP, et al., eds. Pregnancy

and childbirth module. Cochrane pregnancy and childbirth database [revised March 24, 1993]. Cochrane Collaboration, issue 2. Oxford, UK: 1995. Update software available from BMJ Publishing Group, London.

57. Fletcher SE, Fyfe DA, Case CL, et al. Myocardial necrosis in the newborn following long-term low dose subcutaneous terbutaline infusion for suppression of preterm labor. *Am J Obstet Gynecol* 1991;165:1401–1404.

58. Newman RB, Hamer C, Miller MC. Outpatient triplet management: a contemporary review. *Am J Obstet Gynecol* 1989;161: 547–555.

59. Crowther CA, Verkuyl DAA, Neilson JP, et al. The effects of hospitalization for rest on fetal growth, neonatal morbidity and length of gestation in twin pregnancy. *Br J Obstet Gynaecol* 1990;97: 872–877.

60. MacLennan AH, Green RC, O'Shea R, et al. Routine hospital admission in twin pregnancy between 26 and 30 weeks gestation. *Lancet* 1990;335:267–269.

61. Saunders MC, Dick JS, Brown IM, et al. The effects of hospital admission for bed rest on duration of twin pregnancy: a randomized trial. *Lancet* 1985;2:793–795.

62. Hartikainen-Sorri AL, Jouppila P. Is routine hospitalization needed in antenatal care of twin pregnancy? *J Perinat Med* 1984; 12:31–34.

63. Crowther CA. Hospitalization for bed rest in multiple pregnancy. In: Neilson JP, Crowther CA, Hodnett ED, et al., eds. Pregnancy and childbirth module, Cochrane Database of Systematic Reviews. Issue 3. Oxford, UK: Cochrane Collaboration, 1997 [updated June 3, 1997].

64. Andrews WW, Leveno KJ, Sherman ML, et al. Elective hospitalization in the management of twin pregnancies. *Obstet Gynecol* 1991;77:826–831.

65. Crowther CA, Neilson JP, Verkuyl DAA, et al. Preterm labour in twin pregnancies: can it be prevented by hospital admission? *Br J Obstet Gynaecol* 1989;96:850–854.

66. Crowther CA, Verkuyl DAA, Ashworth MF, et al. The effects of hospitalization for bed rest on duration of gestation, fetal growth and neonatal morbidity in triplet pregnancy. *Acta Genet Med Gemellol (Roma)* 1991;40:63–68.

67. Adams DM, Scholl JS, Haney EL, et al. Perinatal outcome associated with outpatient management of triplet pregnancy. *Am J Obstet Gynecol* 1998;178:843–847.

68. Jeffrey RL, Bowes WA, Delaney JJ. Role of bed rest in twin gestation. *Obstet Gynecol* 1974;6:822–826.

69. Moore TR, Iams JD, Creasy RK, et al. Diurnal and gestational patterns of uterine activity in normal human pregnancy. *Obstet Gynecol* 1994;83:517–523.

70. Vergani P, Ghidini A, Bozzo G, et al. Prenatal management of twin gestations: experience with a new protocol. *J Reprod Med* 1991;36:667–671.

71. Tafforeau J, Papiernik E, Richard A, et al. Is prevention of preterm birth in twin pregnancies possible? Analysis of the results of a prevention program in France (1988–91). *Eur J Obstet Gynecol Reprod Biol* 1995;59:169–174.

72. Syrop CH, Varner MW. Triplet gestation: maternal and neonatal implications. *Acta Genet Med Gemellol (Roma)* 1985;34:81–88.
73. Newman RB, Gill PJ, Katz M. Uterine activity during pregnancy in ambulatory patients: comparison of singleton and twin gestations. *Am J Obstet Gynecol* 1986;154:530–531.
74. Garite TJ, Bentley DL, Hamer CA, et al. Uterine activity characteristics in multiple gestations. *Obstet Gynecol* 1990;76:56S–59S.
75. Newman RB, Gill PJ, Campion S, et al. The influence of fetal number on antepartum uterine activity. *Obstet Gynecol* 1989;73: 695–699.
76. Newman RB, Gill PJ, Wittreich P, et al. Maternal perception of prelabor uterine activity. *Obstet Gynecol* 1986;68:765–769.
77. Knuppel RA, Blake MF, Watson DL, et al. Preventing preterm birth in twin gestation: home uterine activity monitoring and perinatal nursing support. *Obstet Gynecol* 1990;76:24S–27S.
78. Dyson DC, Crites YM, Ray DA, et al. Prevention of preterm birth in high risk patients: the role of education and provider contact versus home uterine monitoring. *Am J Obstet Gynecol* 1991;164: 756–762.
79. Dyson DC, Danbe KH, Bamer JA, et al. Monitoring women at risk for preterm labor. *N Engl J Med* 1998;338:15–19.

8

Obstetrical Complications Unique to Multiple Gestations

Multifetal gestations are the quintessential obstetrical challenge in that virtually every conceivable fetal or maternal complication occurs with increased frequency. One who has anticipated and managed all of the risks presented by a multiple pregnancy likely will have mastered all of obstetrics. In addition to an increased frequency of most obstetric complications, multiple gestations also present a variety of obstetric complications that are unique to those pregnancies. This chapter addresses a number of complications that are encountered only in multiple gestation.

VANISHING TWIN PHENOMENON

With the advent of ultrasonography and its extension to the first trimester, multiple gestations are being diagnosed earlier and more frequently. As a consequence of first-trimester diagnosis, a large number of multiple pregnancies are identified that do not result in successful delivery of two or more live infants. The precise frequency with which the vanishing twin phenomenon occurs is difficult to ascertain. Depending on how early the multiple pregnancy is identified, reported frequencies vary from as low as 13% to as high as 50% to 70% for twins identified in the first trimester (1,2). The Norfolk *in vitro* fertilization experience helps estimate the occurrence of this event, although the data are limited by the fact that all the pregnancies were the result of assisted reproductive technology. In the Norfolk experience, spontaneous loss of all fetuses with previously documented fetal cardiac activity occurred in 17 of 165 twin (10.3%), 2 of 26 triplet (7.7%), and 1 of 5 quadruplet (20%) pregnancies. In addition, 33 twin gestations spontaneously reduced to a singleton and 9 triplet gestations spontaneously reduced to twins. The overall early pregnancy loss rate, considering both spontaneous abortion and the vanishing twin phenomenon, becomes 50 of 165 twins (30.3%), 11 of 26 triplets (30.3%), and 1 of 5 quadruplets (20%) (3).

When a twin does vanish, it is usually silently absorbed or in some cases causes uterine bleeding. It has been estimated that 5% of all patients with first-trimester bleeding may be experiencing vanishing twin phenomenon (4). Although first-trimester bleeding is always concerning, maternal reassurance should be given because the prognosis for the surviving fetus or fetuses is excellent when the demise occurs in the first trimester (1,5,6).

It is essential that the diagnosis of vanishing twin phenomenon be preceded by identification of specific embryonic parts and not simply by visualization of an anembryonic cavity. Numerous other sonographic findings can mimic a second anembryonic cavity, including subchorionic blood clots, chorioamnionic separation, decidual pseudosac in the contralateral horn of a bicornuate or didelphic uterus, or even excessive transducer pressure on a thin woman. The diagnosis "vanishing twin" is uttered too frequently in ultrasound suites without full consideration of the psychological effect that this diagnosis may have. From the mother's and father's perspective, the diagnosis of vanishing twin phenomenon will always be remembered as the loss of a child; the life of a surviving "twin" will always be shaded by the loss of a "sibling."

FETAL ANOMALIES

Of the congenital malformations that can occur in multiple gestations, only conjoined and acardiac twins can be considered unique to multiple pregnancies. Overall however, fetal structural defects occur more frequently in multiple gestations than they do in singletons. Kohl and Casey (7) reported that twins had a 2.1% rate of major malformation and a 4.1% rate of minor malformations. Baldwin (8) reviewed 112,384 twin pregnancies from 14 series and highlighted the following four features of congenital malformations among multiples. First, the prevalence of congenital malformation is 1.2 to 2.0 times higher among fetuses from twin pregnancies than among singletons. Second, the higher prevalence occurs primarily among like-sex twin sets or among monozygotic and monochorionic twins when those analyses have been adequately provided. Third, in 80% to 90% of twin sets, the fetuses are discordant for any structural defect. This discordance persists regardless of zygosity, although the concordance rate is slightly higher among monozygotic twins. Fourth, the most common defects are cardiac malformations, neural tube defects, facial clefting, gastrointestinal anomalies, and anterior abdominal wall defects, including cloacal and bladder exstrophy.

Congenital anomalies in multiple gestations are frequently categorized as occurring by one of three mechanisms. The first are midline structural defects believed to be a consequence of the underlying stimulus to zygote splitting. Examples include conjoined twins, sirenomelia, holoprosencephaly, neural tube defects, and cloacal exstrophy. Symmetry and laterality defects also can occur as a consequence of the twinning process. The second category are defects that are a consequence of abnormal placentation with resulting vascular interchange. The classic example is acardiac twin, or twin reversed arterial perfusion (TRAP) sequence as it is now known. Vascular interchange also is involved in the genesis of malformations associated with the demise of a monochorionic twin. Demise of a twin is believed to cause hypotension, vascular thrombosis, or ischemia in the surviving twin. Congenital abnormalities caused by ischemic injury include microcephaly, hydrocephalus, intestinal atresia, renal dysplasia, aplasia cutis, and limb amputation. The third category of defects are those resulting from intrauterine crowding associated with the presence of multiple fetuses. These include foot deformities, dislocation of the hip, and asymmetry of the skull.

Obstetric intervention cannot be provided for fetal anomalies unless the anomalies are detected. In 245 consecutive twin gestations (490 liveborn infants), Edwards et al. (9) identified 21 of 24 anomalous fetuses for a sensitivity of 88%. The overall incidence of congenital anomalies in the cohort was 4.4%, and the mean gestational age at diagnosis was 22.3 ± 5.4 weeks. There were no false-positive diagnoses, and the specificity and positive predictive value both were 100% (Table 8-1).

Table 8-1. Single-center experience: Predictive value of antepartum ultrasound examination for anomalies in 245 consecutive twin gestations (1988–1994)

Number	490 liveborn twins
Infants with anomalies	24 (4.9)
Isolated anomaly	14 (58)
Multiple anomalies	10 (42)
Concordancy	1 (4.2)
Zygosity	
Monochorionic	10 (42)
Same-sex infants	19 (79)
Gestational age (wk)	
First ultrasound examination	17.1 ± 5.8
Diagnosis	22.3 ± 5.4
Validity	
Sensitivity	21/24 (88)
Specificity	466/466 (100)
Positive predictive value	21/21 (100)
Negative predictive value	466/469 (99)

Note: Values in parentheses are percentages.
Adapted from Edwards MS, Ellings JM, Newman RB, et al. Predictive value of antepartum ultrasound examination for anomalies in twin gestation. *Ultrasound Obstet Gynecol* 1995;6:43–49, with permission.

Prenatal diagnosis of congenital malformation in a multiple pregnancy allows for interventions that may include increased antepartum fetal surveillance; a change in the timing, location, or mode of delivery; consultation with various neonatal and pediatric subspecialists; and in some cases, interventions such as fetal therapy, selective feticide of the abnormal twin, or termination of the pregnancy. Selective feticide versus expectant management becomes an issue in multiple pregnancies discordant for a serious fetal structural abnormality.

Acardiac Twins

Acardiac twins or TRAP sequence is an extremely rare anomaly. It occurs in 1 in 100 monozygotic twin pregnancies and 1 in 35,000 pregnancies overall (10). Acardia likely results from umbilical artery-to-artery anastomoses between monochorionic twin fetuses. The acardiac twin, which is typically only partially developed, relies on the normal, or pump, twin to provide circulation through reversal of arterial flow in the umbilical anastomosis (11). Moore et al. (12) reviewed 40 cases of acardiac twins and found that perinatal outcome correlated best with the ratio between the weight of the acardiac twin and that of the pump twin. When the weight of the acardiac twin was 70% or more of that of the normal pump twin, the pregnancy was at high risk. If the twin weight ratio was more than 70%, almost all were delivered prematurely, hydramnios complicated 40% of births, and 30% of the pump twins developed hydrops fetalis. When the birth weight ratio was less than 70%, the preterm delivery rate was still a high 75%, hydramnios occurred in 30% of births, but hydrops fetalis occurred in only 10%

(12). Management options include invasive procedures designed to interrupt the cardiovascular anastomosis and conservative management allied with close fetal observation.

Selective delivery of the acardiac twin by means of hysterotomy has been reported, but high maternal morbidity and risk of subsequent premature rupture of the membranes and preterm delivery make less invasive options preferable (13,14). Fetoscopic cord occlusion has been achieved by means of both ligation (15) and application of an yttrium-aluminum-garnet (YAG) laser (16). Unfortunately, these techniques have proved to be effective only on small umbilical cords (fetuses at less than 21 weeks' gestation).

Ultrasound-guided techniques have been used successfully to occlude the vascular communication between two fetuses. The advantages of these techniques over umbilical cord ligation are the use of much smaller needles, less operative time, and the lack of need for general anesthesia. Successful techniques have included injection of 1 mL absolute ethanol into the intraabdominal portion of a single umbilical artery (17) and injection of helical thrombogenic metal coils into the umbilical artery of the acardiac twin (18). Even with ultrasound-guided needle procedures, there continues to be a risk of premature rupture of the membranes and failure of the ultrasound-guided method.

At present, it seems that close observation is the management of choice when the twin weight ratios are substantially less than 70%. Invasive techniques should be considered when there is ultrasound evidence of polyhydramnios or congestive failure of the pump twin at a previable gestational age (19). If they are to be used aggressively, invasive ultrasound-guided procedures should be considered only for the high-risk group (acardiac twin weight 70% or more of pump twin weight). As experience and technology improve, intrauterine YAG laser therapy may become the optimal mode of management of this disorder if the diagnosis is made early enough in gestation.

Conjoined Twins

Conjoined twins are another exceedingly rare but unique complication associated with monozygotic twinning. It has a reported incidence of between 1 in 50,000 and 1 in 100,000 deliveries (20–22). Although rare, conjoined twins are reliably detected with ultrasonography as a result of failure to identify separation between the fetuses in a monoamnionic-monochorionic twin gestation. Other signs include unusual extension or proximity of the spines, more than three vessels in the umbilical cord, single cardiac motion, and polyhydramnios, particularly in thoracopagus twins. Complete examination of the twins also is indicated because of a high frequency of associated anomalies not associated with the fusion. Common associated malformations include neural tube defects, orofacial cleft, imperforate anus, and diaphragmatic hernia. Echocardiography is important because delineation of any congenital heart disease is important in evaluating the survival prognosis. The main types of conjoined twins are thoracoomphalopagus (25%), thoracopagus (18%), pygopagus (20%), omphalopagus (10%), incomplete duplication (duplicata incompleta; 10%), craniopagus (6%), and ischiopagus (5%).

The combination of ultrasonography and magnetic resonance imaging can be useful to define the extent of organ involvement and the possibility of extrauterine separation and survival. Forty percent of conjoined twins are stillborn and another 35% die within the first 48 hours (21). The prognosis for the survivors depends on the degree of shared organs, the vital nature of the organs, and amenability to surgical separation. Among thoracopagus twins, the degree of fusion of the heart determines the outcome. Congenital heart disease is found among 75% of thoracopagus twins, and a common ventricle is incompatible with survival of either fetus.

Omphalopagus twins have a reasonable chance of survival with surgical separation unless severe associated anomalies are found. An omphalocele is present in one-third of these twins, and congenital heart defects are present in about one-fourth. The liver is shared in approximately 80% of sets. The best situation is when only a skin or muscle bridge connects the fetuses and there are no shared organs. Omphalopagus twins usually have the best chance for separation and survival.

Craniopagus twins have an unpredictable outcome because it is difficult to assess the degree of intracranial fusion and the extent of venous connection before delivery (23). Bucholz et al. (23) described a cerebral connection in 43% of the cases they reviewed. They determined that the site of connection was an important prognostic factor. Temporoparietal and occipital connections had a worse prognosis than did frontal and parietal connections. The perioperative mortality was high (36%), but only 1 of 9 survivors had a severe neurologic deficit.

Pygopagus twins have a fairly good outcome because sharing of vital organs does not occur. These twins usually are joined at the buttocks and lower spine, often sharing a common rectum, anus, and external genitalia. Ischiopagus twins present more complex problems because they are technically more difficult to separate and often share abdominal and pelvic viscera. These twins often have a common pelvic ring and may have four legs (ischiopagus tetrapus) or three legs (ischiopagus tripus). Their lower gastrointestinal tracts join at the terminal ileum and empty into a single colon. They also usually share a bladder and urethra and frequently have rectovaginal anomalies. Incompletely duplicated twins have no survival potential.

Delivery of conjoined twins in a tertiary care center is recommended because the postdelivery evaluation and care of these infants is multidisciplinary and complex. Unless an emergency exists, attempts at separation should be delayed to allow the twins to become larger, other abnormalities to be detected, and the operation to be carefully planned.

If there is a possibility of extrauterine survival, conjoined twins should be delivered by means of elective cesarean section (24). Even if the conjoined twins are not expected to survive, cesarean section usually is needed to avoid maternal trauma. A low vertical uterine incision usually is needed for delivery. Before viability, induced delivery of conjoined twins may be possible because of the smaller fetal size. When the diagnosis of conjoined twins is made in the first or early second trimester, the option of pregnancy termination should be discussed with the family. Although vaginal delivery is possible later in gestation (25), dystocia occurs in a high percentage of cases (22,26).

Postpartum support of the family also is an important concern (27). The planned attempt at separation can present difficult family decisions. An obstetrician who has been interacting with the family prenatally can offer great assistance during the postpartum period. Survivors of separation are likely to need long-term rehabilitation for orthopedic, neurologic, gastrointestinal, genitourinary, and gynecologic disabilities. The parents must be reassured that conjoined twinning is a random event with negligible risk of recurrence and that there are no reported cases of a conjoined twin's having conjoined offspring (28).

INTERTWIN GROWTH DISCORDANCE

Although intrauterine growth retardation (IUGR) is more common in multifetal gestations, it is not truly unique. However, because of the presence of two or more fetuses, the problem of intertwin growth discordance is a unique consideration in multiple gestations. In a 1975 review, Kohl and Casey (7) found that birth weights differed by 500 to 999 g in 18% of twin sets and that the difference was more than 1,000 g in 3% of sets. In a 1987 review, Yarkoni et al. (29) found that the mean intertwin birth weight difference was 10.3%. Between 15% and 20% of twins are 20% or more discordant at birth, and 5% of twin pairs display 25% or more birth weight discordance (30,31). Among triplets, discordance between the smallest and largest triplet is even more remarkable. Jones et al. (32) reviewed 196 triplet gestations with a mean intertriplet birth weight difference of 20%. Thirty percent of sets had an intertriplet discordance of 25% or more, and 7% displayed 40% or more discordance.

Much of the discordance in birth weight is caused by constitutional factors such as genetic dissimilarity of dizygotic twins. More severe discordance, however, raises the possibility of pathologic conditions such as twin–twin transfusion syndrome, fetal anomaly with a normal twin, congenital infection with growth retardation affecting only one twin, or local placental factors. The presence of a placental factor implies inability of the uteroplacental circulation to provide for the increased demands of multiple fetuses. Why this preferentially affects one member of the twin pair more than the other is not always understood. Inadequate uteroplacental circulation may lead to chronic malnutrition and growth retardation of one or both fetuses. The percentage of discordance is calculated by means of dividing the actual or estimated weight difference by the actual or estimated weight of the larger twin.

Intertwin weight differences of 25% to 30% usually are cited as values that differentiate normal birth-weight discordance from fetuses at risk of intrauterine or newborn complications. Evidence suggests that the smaller infant of a discordant twin pair is at increased risk of both neonatal morbidity and mortality (33,34). Cheung et al. (35) looked specifically at preterm twins and found no differences in the incidence of prematurity associated neonatal complications such as respiratory distress syndrome, intraventricular hemorrhage, or neonatal jaundice among twins with increasing degrees of birth-weight discordance. It was only among a small group of preterm twins with more than 30% discordance that there were increased incidences of infant death (25%), smallness for gestational age (32%), low Apgar scores (33%), and periventricular leukomalacia (17%). These findings were confounded, however, by the authors' inclusion of infants with congenital anomalies—9 of the 24 infants with a birth weight discordance of more than 30%.

Twin birth-weight discordance and IUGR are interrelated variables. O'Brien et al. (36) found that with birth-weight differences of 20% or more, one small-for-gestational-age twin was present in more than 50% of cases. Blickstein et al. (37) found no significant differences in perinatal outcome among discordant twins at term as long as they were all appropriate for gestational age. Patterson and Wood (38) reported that neither neonatal death nor combined morbidity could be related to birth-weight discordance. Both prematurity and birth weight less than tenth percentile were a greater threat to the fetus than was degree of discordance. Bronsteen et al. (39) also identified IUGR as being more predictive of neonatal morbidity than was birth weight discordance. In a multiple logistic regression analysis involving 1,145 twin pairs, Fraser et al. (40) found that birth-weight discordance was an independent risk factor only for neonatal hypoglycemia.

Another concern is that divergence in twin growth may identify smaller twins at a disadvantage for long-term physical and intellectual development. Sixteen twin pairs with at least 25% discordance in birth weight were observed until 18 years of age; both physical and intellectual differences persisted in most cases (41). A follow-up study by the same investigators (42) showed a significant difference in IQ (6.75 points) between the larger and smaller dissimilar twins at 8 years of age. Drillien (43) also found a lower IQ among the smaller of male monozygotic twins and among the smaller of dizygotic twins when birth-weight discordance exceeded 25%. Hohenauer (44) studied 18 same-sex twins with a birth-weight discordance of more than 300 g. He found mean IQ differences of 7.0 and 8.4 points for monozygotic and dizygotic twins, respectively. The smaller infant of each discordant pair had evidence of intellectual deficit. The suggestion was that insufficient intrauterine perfusion or nutrition may be a cause of suboptimal intellectual development.

The data suggest that intertwin growth discordance is probably of greatest relevance when it is associated with IUGR or with another pathologic condition. Intertwin growth discordance should be evaluated simultaneously with gestational age, individual fetal growth, and testing of fetal health and well-being. In the absence of fetal anomalies or marked IUGR and in the presence of reassuring fetal test results, birth-weight discordance of 25% or more among preterm twins should be managed expectantly in anticipation of achieving a more advanced gestational age or enhanced fetal maturity. It should be cautioned that both the degree of intrauterine growth discordance and the presence or absence of IUGR are not reliably detected with antenatal ultrasonography. That the sensitivity of ultrasonography for substantial intertwin discordance is at best only 60% is one justification for routine antepartum fetal assessment of all twins as they approach term (Table 8-2). On the other hand, ultrasound evidence suggesting a birth-weight discordance of 25% or more or IUGR of either twin at term (more than 35 weeks' gestation) would justify consideration of

Table 8-2. Literature review of the accuracy of ultrasonographic prediction of intertwin birth-weight discordance of 25% or more

Reference	n	Prevalence (%)	Diagnostic Study	Sensitivity	Specificity (%)	Positive Predictive Value (%)	Negative Predictive Value (%)
Blickstein et al., 1996 (110)	92	14	AC, FL	23	96	50	88
Chamberlain et al., 1991 (111)	85	9	AC, FL	37	98	75	93
			AC Δ >20 mm	43	91	53	77
Caravello et al., 1997 (112)	241	8	AC, FL	33	94	33	94
Gernt, 1999[a]	192	10	BPD, HC AC, FL	55	97	82	91

[a] Unpublished data from our institution.

AC, abdominal circumference; FL, femur length; BPD, biparietal diameter; HC, head circumference.

delivery. However, it is again cautionary that this degree of discordance may be incorrectly diagnosed in as many as 20% of cases. Because ultrasound prediction is not perfect, each patient's case must be individually assessed and ultrasound findings used as one part of the entire clinical evaluation.

MONOAMNIONIC TWINS

The presence of monoamnionic twins is extremely rare. It complicates fewer than 1% of monozygotic gestations and occurs approximately once in every 25,000 to 30,000 pregnancies. The importance, however, is found in the almost 50% fetal mortality rate associated with this type of placentation (45,46). Umbilical cord occlusion is believed to be the primary cause of fetal death among monoamnionic twins. It is caused by cord entanglement, which is present among 70% of sets of monoamnionic twins (47) (Fig. 8-1). Other causes of perinatal morbidity and mortality include congenital anomalies and twin–twin transfusion syndrome (48–50).

In terms of antepartum management, some obstetricians have recommended enhancement of lung maturity with glucocorticoid therapy followed by elective cesarean section at 32 weeks or earlier if obstetrically indicated (51). Other investigators have suggested that spontaneous intrauterine demise as a result of cord entanglement is uncommon in the third trimester. In two studies with small sample sizes, no fetal deaths occurred after 32 weeks (52) and 30 weeks (53), respectively. However, a review of 202 sets of nonconjoined, monoamnionic twins by Rodis et al. (54) showed that fetal deaths occurred throughout pregnancy, a large percentage occurring after 32 weeks. Of the 202 twin sets identified in a literature search, 52 were detected prenatally, and information on outcomes was available. Eighty-two of these 104 infants (79%) survived. To this total, Rodis added 13 more prenatally diagnosed monoamnionic twin pregnancies managed over a 10-year period at their institution. All 26 infants were liveborn, and only 2 died during the neonatal period (92% perinatal survival rate).

Antenatal fetal surveillance was performed with a nonstress test performed daily or two to three times a week beginning at viability. All 13 sets of monoamnionic twins described by Rodis et al. (54) had cord entanglement at birth, and for 8 the sole indication for delivery was nonreassuring results of fetal heart rate tests. The nature of these test results included persistent moderate-to-severe variable deceleration (4 cases), persistent fetal bradycardia (1 case), and a persistently nonreactive nonstress test result with a nonreassuring fetal biophysical profile (2 cases). Two other sets of twins were delivered because of premature labor, one as a consequence of intrauterine growth restriction, and two electively after documentation of fetal lung maturity. It appears that with accurate prenatal diagnosis, intensive fetal surveillance, glucocorticoid induction of fetal lung maturity, and appropriately timed delivery, perinatal survival of monoamnionic twins can be greatly improved from what has been historically reported (Table 8-3).

Route of delivery has typically been cesarean for fear of intrapartum complications (54). Entanglement of the umbilical cords is the main reason that cesarean delivery is preferred by most obstetricians (47,55,55a). Intimate entanglement of the first twin's

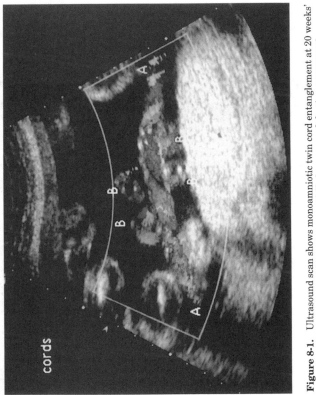

Figure 8-1. Ultrasound scan shows monoamniotic twin cord entanglement at 20 weeks' gestation. The twins were delivered uneventfully by means of elective cesarean at 34 weeks' gestation with multiple loops of entangled cord.

Table 8-3. Management strategy for monoamniotic tv

Ultrasonographic confirmation of monoamnionicity (carefully excl
  stuck twin syndrome)
Ultrasonographic evaluation at 18–20 wk to rule out congenital
  anomalies
Serial ultrasonography for fetal growth every 2–4 wk
Daily kick counts beginning at 26 wk
Nonstress test every other day beginning at 26 wk
Weekly antenatal administration of glucocorticoid beginning at 26 wk
Amniocentesis for fetal lung maturity beginning at 32 wk
Elective delivery between 34 and 35 wk if fetal lung maturity not
  previously documented
Delivery by cesarean section

umbilical cord with that of the second has resulted in unintentional cramping of its umbilical cord after delivery of the first twin (56). If vaginal delivery is anticipated, continuous fetal monitoring during labor is a prerequisite because acute fetal distress may be caused by constriction of a Gordian knot of the umbilical cords. If at delivery both twins are cephalic and ultrasound examination reveals no evidence of considerable cord entanglement, vaginal delivery can be attempted in the absence of other contraindications (49,57).

ACUTE INTERTWIN TRANSFUSION

Acute intertwin transfusion occurs in monochorionic twin gestations with the intrauterine death of one of the twin pair. Excluding first-trimester losses, intrauterine demise of one fetus occurs in 2% to 5% of twin gestations (58,59) and 14% to 17% of triplet gestations (60,61). The risk of second- and third-trimester fetal loss is many times higher for monochorionic twins than for dichorionic twins and for gestations in which one twin has a structural malformation (59).

When intrauterine fetal demise occurs in a multiple gestation, almost all of the adverse sequelae for the surviving twin occur in monochorionic gestations (62,63). Rydhstrom and Ingemarsson (64) and Nijhuis et al. (65) reported approximately a 25% mortality rate for the surviving twin after the antenatal death of the other twin.

Even more insidious is the high incidence of neurologic, gastrointestinal, and renal injuries experienced by the surviving twin. In a retrospective study of 206 twin gestations in which one twin died before delivery, 4.6% of the surviving children located for at least 8-year follow-up data collection had a neurologic deficit (64). All the affected twins were the second born and of the same sex as their sibling, suggesting monozygosity. Comparison with data on 4,000 low-birth-weight twins whose twin did not die *in utero* showed a neurologic deficit in only 1.9% of the children. A review of data from the National Collaborative Perinatal Project found that all cases in which the survivor had damage after intrauterine death of a twin were associated with monochorionic placentas (66). Anderson et al. (67), in San Francisco, documented a monochorionic

nta in 3 of 4 cases of second-trimester fetal death in a multi-
gestation with subsequent neurologic damage to the survivor .
n prospective studies, 5% to 25% of surviving twins have
chemic organ injury, including neurologic deficits (58,63,66–70).
lost reported cases of fetal demise or neurologic injury have
involved third-trimester fetal death *in utero*. However, neurologic
deficit of the surviving twin has been reported with demise of the
other twin as early as 18 weeks' gestation.

Neurologic abnormalities reported among surviving twins include necrosis and cavitation of the cerebral white matter, cerebellar necrosis, multicystic encephalomalacia, hydranencephaly,
hydrocephalus, porencephaly, microcephaly, and hemorrhagic infarction. Bejar et al. (71) examined echoencephalograms of
89 twins and 12 triplets born at less than 36 weeks' gestation and
showed cerebral white matter lesions within 3 days of birth in
14 of the infants. Magnetic resonance imaging and pathologic
study of the affected infants detected cavitation, gliosis, and calci-
fication of the white matter. Although the incidence of antenatal
necrosis of the white matter among infants from multiple gestations
(13.8%) was not significantly higher than the incidence of antenatal necrosis previously found among singletons (8.8%), monochorionic infants had a significantly higher incidence (30%) than did
either singleton or dichorionic infants. In addition to neurologic
injury, a variety of other abnormalities occur among surviving
twins, including ischemic bowel lesions, intestinal atresia, renal
cortical necrosis, and cystic renal dysplasia.

Acute intertwin transfusion is believed to be the cause of most
of the morbidity and mortality associated with single intrauterine fetal demise in a monochorionic twin gestation. Previous theo-
ries suggested that the reported morbidity and mortality were
caused by embolization of tissue thromboplastins from the circulation of the dead fetus to that of the surviving twin through placental anastomoses. The passage of thromboplastins results in
embolic ischemic organ injury or development of disseminated
intravascular coagulation in the survivor. Recent theory suggests
that the surviving twin transfuses blood acutely into the dead
twin's circulation through ubiquitous placental anastomoses. The
result is severe fetal hypotension and subsequent ischemic injury.
This acute intertwin transfusion can result in hypoxic neurologic
or other end-organ injury and in some cases fetal exsanguination
and possible death. Evidence of this more recent theory is found,
first, in fetal heart rate tracings that suggest the presence of fetal
anemia in the survivor soon after demise of the other twin and,
second, in hematologic information obtained through fetal blood
sampling of the surviving twin that reveals marked anemia
rather than clotting abnormalities (72). Other indirect evidence
is that immediate delivery has not prevented the finding of multicystic encephalomalacia in the surviving twin (70).

Pregnancy management after one fetus has died *in utero* depends
on gestational age, chorionicity, maternal status, and the status of
the living fetus. Knowledge of chorionicity is essential because the
sequelae of acute intertwin transfusion depend on placental anastomoses that occur only in monochorionic placentas. Although
anastomoses have been described in dichorionic placentas, they are
so rare that one may assume that the risk of acute intertwin trans-

fusion is clinically insignificant and that dichorionic twins
be treated expectantly. If expectant management is under
close surveillance of the surviving fetus is recommended. Pro
the greatest risk to the surviving twin is premature labor or
mature rupture of the membranes (58,68).

In monochorionic pregnancies, actual or impending intrauterir
fetal death is a much more complicated management issue. Intrauterine demise of one fetus at a point at which maturity of the
other twin can be presumed from gestational age or documented
by means of amniocentesis would justify immediate delivery. As a
generalization, this would be at about 34 weeks for a twin pregnancy. Delivery of the surviving twin between 30 and 34 weeks'
gestation would be associated with a very high survival rate in
most level III centers but would expose the newborn to some of
the morbidity associated with iatrogenic prematurity. However,
the morbidity expected as a consequence of delivery between 30
and 34 weeks' gestation appears to be less than that anticipated
with acute intertwin transfusion.

The maternal or obstetric condition that may have predisposed
to the loss of a twin should be considered, as should careful evaluation of the well-being of the surviving twin. It is unclear whether
the time from loss of a twin is of any significance in decisions
regarding preterm delivery. In the face of an impending intrauterine fetal demise of one twin, the decision regarding delivery should
be based primarily on gestational age. If both twins have a reasonable chance of survival, delivery of both fetuses is appropriate. If
the fetus at risk of demise is not viable, decisions regarding delivery should be based on the anticipated neonatal outcome for the
fetus at that particular hospital and whether or not it is superior
to the anticipated sequelae of acute intertwin transfusion (approximately 25% fetal mortality and as high as 25% risk of ischemic
injury among survivors). If the risks of delivery are believed to be
greater than the risk of acute intertwin transfusion, expectant
management is chosen. Close fetal surveillance of the surviving
twin should be undertaken. If fetal distress caused by partial
exsanguination of the surviving twin is identified within 24 to
48 hours of death of the other twin, an extremely high likelihood
of death or injury is anticipated. Options at that point would
include delivery or potentially fetal blood sampling with transfusion for fetal anemia. Unfortunately, neither of these interventions has proved successful in preventing an adverse outcome. In
the absence of acute intertwin transfusion, expectant management
had the advantage of greater gestational age for the healthy twin,
although subsequent preterm birth is an increased risk in this
scenario.

Another alternative to consider in the face of previable gestation with impending demise of one twin is selective feticide.
Intrauterine endoscopic occlusion of the umbilical cord of the compromised fetus has been successfully performed, although this
technique is still considered investigational. Selective delivery
of the compromised fetus has been performed, although both
short-term and long-term complications of intrauterine surgery
in continuing pregnancies are a problem. It seems likely that
endoscopic procedures will ultimately be associated with lesser
morbidity.

al concern associated with intrauterine fetal demise of one
s the possibility of maternal consumptive coagulopathy (67).
y and Weingold (73) estimated that there is an approximately
incidence of maternal disseminated intravascular coagulation
en a single fetal demise occurs in a multiple gestation and the
etus is retained for at least 4 weeks. However, in the previously
cited reviews maternal coagulopathy has been only infrequently
reported, and the 25% incidence seems to be a marked overestimation (58,63,67,68). Although uncommon, if expectant management is undertaken after intrauterine fetal demise, a baseline
maternal coagulation profile is recommended with periodic follow-up evaluations to detect developing coagulopathy. If hypofibrinoginemia is detected, treatment with heparin has been reported to
reverse the coagulation abnormality. Subsequent delivery of the
infant after remote intrauterine fetal demise of one twin should
probably include a consideration of maternal coagulation status.

CHRONIC INTERTWIN TRANSFUSION
(TWIN–TWIN TRANSFUSION SYNDROME)

Chronic intertwin transfusion is a complication of monozygotic-monochorionic twin pregnancies in which intraplacental arteriovenous shunts are uncompensated and preferential blood flow
occurs. Vascular communications are present in all monochorionic placentas, and as many as one-third of monochorionic twins
have clinical evidence of the syndrome to various degrees (74–76).
The severity of chronic intertwin transfusion syndrome is determined in large part by how early it is detected. The most severely
affected pregnancies usually are identified in the second trimester.
If the patient is untreated, the loss rate for both twins approaches
100% (77–79). Overall, chronic intertwin transfusion syndrome or
twin–twin transfusion syndrome, as it is more commonly known,
accounts for 15% to 17% of all perinatal mortality in twin gestations (80,81) .

In the classic model, an artery from one twin (donor) perfuses
a placental cotyledon which is drained by a vein to the other twin
(recipient) through a complex placental vascular anastomosis.
This model is complicated by the fact that reanastomoses are the
rule rather than the exception in monochorionic placentas. Vascular anastomoses can be superficial or deep and can be artery to
artery, vein to vein, or arteriovenous. Detailed characterization
of the angioarchitecture of monochorionic placentas has revealed
that patients with twin–twin transfusion syndrome were found to
have significantly fewer vascular anastomoses overall and for each
of the different subtypes (arterial-arterial, venous-venous, or
arteriovenous). When an anastomosis was present, it was more
likely to be deeper compared with monochorionic placentas in
pregnancies without twin–twin transfusion syndrome. These control placentas were characterized by multiple anastomoses, which
were both superficial and deep (82). As opposed to what may be
intuitive, twin–twin transfusion syndrome is associated not with
multiple vascular anastomoses but with fewer or, more commonly,
even a single arteriovenous anastomosis deep within the placenta. Multiple anastomoses tend to restore a balance of bidirectional flow in a monochorionic placenta, and a limited number
predispose to preferential flow (Fig. 8-2).

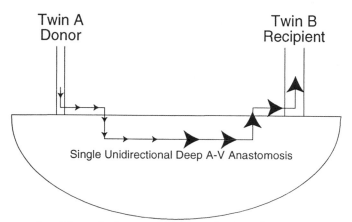

A. Chronic Intertwin Transfusion Syndrome

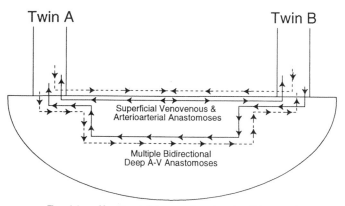

B. Unaffected Monochorionic Placenta

Figure 8-2. Angioarchitectural differences in the monochorionic placentation typically affected by chronic intertwin transfusion syndrome (**A**) and the unaffected monochorionic placenta (**B**). Chronic intertwin transfusion syndrome is associated with markedly fewer vascular anastomoses overall and a greater likelihood that anastomoses that do exist will be located deep within the placenta rather than superficially. The more limited number of vascular anastomoses predisposes to preferential flow from donor to recipient twin.

The arterial donor experiences anemia, hypovolemia, and growth restriction. The anemia and hypovolemia reduce renal blood flow and fetal urinary output. The resultant oligohydramnios can cause the amnionic membranes to lie in close apposition and enshroud the smaller fetus. The enveloping membrane restricts the fetus to the side of the uterine wall, causing what is referred to as a stuck twin. The stuck twin often appears to defy gravity and is sometimes misidentified as a monoamnionic twin. The organs of the donor twin are proportionately smaller and the fetus may also sustain ischemic injury involving the brain, kidneys, or intestine.

The venous recipient is hypervolemic, hyperviscous, and poly-hydramnionic because of increased urination. The recipient twin has much higher circulating levels of arterial natriuretic peptide, which promotes diuresis and other vascular changes (83). The recipient twin may have cardiohypertrophy, tricuspid insufficiency, and congestive heart failure, which cause fetal hydrops. The poly-hydramnios of the venous recipient also predisposes the fetus to complications such as premature labor and amniorrhexis.

The diagnostic criteria for chronic intertwin transfusion syndrome are controversial. The older neonatal diagnostic criteria for chronic intertwin transfusion syndrome (cord blood hemoglobin difference of 5 g/dL of more and a birth-weight difference of 20% or more) have been largely discarded. Hemoglobin differences of 5 g/dL or more and birth-weight differences of 20% or more occur at similar rates among both dichorionic and monochorionic gestations (84). Wenstrom et al. (85) reviewed 97 monochorionic twin pregnancies and observed all conceivable combinations of birth weight and hemoglobin discordance, including smaller twins with higher hemoglobin levels. Hemoglobin levels probably fluctuate with volume shifts during the course of pregnancy and can shift even more remarkably as a result of intrapartum shunting so as to make the neonatal diagnostic criteria entirely unsatisfactory.

Chronic intertwin transfusion syndrome is now diagnosed according to ultrasonographic criteria. These criteria include the following: (a) marked size disparity in fetuses of the same sex, (b) disparity in size between two amnionic sacs, (c) disparity in size of the umbilical cords, (d) single placenta, (e) evidence of hydrops in either fetus or findings of congestive heart failure in the recipient (86,87).

The prenatal diagnosis of chronic intertwin transfusion syndrome often is presumptive. The differential diagnosis includes other pathologic conditions, such as chromosomal or congenital anomaly, congenital infection, or most commonly IUGR that affects only one of the fetuses as a consequence of a placental factor. Even visualization of what appears to be the stuck twin phenomenon is not pathognomonic of chronic intertwin transfusion syndrome. A similar finding can be caused by structural fetal abnormalities, particularly those causing oliguria, such as renal agenesis. Ruptured membranes, congenital infection, umbilical cord abnormality, such as velamentous insertion or single umbilical artery, and severe IUGR are other diagnostic possibilities to be considered.

Some investigators have suggested that Doppler ultrasound examination of the umbilical arteries may help to improve diagnostic accuracy. Giles et al. (88) described 11 like-sexed twin pairs with monochorionic placentas and cord blood hemoglobin differ-

ences of more than 5 g/dL at delivery. The mean differer
systolic to diastolic (S/D) ratios was 0.4, leading the invest
to conclude that in confirmed chronic intertwin transfusio.
drome there is concordance of the umbilical artery S/D ratio.
spite discordant fetal growth. Other investigators have not fou
significant intertwin differences in umbilical artery Doppler fin
ings (89,90). In the assessment by Giles et al., abnormal Doppler
findings more likely reflected placental abnormalities associated
with fetal growth retardation as opposed to chronic intertwin transfusion syndrome. In the latter the pathologic process is hematologic
not placental. The normal placental structure present in chronic
intertwin transfusion syndrome produces normal, nondiscordant
S/D ratios (91). Giles et al. suggested that Doppler velocimetry is
helpful in differentiating chronic intertwin transfusion syndrome
from fetal growth restriction. They hypothesized that the concordance in waveforms was caused by an absence of underlying placental vascular lesions.

Other investigators have seen abnormal findings at Doppler
velocimetry in well-established cases of chronic intertwin transfusion syndrome (92,93). These conflicting results are confusing but
may be explained by differences in diagnostic criteria used by the
different investigators and, importantly, differences in the severity of disease expression. More severe cases of chronic intertwin
transfusion syndrome, such as those with onset early in the second
trimester or with the development of a stuck twin, may be more
likely to manifest abnormal Doppler flow findings in the umbilical
artery of the smaller twin.

Some investigators have chosen to categorize chronic intertwin
transfusion syndrome as mild, moderate, or severe on the basis of
anticipated outcome. Severe intertwin transfusion usually is identified before 20 weeks' gestation and is frequently associated with
the stuck twin phenomenon. The stuck twin has severe growth
retardation, and the recipient twin has progressive polyhydramnios, which causes premature labor or rupture of the membranes.
Without intervention, delivery usually occurs before 26 weeks' gestation, and the mortality approaches 100%. In moderate twin–twin
transfusion syndrome, the diagnosis usually is made after 20 weeks'
gestation, in the late second or early third trimester. The degree of
birth-weight discordance is less than in severe intertwin transfusion syndrome, and the fluid shifts are variable and less severe.
Without intervention, the mortality rate for moderate intertwin
transfusion still approaches 50% to 70%. Mild intertwin transfusion syndrome has the most benign expression. The diagnosis usually is made in the third trimester or neonatal period. The diagnosis usually is based on a discrepancy in birth weights and a
hemoglobin discrepancy of 5 g/dL or more. The anticipated outcome
in mild intertwin transfusion usually is good, similar to that of
other twin pregnancies with discordant growth (94).

A mainstay of therapy for both moderate and severe intertwin
transfusion syndrome is large-volume reduction amniocentesis.
Reduction amniocentesis is indicated for (a) amnionic fluid index
of 40 cm or more; (b) deepest vertical pocket 12 cm or greater;
(c) maternal respiratory embarrassment; (d) cervical shortening
or cervical score suggestive of an increased risk of prematurity; or
(e) stuck twin phenomenon. An 18-gauge spinal needle is placed

polyhydramnionic sac and amnionic fluid is removed as
as possible with a 50-mL syringe. Amnionic fluid is removed
ate of approximately 1 L every 10 to 15 minutes. The average
me of amnionic fluid removed is 1,500 to 2,000 mL. The goal
restitution of normal amnionic fluid volume (deepest vertical
ocket less than 8 cm).

Initial fears that large volume reduction amniocentesis may pre-
cipitate abruptio placentae, amnionic rupture, and chorioamnionic
separation have not been borne out. Elliott et al. (95) found a
complication rate of only 1.5% in a review of more than 200 large-
volume reduction amniocenteses. In addition to reducing excessive
amnionic fluid volume, reduction amniocentesis also appears to
improve uteroplacental circulation. A study of Doppler examinations of patients undergoing large-volume reduction amniocentesis
showed a 74% increase in uterine artery blood flow (96). Increased
uteroplacental blood flow may improve circulation to the stuck twin,
increase urine production, normalize amnionic volume differences,
and in some cases resolve hydrops fetalis (97–99). The overall perinatal survival rate gleaned from the available literature on large-
volume reduction amniocentesis is 60% to 65% (100).

Another treatment approach is a technique in which a fetoscopic neodymium:YAG laser is used to occlude superficial placental vessels and ablate the vascular communication between
the two fetuses (101). DeLia et al. (101) and Ville et al. (102) have
reported findings for two series totaling 71 patients with an overall fetal survival rate of 53%. In about one-third of the pregnancies, both twins survived. In the others either one or both of the
twins died, usually within the first 24 hours after laser ablation.
Although ablation of vascular communications between the twins
has appeal as the most direct therapy for the underlying patho-
physiologic condition, there remain a number of concerns. Does
laser ablation of superficial vessels on the chorionic plate affect
the deep vascular anastomoses believed to be typical of chronic
intertwin transfusion syndrome? Are the fetal losses that occur
so soon after laser ablation a result of necrosis of the cotyledons
or possibly occlusion of superficial vascular connections that had
the protective function of providing a unidirectional shunt in the
opposite direction? These questions need to be addressed.

Berry et al. (103) reported on nine pregnancies complicated by
chronic intertwin transfusion syndrome managed with amnionic
septostomy. The survival rate was more than 80%. With fenestra-
tion of the intertwin membrane, the amnionic fluid volumes equal-
ize. The donor fetus is then able to swallow the amnionic fluid.
This corrects the hypovolemic state and increases urine production. The main theoretical disadvantage of this procedure is iatrogenic monoamnionicity with resultant cord entanglement.

Selective feticide has been described but is limited as an option
because of the inevitable loss of the first twin and because of an
increased risk of death or neurologic impairment of the second
twin. Techniques that allow percutaneous vascular occlusion of
the cord of one twin may ultimately have potential if they prevent
subsequent acute injury to the other twin.

Both digoxin and indomethacin have been used for medical therapy for chronic intertwin transfusion syndrome. DeLia et al. (104)
reported successful use of digoxin for intrauterine treatment of a

27-week recipient fetus with hydrops and polyhydr
digoxin therapy, heart failure resolved, and the twin
tively delivered at 34 weeks with a normal outcome. Ind.
has been proposed because of its ability to reduce fetal uri
put. Unfortunately, although it may have potential to red
degree of polyhydramnios in the sac of the recipient twin,
methacin may also cause unwanted renal failure in the alre.
oliguric arterial donor (105).

The long-term outcome among survivors has been poorly stud
ied. Concerns have been expressed over the possibility of ischemic
brain injury to the donor twin and cardiomyopathy among surviving recipient twins (106–108). Neonatal hypertension also has
been associated with discordant twin syndrome. Question also
exists about the impact of this syndrome on hypertension later in
childhood and adulthood (109). More information is needed about
the long-term complications of chronic intertwin transfusion syndrome. Of all the management options, it appears that large-
volume reduction amniocentesis is an efficacious and minimally
invasive therapy that is probably the treatment of choice after
20 weeks' gestation. For patients found to have chronic intertwin
transfusion syndrome before 20 weeks' gestation, the prognosis is
extremely poor even with large-volume reduction amniocentesis.
For those patients, consideration should be given to intrauterine
laser ablation of vascular communications or to fetoscopic cord
clamping.

REFERENCES

1. Samuels P. Ultrasound in the management of the twin gestation. *Clin Obstet Gynecol* 1988;31:110–122.
2. Landy HJ, Keith L, Keith D. The vanishing twin. *Acta Genet
   Med Gemellol (Roma)* 1982;31:179–183.
3. Seoud MAF, Toner JP, Kruithoff C, et al. Outcome of twin,
   triplet, and quadruplet in vitro fertilization pregnancies: the
   Norfolk Experience. *Fertil Steril* 1992;57:825–834.
4. Jauniaux E, Elkazen N, Leroy F, et al. Clinical and morpholog-
   ical aspects of the vanishing twin phenomena. *Obstet Gynecol*
   1988;72:577–581.
5. Landy HJ, Weiner S, Corson SL, et al. The "vanishing twin":
   ultrasonic assessment of fetal disappearance in the first trimester.
   Am J Obstet Gynecol 1986;155:14–19.
6. Prompeler HJ, Madjar H, Klosa W, et al. Twin pregnancies with
   single fetal death. *Acta Obstet Gynecol Scand* 1994;73:205–208.
7. Kohl SG, Casey G. Twin gestation. *Mt Sinai J Med* 1975;42:
   523–529.
8. Baldwin VJ. Anomalous development of twins. In: Baldwin VJ,
   ed. *Pathology of multiple pregnancy*. New York: Springer-Verlag,
   1994:169–197.
9. Edwards MS, Ellings JM, Newman RB, et al. Predictive value of
   antepartum ultrasound examination for anomalies in twin gestations. *Ultrasound Obstet Gynecol* 1995;6:43–49.
10. Gillim DL, Hendricks CH, Holocardius: review of the literature
    and case report. *Obstet Gynecol* 1953;2:647–653.
11. VanAllen MI, Smith DW, Shepard TH. Twin reversed arterial
    perfusion (TRAP) sequence: a study of 14 twin pregnancies with
    acardius. *Semin Perinatol* 1983;7:285–293.

    R, Gale S, Benirschke K. Perinatal outcome of 49 preg-
    s complicated by acardiac twinning. *Am J Obstet Gynecol*
    ;163:907–912.
    ie GF, Payne GG Jr, Morgan MA. Selective delivery of an
    cardiac, acephalic twin. *N Engl J Med* 1989;320:512–513.
    Fries MH, Goldberg JD, Golbus MS. Treatment of acardiac-
    acephalus twin gestations by hysterotomy and selective deliv-
    ery. *Obstet Gynecol* 1992;79:601–604.

15. Quintero RA, Rich H, Puder K, et al. Brief report: umbilical-cord ligation of an acardiac twin by fetoscopy at 19 weeks gestation. *N Engl J Med* 1994;330:469–471.

16. Hecher K, Reinhold U, Gbur K, et al. Unterbrechung des umbilikalen Blutflusses bei einem akardischen Zwilling durch endoskopische Laserkoagulation. *Geburtshilfe Frauenheilk* 1996; 56:97–100.

17. Sepulveda W, Bower S, Hassan J, et al. Ablation of acardiac twin by alcohol injection into the intraabdominal umbilical artery. *Obstet Gynecol* 1995;84:680–681.

18. Porreco RP, Barton SM, Haverkamp AD. Occlusion of umbilical artery in acardiac, acephalic twin. *Lancet* 1991;337:326–327.

19. Platt LB, DeVore GR, Bieniarz A, et al. Antenatal diagnosis of acephalus acardia: a proposed management scheme. *Am J Obstet Gynecol* 1983;146:857–859.

20. Hanson JW. Incidence of conjoined twinning. *Lancet* 1975;2:1257.

21. Edmonds LD, Layde PM. Conjoined twins in the United States, 1970–1977. *Teratology* 1982;25:301–306.

22. Harper RG, Kenigsberg K, Sia CG, et al. Xiphopagus conjoined twins: a 300 year review of the obstetric morphopathologic, neonatal and surgical parameters. *Am J Obstet Gynecol* 1980;137: 617–629.

23. Bucholz RD, Yoon KW, Shively RE. Temporoparietal craniopagus: case report and review of the literature. *J Neurosurg* 1987; 66:72–78.

24. Filler RM. Conjoined twins and their separation. *Semin Perinatol* 1986;10:82–91.

25. Rudolph AJ, Michaels JP, Nichols BL. Obstetric management of conjoined twins. *Birth Defects* 1967;3:28–32.

26. Nichols BL, Blattner RJ, Rudolph AJ. General clinical management of thoracopagus twins. *Birth Defects* 1967;3:38–40.

27. Sakala EP. Obstetric management of conjoined twins. *Obstet Gynecol* 1986;67:21S–25S.

28. Ellis JW, Keith LG, Keith DM. Conjoined twins. *Curr Probl Obstet Gynecol* 1983;6:55–60.

29. Yarkoni S, Reece A, Holford T, et al. Estimated fetal weight in the evaluation of growth in twin gestations: a prospective longitudinal study. *Obstet Gynecol* 1987;69:636–639.

30. Chitkara U, Berkowitz GS, Levine R. Twin pregnancy: routine use of ultrasound examinations in the prenatal diagnosis of IUGR and discordant growth. *Am J Perinatol* 1985;2:49–53.

31. Carlson N. Discordant twin pregnancy: a challenging condition. *Contemp Ob/Gyn* 1989;34:100–116.

32. Jones JS, Newman RB, Miller MC. Cross-sectional analysis of triplet birth weight. *Am J Obstet Gynecol* 1991;168:135–140.

33. Guaschino S, Spinillo A, Stola E, et al. Growth retardation, size at birth, and perinatal mortality in twin pregnancy. *Int J Gynecol Obstet* 1987;25:399–403.

34. Erkkola R, Ala-Mello S, Piiroinen O, et al. Growth discordar in twin pregnancies: a risk factor not detected by measuremen of biparietal diameter. *Obstet Gynecol* 1985;66:203–206.

35. Cheung VYT, Bocking AD, Dasilva OP. Preterm discordant twins: what birth weight difference is significant? *Am J Obstet Gynecol* 1995;172:955–959.

36. O'Brien WF, Knuppel RA, Serbo JC, et al. Birth weight in twins: analysis of discordancy and growth retardation. *Obstet Gynecol* 1986;67:483–486.

37. Blickstein I, Shoham-Schwartz Z, Lancet M. Growth discordancy in appropriate for gestational age, term twins. *Obstet Gynecol* 1988;72:582–584.

38. Patterson RM, Wood RC. What is birth weight discordance? *Am J Perinatol* 1990;7:217–219.

39. Bronsteen R, Goyert G, Bottoms S. Classification of twins and neonatal morbidity. *Obstet Gynecol* 1989;74:98–101.

40. Fraser D, Picard R, Picard E, et al. Birth weight discordance, intrauterine growth retardation, and perinatal outcome in twins. *J Reprod Med* 1994;39:504–508.

41. Babson GS, Kangas J, Young N, et al. Growth and development of twins of dissimilar size at birth. *Pediatrics* 1964;33:327–333.

42. Babson GS, Phillips DS. Growth and development of twins of dissimilar size at birth. *N Engl J Med* 1973;289:937–940.

43. Drillien CM. The small for date infant: etiology and prognosis. *Pediatr Clin North Am* 1970;17:9–24.

44. Hohenauer L, Studien zur intrauterinen Dystrophie, II: Folgen intrauterinen Mangelernaehrung beim Menschen: eine vergleichende Studie von zwillingspaaren mit unterschiedlichem Geburtsgewicht. *Paediatr Paedol* 1971;6:17–30.

45. Mantoni M, Peterson JF. Monoamniotic twins diagnosed by ultrasound in the first trimester. *Acta Obstet Gynecol Scand* 1980;59:551–553.

46. Benirschke K, Kim CK. Multiple pregnancy, I. *N Engl J Med* 1973;288:1276–1284.

47. Lee CY. Management of monoamniotic twins diagnosed antenatally by ultrasound. *Am J Gynecol Health* 1992;6:25–29.

48. Sutter J, Arab H, Manning FA. Monoamniotic twins: antenatal diagnosis and management. *Am J Obstet Gynecol* 1986;155:836–837.

49. Dubecq F, Dufour D, Vinatier D, et al. Monoamniotic twin pregnancies: review of the literature and a case report with vaginal delivery. *Eur J Obstet Gynecol Reprod Biol* 1996;66:183–186.

50. Timmons, JD, DeAlvarez RR. Monoamniotic twin pregnancy. *Am J Obstet Gynecol* 1963;86:875–881.

51. Beasley E, Megerian G, Gerson A, et al. Monoamniotic twins: case series and proposal for antenatal management. *Obstet Gynecol* 1999;93:130–134.

52. Tessen JA, Zlatnik FJ. Monoamniotic twins: a retrospective controlled study. *Obstet Gynecol* 1991;77:832–834.

53. Carr SR, Aronson MP, Coustan DR. Survival rates of monoamniotic twins do not decrease after 30 weeks gestation. *Am J Obstet Gynecol* 1990;163:719–722.

54. Rodis JF, McIlveen PF, Egan JFX, et al. Monoamniotic twins: improved perinatal survival with accurate prenatal diagnosis and antenatal fetal surveillance. *Am J Obstet Gynecol* 1997;177:1046–1049.

5. Colburn DW, Pasquale SA. Monoamniotic twin pregnancy. *J Reprod Med* 1982;27:165–168.
55a. Trofatter KF. Management of delivery. *Clin Perinatol* 1988;15: 93–106.
56. McLeod FN, McCoy DR. Monoamniotic twins with an unusual cord complication. *Br J Obstet Gynaecol* 1981;88:774–775.
57. Ritossa M., O'Loughlin J. Monoamniotic twin pregnancy and cord entanglement: a clinical dilemma. *Aust N Z J Obstet Gynaecol* 1996;36:309–312.
58. Eglowstein M, D'Alton ME. Intrauterine demise in multiple gestation: theory and management. *J Matern Fetal Med* 1993;2: 272–275.
59. Kilby MD, Govind A, O'Brien PM. Outcome of twin pregnancies complicated by single intrauterine death: a comparison with viable twin pregnancies. *Obstet Gynecol* 1994;84:107–109.
60. Gonen R, Heyman E, Asztalos E, et al. The outcome of triplet gestations complicated by fetal death. *Obstet Gynecol* 1990;75: 175–178.
61. Borlum KG. Third trimester fetal death in triplet pregnancies. *Obstet Gynecol* 1991;77:6–9.
62. Enbom JA. Twin pregnancy with intrauterine death of one twin. *Am J Obstet Gynecol* 1985;152:424–429.
63. Carlson NJ, Towers CV. Multiple gestation complicated by the death of one fetus. *Obstet Gynecol* 1989;73:685–689.
64. Rydhstrom H, Ingemarsson I. Prognosis and long-term follow-up of a twin after antenatal death of the co-twin. *J Reprod Med* 1993;38:142–146.
65. Nijhuis J, van Hetren C, Semmekrot B, et al. What is the risk for the surviving twin after death of the co-twin in twin-twin transfusion syndrome? *Am J Obstet Gynecol* 1997;176: S116(abst).
66. Melnick M. Brain damage in survivors after in utero death of monozygous co-twin. *Lancet* 1977;2:1287.
67. Anderson RL, Golbus MS, Curry CJR, et al. Central nervous system damage and other anomalies in surviving fetus following second trimester antenatal death of co-twin. *Prenat Diagn* 1990; 10:513–518.
68. Fusi L, Gordon H. Twin pregnancy complicated by single intrauterine death: problems and outcome with conservative management. *Br J Obstet Gynaecol* 1990;97:511–516.
69. Yoshida K, Matayoshi K. A study on prognosis of surviving co-twin. *Acta Genet Med Gemellol (Roma)* 1990;39:383–387.
70. D'Alton ME, Newton ER, Cetrulo CL. Intrauterine fetal demise in multiple gestation. *Acta Genet Med Gemellol (Roma)* 1984; 33:43–49.
71. Bejar R, Vigliocco G, Gramajo H, et al. Antenatal origin of neurologic damage in newborn infants. II. Multiple gestations. *Am J Obstet Gynecol* 1990; 162:1230–1236.
72. Okamura K, Murotsuki J, Tanigawara F, et al. Funipuncture for evaluation of hematologic and coagulation indices in the surviving twin following co-twin's death. *Obstet Gynecol* 1994;83: 975–978.
73. Landy HJ, Weingold AB. Management of a multiple gestation complicated by an antepartum fetal demise. *Obstet Gynecol Surv* 1989;44:171–176.
74. Robertson EG, Neer KJ. Placental injection studies in twin gestation. *Am J Obstet Gynecol* 1983;147:170–174.

75. Patten RM, Mack LA, Harvey D, et al. Disparity of amnic volume in fetal size: problem of the stuck twin—U.S. s *Radiology* 1989;172:153–157.

76. Rausen AR, Seki M, Strauss L. Twin transfusion syndro *J Pediatr* 1965;66:613–628.

77. Chescheir NC, Seeds JW. Polyhydramnios and oligohydramnic in twin gestations. *Obstet Gynecol* 1988;71:882–884.

78. Reisner DP, Mahoney BS, Petty CN, et al. Stuck twin syndrome: outcome in 37 consecutive cases. *Am J Obstet Gynecol* 1993;169: 991–995.

79. Saunders NJ, Snijders RJ, Nicolaides KH. Therapeutic amniocentesis in twin-twin transfusion syndrome appearing in the second trimester of pregnancy. *Am J Obstet Gynecol* 1992;166:820–824.

80. Weir PE, Ratten GJ, Beischer NA. Acute polyhydramnios: a complication of monozygous twin pregnancy. *Br J Obstet Gynaecol* 1979;86:849–853.

81. Steinberg LH, Hurley EA, Desnedt E, et al. Acute polyhydramnios in twin pregnancies. *Aust N Z J Obstet Gynaecol* 1990;30: 196–200.

82. Bajoria R, Wigglesworth J, Fisk NM. Angioarchitecture of monochorionic placentas in relation to the twin-twin transfusion syndrome. *Am J Obstet Gynecol* 1995;172:856–863.

83. Rosen DJ, Rabinowitz R, Beyth Y, et al. Fetal urine production in normal twins and in twins with acute polyhydramnios. *Fetal Diagn Ther* 1990;5:57–60.

84. Danskin FH, Neilson JP. Twin-twin transfusion syndrome: what are appropriate diagnostic criteria? *Am J Obstet Gynecol* 1989;161:365–368.

85. Wenstrom KD, Tessen JA, Zlatnik FJ, et al. Frequency, distribution, and theoretical mechanisms of hematologic and weight discordance in monochorionic twins. *Obstet Gynecol* 1992;80:257–261.

86. Wittmann BK, Baldwin VJ, Nichol F. Antenatal diagnosis of twin transfusion syndrome by ultrasound. *Obstet Gynecol* 1981;58: 123–127.

87. Brennan JN, Diwan RJ, Rosen MG, et al. Fetofetal transfusion syndrome: prenatal ultrasonographic diagnosis. *Radiology* 1982; 143:535–536.

88. Giles WB, Trudinjer BJ, Cook CM. Doppler umbilical artery studies in twin-twin transfusion syndrome. *Obstet Gynecol* 1990; 76:1097–1099.

89. Ishimatsu J, Yoshimura O, Manabe A, et al. Ultrasonography and doppler studies in twin-twin transfusion. *Asia Oceania J Obstet Gynecol* 1992;18:325–331.

90. Rizzo G, Arduini D, Romanini C. Cardiac and extracardiac flows in discordant twins. *Am J Obstet Gynecol* 1994;170:1321–1327.

91. Fries MH, Goldstein RB, Kilpatrick FJ, et al. The role of velamentous cord insertion in the etiology of twin-twin transfusion syndrome. *Obstet Gynecol* 1993;81:569–574.

92. Pretorius DH, Manchester D, Barkin S, et al. Doppler ultrasound of twin transfusion syndrome. *J Ultrasound Med* 1988;7:117–124.

93. Castaner J, Baker E, Cetrulo CL, et al. Umbilical artery Dopplers in twin-twin transfusion syndrome. *J Ultrasound Med* 1992;11:S51.

94. Elliott JP. Amniocentesis for twin-twin transfusion syndrome. *Contemp Ob/Gyn* 1992;Aug:30–47.

..liott JP, Sawyer AT, Radin TG, et al. Large volume therapeu
..ic amniocentesis in the treatment of hydramnios. *Obstet Gynecol* 1994;84:1025–1027.

.. Bower SJ, Flack NJ, Sepulveda W, et al. Uterine artery blood flow response to correction of amniotic fluid volume. *Am J Obstet Gynecol* 1995;173:502–507.

97. Elliott JP, Urig MA, Clewell WH. Aggressive therapeutic amniocentesis for treatment of twin-twin transfusion syndrome. *Obstet Gynecol* 1991;77:537–540.

98. Pinette MG, Pan Y, Pinette SG, et al. Treatment of twin-twin transfusion syndrome. *Obstet Gynecol* 1993;82:841–846.

99. Wax JR, Blakemore KJ, Blohm P, et al. Stuck twin with co-twin non-immune hydrops: successful treatment by amniocentesis. *Fetal Diagn Ther* 1991;6:126–131.

100. Fisk NM, Denbow ML. Feto-fetal transfusion syndrome: amnioreduction as optimal treatment. In: Donnez J, Brosens L, eds. Proceedings of the Fourth European Society for Gynecological Endoscopy, Brussels, Belgium. Bologna, Italy: Monduzzi Editore, 1996:9–18.

101. DeLia JE, Cruikshank DP, Keye WR Jr. Fetoscopic neodymium:YAG laser occlusion of placental vessels in severe twin-twin transfusion syndrome. *Obstet Gynecol* 1990;75:1046–1053.

102. Ville Y, Hyett J, Hecher K, et al. Preliminary experience with endoscopic laser surgery for severe twin-twin transfusion syndrome. *N Engl J Med* 1995;332:224–227.

103. Berry D, Montgomery A, Johnson A, et al. Amniotic septostomy for the treatment of the stuck twin sequence. *Am J Obstet Gynecol* 1997;176:S19(abst).

104. DeLia JE, Emery MG, Sheafor SA, et al. Twin transfusion syndrome: successful in utero treatment with digoxin. *Int J Gynaecol Obstet* 1985;23:197–201.

105. Buderus S, Thomas B, Fahnenstich H, et al. Renal failure in two preterm infants: toxic effects of prenatal maternal indomethacin treatment? *Br J Obstet Gynaecol* 1993;100:97–98.

106. Naeye RL. Human intrauterine parabiotic syndrome and its complications. *N Engl J Med* 1963;268:804–809.

107. Reisner SH, Forbes AE, Cornblath M. The smaller of twins in hypoglycemia. *Lancet* 1965;1:524–526.

108. Zosner N, Bajoria R, Weiner E, et al. Clinical and echocardiographic features of in utero cardiac dysfunction in the recipient twin in twin-twin transfusion syndrome. *Br Heart J* 1994;72:74–79.

109. Tolosa J, Zoppini C, Ludomirsky A, et al. Fetal hypertension and cardiac hypertrophy in the discordant twin syndrome. *Am J Obstet Gynecol* 1993;168:292(abst).

110. Blickstein I, Manor M, Levi R, et al. Is intertwin birth weight discordance predictable? *Gynecol Obstet Invest* 1996;42:105.

111. Chamberlain P, Murphy M, Comerford FR. How accurate is antenatal sonographic identification of discordant birth weight in twins? *Eur J Obstet Gynecol Reprod Biol* 1991;40:91–96.

112. Caravello JW, Chauhan SP, Morrison JC, et al. Sonographic examination does not predict twin growth discordancy accurately. *Obstet Gynecol* 1997;89:529–533.

9

Maternal Complications

Women pregnant with multiple fetuses are more likely to need intensive prenatal care (1), to be hospitalized antenatally (2), to have longer hospitalizations (3) and to experience significantly greater and more severe pregnancy-related complications. A portion of this risk is linked to maternal characteristics present at the onset of pregnancy, including older maternal age, extremes of parity and pregravid weight, and conception with assisted reproductive techniques. The majority of this excess risk, though, is due to higher plurality and an exaggeration of maternal adaptations to pregnancy and associated obstetrical interventions. Even with multifetal pregnancy reduction (see Chapter 4), there is still residual higher risk for complications. In a recent case–control study of causes for admission of pregnant women to intensive care units, multiple pregnancy was found to be an independent risk factor, with an odds ratio of 2.3 (95% confidence interval [CI], 1.2–4.5) (4).

PRECONCEPTION AND EARLY PREGNANCY RISKS

Maternal Age

Maternal age is a known risk factor for many obstetric complications, as well as maternal mortality (5). Older maternal age is associated with histories of spontaneous and induced abortions and chronic medical conditions (6). In a study of singleton pregnancies, Berkowitz et al. (6) demonstrated a significantly higher risk of antepartum complications, including gestational diabetes, pregnancy-induced hypertension, bleeding, abruptio placentae, and placenta previa (adjusted odds ratio [AOR], 2.0; 95% CI, 1.6–2.5), and cesarean delivery (AOR, 1.8; 95% CI, 1.5–2.2) among women 35 years and older, particularly among those who were primiparous. Other studies have confirmed these associations, reporting higher rates of medical complications (diabetes, chronic hypertension, and antepartum bleeding), antenatal admissions, intrapartum complications and labor abnormalities, and cesarean delivery (7–13). Maternal age has been found to be an independent risk factor for placenta previa (14,15), with the highest risk for older women at extremes of parity (AOR 5.6; 95% CI, 1.6–19.6 for parity of 0 and AOR 5.8; 95% CI, 2.7–12.6 for parity of 4 or more) (15). Population-based studies using vital statistics data have reported an increased risk of stillbirth, low birth weight, and preterm birth among older women, particularly if they are primiparous (16–21).

About 40% of childless women 35 to 44 years of age in the United States have impaired fecundity (22,23). Because of advances in assisted reproductive technology, an increasing number of women are giving birth in their late forties and even early fifties. According to the most recent vital statistics, the number of births to women 50 years and older totaled 135 and 158 births, respectively, in 1997 and 1998 (24,25). Older maternal age is a challenge for reproductive endocrinologists, often necessitating transfer of a higher number of oocytes or embryos to achieve a clinical pregnancy

1). Most pregnancies among women 40 years and older occur n four or more embryos are transferred (27,28). In a study of pregnancies among women 50 years and older using oocyte onation, more than one-half resulted in multiple gestations (29). When donor oocytes are used, the recipient's age has been found not to adversely affect the pregnancy (30). In a recent analysis of trends over a 10-year period regarding maternal age and multifetal pregnancy reduction, Evans et al. (31) found that between 1986 and 1996, the proportion of women who underwent this procedure at their site increased from 0 to 12%. These researchers found that these older women are much more likely to use donor eggs and to reduce the pregnancy to a singleton.

Assisted versus Spontaneous Conception

There is inconsistent evidence regarding the effect of infertility status on the course and outcome of pregnancies. Several investigators have shown that multiple gestations from infertility treatments are at significantly higher risk for low birth weight, small-for-gestational-age birth weight, and morbidities associated with prematurity compared to non-assisted reproductive techniques (ART) controls (32–34). Others have reported that spontaneously-conceived multiples have shorter gestations (35,36), lower average birth weights, and higher rates of intrauterine growth retardation, neonatal death, and maternal preeclampsia (36). Others have shown no significant differences, except that spontaneously-conceived multiples have slightly higher neonatal and perinatal mortality, probably due to higher rates of monochorionicity (37). Because pregnancies resulting from infertility treatments have higher serum relaxin concentrations than either singleton or multiple pregnancies achieved spontaneously (32,38), these pregnancies may be at increased risk for preterm birth (39,40). It has been hypothesized that the increase in serum relaxin levels may increase the risk for preterm birth by weakening the cervical tissue (41,42).

The results of six recent studies comparing the course and outcomes of assisted versus spontaneously conceived pregnancies are shown in Table 9-1. Among singleton pregnancies, those resulting from infertility treatments had significantly more bleeding, pregnancy-induced hypertension, placenta previa, cesarean deliveries, and prematurity, and the infants were more likely to have very low birth weight or low birth weight, have congenital anomalies, and need admission to a neonatal intensive care unit (NICU). For singleton and twin pregnancies from infertility treatments, the rates of stillbirth and perinatal death were significantly higher. Because of small numbers, most differences in twin and triplet pregnancies according to method of conception were not significant. There may be differences in assisted versus spontaneous conceptions that confound these results, such as maternal differences in age, pregravid weight, parity, smoking and alcohol use, entry to care, weight gain, and iron status. Two recent large studies of twin pregnancies reported significant differences in assisted versus spontaneous conception, including racial distribution, parity, smoking habits, height and pregravid weight, chorionicity and length of gestation (43,44).

Table 9-1. Comparison of obstetric and neonatal outcomes by assisted versus spontaneous conception

Factor	Singletons			Twins			Triplets		
	ART	Spontaneous	Significance[a]	ART	Spontaneous	Significance	ART	Spontaneous	Significance
Maternal & Obstetric (n)	**3,551**	**4,035**		**1,366**	**129**		**16**	**16**	
Nulliparity (%)	10.7	7.1	NS	73.2	74.1	NS			
Prenatal hospitalization (%)							75	50	NS
Bleeding (%)	15.5	10.3	.001	18.4	14.3	NS	31.3	37.5	NS
PPROM (%)				14.3	19.4	NS	18.8	12.5	NS
PIH (%)	11.7	7.2	.001	16.6	18.6	NS	18.8	62.5	NS
Preterm labor (%)				35.7	26.9	NS			
Gestational diabetes (%)				14.2	14.8	NS	6.3	18.8	NS
Cerclage (%)				5.4	4.6	NS	31.3	0	NS
Placenta previa (%)	3	1.3	.01	0	0	NS	0		
Cesarean delivery (%)	24.8	16.3	$p < .0001$	46.8	61.9	NS			
Gestation <37 weeks (%)	12.3	6.9	$p < .0001$	56	37.8	$p = .05$	100	75	NS
Neonatal (n)	**3,258**	**3,258**		**2,594**	**2,698**		**48**	**48**	
NICU admission (%)	20.7	16.3	$p < .0001$	7	6.8	NS	48		

continued

Table 9-1. Continued

Factor	Singletons			Twins			Triplets		
	ART	Spontaneous	Significance[a]	ART	Spontaneous	Significance	ART	Spontaneous	Significance
Anomalies (%)	2.8	2.0	p = .04	3.5	2.9	NS			
Birth weight <1,500 g (%)	2.4	0.7	p < .0001						
Birth weight <2,500 g (%)	10.2	5.5	p < .0001	46.9	37.5	NS	100	100	NS
Stillbirth rate[b]	9.8	1.97	p = .0001	12.1	21.9	p = .006	41.7	0	NS
Perinatal death rate[b]	13.5	6.3	p = .006	24.3	39.3	p = .002	62.5	62.5	NS

Singletons, ART versus spontaneous[c]

Bleeding	1.59	(1.18–2.15)
PIH	1.69	(1.20–2.39)
Placenta previa	2.44	(1.16–5.17)
Cesarean delivery	1.69	(1.51–1.90)
Gestation <37 weeks	1.89	(1.38–2.60)

[a] $p < .05$, two-sided.
[b] Per 1,000 conceptions.
[c] Odds ratios and 95% confidence intervals.
ART, assisted reproductive technology; NS, not significant; PPROM, preterm premature rupture of membranes; PIH, pregnancy-induced hypertension; NICU, neonatal intensive care unit.
From Tallo et al., 1995 (33); Fitzsimmons et al., 1998 (37); Dhont et al., 1999 (98); Petersen et al., 1995 (99); Verlaenen et al., 1995 (100).

Residual Effects of Multifetal Pregnancy Reduction

As discussed in Chapter 4, even after reduction, there is some residual high risk, including shorter gestation, lower birth weight, and higher incidence of growth retardation, possibly related to a reduction in total endometrial function, with declines in insulin-like growth factor binding protein 1 (IGFBP-1), placental protein 14 (PP14), human chorionic gonadotropin, estradiol, and progesterone (45,46). In addition, there is a small risk to the mother of developing disseminated intravascular coagulopathy (47). This rare complication is thought to be caused by the release of thromboplastic material into the maternal circulation.

ANTENATAL ADAPTATIONS AND RISKS

Cardiovascular

Cardiac Function

Adaptations to a multiple pregnancy include a significant expansion of the plasma volume above singleton levels and an increase in cardiac output that may be 50% or more above normal. In the absence of underlying cardiac disease, such as mitral valve stenosis, these increased cardiac demands are tolerated uneventfully. However, when additional cardiovascular stresses are imposed, such as tocolytic therapy, infection, or iatrogenic fluid overload, serious cardiovascular complications can occur. Tocolytic therapy for multiple gestations increases the risk of pulmonary edema, myocardial ischemia, and maternal tachyarrhythmia. Although all these complications are infrequent, women pregnant with multiples should be carefully monitored while receiving tocolytic therapy, and intravenous fluids should be restricted to less than 2,000 mL per day. The increasing frequency of higher-order multiple pregnancies among older women has also been associated with an increasing risk of cardiomyopathy (48).

Hematologic Profile

Iron Deficiency Anemia. From about 20 weeks' gestation onward, the plasma volume in multiple gestations is about 20% greater than in singleton pregnancies. Total red blood cell volume also increases about 25% above singleton levels in multiple gestation. This is indicative of a markedly increased oxygen-carrying capacity required for the oxygen transfer for more than one fetus. The increase in red blood cell volume is not as great as that of the plasma, resulting in a more exaggerated hemodilution. The hemoglobin concentration of women pregnant with twins averages 10 g/dL from 20 weeks' gestation onward (see Chapter 6). For women with adequate iron stores, hemoglobin and hematocrit values begin to decline during the first trimester, reach a nadir by the end of the second trimester, and gradually rise again during the third trimester. Multiple gestation imposes a special demand for iron, which may not be met among women with low or absent iron stores. Hemoglobin levels below 11 g/dL during the first and third trimesters, when accompanied by a serum ferritin concentration less than 12 µg/dL are characteristic of iron deficiency anemia. As shown in Table 9-2, the incidence of iron deficiency anemia in multiple pregnancy ranges from 21% to 36%, which is two- to threefold higher than in singleton pregnancies.

Table 9-2. Maternal complications by plurality

	Singletons	Twins	Triplets	Quadruplets
No. of pregnancies	63,078	2,000	1,014	165
Antepartum complications				
Hospital admission (%)		27	53	75
Hospital length of stay (d, range of means)		11–16.5	10–42	44.5–56
Hyperemesis (admission, %)		—	46	40
Preterm labor (%)		35	70	94
Anemia (%)		21	36	24
Preeclampsia (%)		14	21	40
PPROM* (%)	3	15	20	14
Cerclage (%)		4	13	26
Gestational diabetes mellitus (%)	4	7	9	11
Urinary tract infections (%)		9	6	20
Acute fatty liver (%)			5	
Pulmonary edema (%)		1	8	6
Postpartum complications				
Hemorrhage (%)		6	12	21
Transfusion (%)			8	13
Endometritis (%)		8	19	11
Readmission (%)			11	

PPROM, preterm premature rupture of membranes.
Data from
Singletons: Gardner et al., 1995 (101); Schwartz et al., 1999 (102).
Twins: Fitzsimmons et al., 1998 (37); Gardner et al., 1995 (101); Porreco et al., 1991 (103); Silver et al., 1997 (104); Boulot et al., 1993 (105); Lipitz et al., 1994 (106); Lipitz et al., 1996 (107); Seoud et al., 1992 (108); Santema et al., 1995 (109); Alexander et al., 1995 (110); Groutz et al., 1996 (111); Macones et al., 1993 (112).
Triplets: Fitzsimmons et al., 1998 (37); Porreco et al., 1991 (103); Boulot et al., 1993 (105); Lipitz et al., 1994 (106); Seoud et al., 1992 (108); Santema et al., 1995 (109); Albrecht and Tomich, 1996 (78); Malone et al., 1998 (80); Thorp et al., 1994 (81); Peaceman et al., 1992 (82); Sassoon et al., 1990 (113); Melgar et al., 1991 (114); Smith-Levitan et al., 1996 (115); Weissman et al., 1991 (116); Newman et al., 1989, 1991 (117,118); Bollen et al., 1993 (119); Gonen et al., 1990 (120); Kaufman et al., 1998 (121); Vervliet et al., 1989 (122); Creinin et al., 1991 (123).
Quadruplets: Elliott and Radin, 1992 (79); Seoud et al., 1992 (108); Groutz et al., 1996 (111); Gonen et al., 1990 (120); Collins and Bleyl, 1990 (124); Pons et al., 1996 (125).

Postpartum Hemorrhage.   Postpartum hemorrhage oft
caused by uterine atony, retention of placental tissue, surgica
mechanical trauma to the uterine tissue, pharmacological effec
at the cellular level, or a combination of these factors. As show
in Figure 9-1, the fundal height of women pregnant with multiples reaches singleton term size at 32 weeks for twins, 28 weeks
for triplets, and 24 weeks for quadruplets. The risk of postpartum
hemorrhage increases with higher plurality, and is compounded by
certain underlying maternal characteristics, such as advanced
maternal age, obesity, and higher parity, as well as associated
obstetrical factors, such as surgical delivery and the use of magnesium sulfate to manage preeclampsia. In a British population-
based study of postpartum hemorrhage, defined as blood loss of
1,000 mL or more in the 24 hours following delivery, significant
risk factors included abruptio placentae, placenta previa, obesity,
multiple pregnancy, retained placenta, induced labor, cesarean
delivery, and birth weight of 4 kg or more (49). The risk ratio (RR)
for multiple pregnancy in this study was 4.46 (99% CI, 3.01–6.61).
Among singletons, the risk of postpartum hemorrhage was about
1.2% (49), compared with 6% among twins, 12% among triplets,
and 21% among quadruplets (Table 9-2). Compared with twins,
the risk of postpartum hemorrhage is twofold higher for triplets
and fourfold higher for quadruplets (Table 9-3).

Pregnancy-induced Hypertension

One of the major complications associated with multiple pregnancy is pregnancy-induced hypertension and preeclampsia. As
shown in Tables 9-1 and 9-2, the incidence of pregnancy-induced
hypertension is about 7% for singletons, 14% for twins, 21% for
triplets, and 40% for quadruplets. Reported frequencies range from
13% to 37% for twin pregnancies and even higher for triplets
(50,51). In a population-based study of singleton and twin births
in the state of Washington, Conrad et al. (52) found a fourfold
higher risk of preeclampsia among women carrying twins; the
risk increased to 14-fold higher among primigravidas. The most
common presentation among higher-order multiples is maternal
symptoms typical of severe preeclampsia associated with laboratory abnormalities consistent with HELLP syndrome (hemolysis,
elevated liver function, and low platelets).

Metabolic and Gastrointestinal Disorders

Carbohydrate Metabolism

During pregnancy an alteration in carbohydrate metabolism
causes a decrease in fasting glucose level and an exaggeration of
the insulin response to eating. In both diabetic and twin gestations,
these changes are magnified, particularly during the second half of
pregnancy, and cause accelerated starvation (53). Women pregnant with multiples have significantly lower blood glucose and
insulin levels, and higher plasma levels of β-hydroxybutyrate than
do women pregnant with singletons (53). These differences indicate
more rapid depletion of glycogen stores and resultant metabolism
of fat between meals and during an overnight fast.

Glucose intolerance also is more common in multiple gestations
due to elevated levels of placental hormones in proportion to the

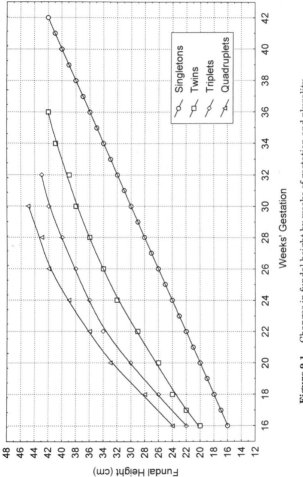

Figure 9-1. Changes in fundal height by weeks of gestation and plurality.

Table 9-3. Risk of maternal complications by plurality as odds ratio and 95% confidence interval

	Singleton	Twins	Triplets	Quadruplets
No. of pregnancies	63,078	2,000	1,014	165
Antepartum complications				
PPROM	1.0	5.8 (4.9–6.8)	7.9 (6.4–9.8)	5.4 (1.4–25.3)
Gestational diabetes mellitus	1.0	1.8 (1.4–2.2)	2.4 (1.5–3.6)	2.7 (1.2–5.9)
Hospital admission		1.0	3.1 (2.1–4.8)	8.2 (0.7–57.2)
Preterm labor		1.0	4.2 (3.4–5.1)	14.1 (8.4–23.9)
Anemia		1.0	2.2 (1.3–3.6)	1.2 (0.6–2.1)
Preeclampsia		1.0	1.6 (1.3–2.1)	4.1 (2.6–6.5)
PPROM		1.0	1.4 (1.1–1.8)	0.9 (0.2–4.4)
Cerclage		1.0	3.7 (1.8–7.9)	8.7 (4.0–19.4)
Gestational diabetes mellitus		1.0	1.3 (0.8–2.2)	1.5 (0.7–3.4)
Pulmonary edema		1.0	7.8 (0.7–88.7)	5.7 (0.6–39.8)
Postpartum complications				
Hemorrhage		1.0	2.0 (0.7–6.5)	4.0 (1.3–13.5)
Endometritis		1.0	2.8 (0.3–20.9)	1.5 (0.2–12.2)

PPROM, preterm premature rupture of membranes.
Source: Same as Table 9-2.

increased placental volume. Sicuranza et al. (54) found a twofold higher incidence of abnormal glucose screen results and a threefold higher incidence of gestational diabetes among multiple than among singleton pregnancies. As shown in Table 9-2, the incidence of gestational diabetes is 4% among singletons, 7% among twins, 9% among triplets, and 11% among quadruplets. It is still recommended that glucose screening (with a 50-g dose) be performed between 24 and 28 weeks' gestation. If these results are 140 mg/dL or greater, the 3-hour oral glucose tolerance test (with a 100-g dose) is performed. Gestational diabetes is also significantly increased among women receiving β-adrenergic agents and corticosteroids for preterm labor (55,56). Terbutaline also significantly increases the basal metabolic rate and decreases insulin sensitivity.

Hyperemesis

Hyperemesis in the first trimester of pregnancy should always suggest the possibility of a multiple pregnancy. An increase in nausea and vomiting is common in twin and triplet pregnancies and may be associated with substantially elevated levels of β human chorionic gonadotropin. The treatment of hyperemesis in a multiple pregnancy is the same as for singletons. For the majority of patients, the symptoms improve spontaneously between 10 and 12 weeks of gestation.

Preterm Labor

Multiples are at very high risk for preterm labor and premature delivery. Gestational age at onset of labor is related to increasing plurality (57). As shown in Table 9-2, 35% of twin, 70% of triplet, and 94% of quadruplet pregnancies are complicated by preterm labor. Heffner et al. (58) reported the risk (AOR) of preterm labor in twin gestations to be 41.1 (95% CI, 9.3–182). On a national basis, 57% of multiple births deliver before 37 weeks' gestation, compared to 10% of singletons (24). The use of β-sympathomimetic tocolytic agents carries the potential risk of maternal complications, often magnified in multiple gestations. The most serious of these is pulmonary edema, which can result in maternal death (59). Predisposing factors that increase the risk of pulmonary edema include prolonged tocolytic therapy, multiple pregnancy, iatrogenic fluid overload, and occult sepsis or chorioamnionitis (60). Because tocolysis is most effective before substantial cervical dilatation occurs (less than 2 cm), early detection of preterm labor is critical. For twins, shortened cervical length (25 mm or less) has been reported to be the best predictor of spontaneous preterm birth before 32 weeks' gestation (61). Programs that have focused on educating women about the signs and symptoms of preterm labor and teaching self-palpation to help women detect the increasing rate of uterine contractions have had mixed results. It has been reported that only 15% of contractions are detected by patients, and that only 11% of pregnant women are able to identify half of their recorded contractions (62).

The results of studies of singleton pregnancies using ambulatory tocodynamometry have been conflicting. Some have shown that preterm labor is diagnosed earlier, tocolysis is more effective, and the pregnancy is more likely to continue to term among women who undergo monitoring (63–68). Others have reported no differences between monitored and unmonitored pregnancies (69–72). In 1993, the U.S. Preventive Services Task Force issued a policy statement concluding that there was insufficient evidence of clinical effectiveness to recommend for or against home uterine activity monitoring (HUAM; 73,74). A metaanalysis of six randomized, controlled trials of HUAM showed that among singleton pregnancies, the use of HUAM was associated with a significant reduction (24%) in risk of preterm birth (RR, 0.76; 95% CI, 0.59–0.98), but not in risk of preterm labor with cervical dilatation more than 2 cm (RR, 0.67; 95% CI, 0.34–1.32) (75). In twin pregnancies, however, the use of HUAM was associated with a 66% reduction in preterm labor with cervical dilation more than 2 cm (RR, 0.44; 95% CI, 0.25–0.78), but not in preterm birth (RR, 1.01; 95% CI, 0.79–1.30).

Newman et al. (76) reported that when HUAM is used, preterm labor in singleton and twin pregnancies but not in triplet pregnancies is preceded by a significant increase in contractions. Knuppel et al. (77) reported that for twin pregnancies, the use of HUAM resulted in earlier detection of preterm labor and fewer deliveries due to failed tocolysis. The use and effectiveness of HUAM with multiple gestations, though, is inconsistent. Some centers routinely use it for all triplet or quadruplet pregnancies (78,79). Others have either discontinued its use (80) or have never used it (81,82). Some of this difference stems from the philosophy of home-based versus hospital-based care of women with multifetal pregnancies, particularly triplet and quadruplet pregnancies, with a more intensive testing and monitoring of the latter on a periodic or continuous basis. For example, Elliott and Radin (79), in their prenatal management of quadruplet pregnancies, report using HUAM starting at 18 weeks, with hospitalization as necessary. In France, Pons et al. (35) treating 21 women with triplet pregnancies, and Papiernik et al. (83) treating 197 women with twin pregnancies, provided a standard of care that included regular home visits by a midwife. Studies of preventive hospitalization of women pregnant with twins, in the absence of preterm labor, have consistently reported no significant therapeutic effect (84–87).

PSYCHOLOGICAL AND SOCIAL RISKS

The diagnosis of multiple pregnancy carries with it a series of physical and emotional stresses that span from conception through several years after the delivery. As discussed in this chapter, the frequency and severity of antepartum and postpartum complications are greater with multiple pregnancies, and increase with higher plurality. The likelihood of repeated and prolonged hospitalizations, early work leave, and bed rest is greater with multiples, leading to feelings of isolation and depression.

Although some women are delighted to receive the news that they are pregnant with multiples, particularly twins, many express feelings of fear, despair, and anxiety about bringing their children home from the hospital (88). As with parents of very low birth weight infants (89,90), depression and psychological stress are common among mothers of multiples (91,92) and are compounded by fatigue, marital, and financial problems (93,94). While many of these problems resolve by the time the children are school age, there is a higher risk for child abuse in these families as a result of the additional stresses (95–97).

In addition to physical help with raising multiples, Goshen-Gottstein (88) recommends psychological intervention to help mothers work through their ambivalence about having more than one baby at a time. It is particularly important to enable mothers to express their fears and negative feelings soon after giving birth. Psychological intervention may also be necessary to enable some mothers to individualize their children, and to help her foster the growth of her multiples as different persons.

CLINICAL CONSIDERATIONS AND KEY POINTS

- Tocolytic therapy for multiple gestations increases the risk of pulmonary edema, myocardial ischemia, and maternal tachyarrhythmia.
- The incidence of iron-deficiency anemia in multiple pregnancy ranges from 21% to 36%, which is two- to threefold higher than in singleton pregnancies.
- The incidence of pregnancy-induced hypertension is about 7% for singleton, 14% for twin, 21% for triplet, and 40% for quadruplet pregnancies.
- The incidence of gestational diabetes is 4% for singleton, 7% for twin, 9% for triplet, and 11% for quadruplet pregnancies.
- The incidence of preterm labor is 35% for twin, 70% for triplet, and 94% for quadruplet pregnancies.
- The likelihood of repeated and prolonged hospitalizations, early work leave, and bed rest is greater for women pregnant with multiples, leading to feelings of isolation and depression.
- As with parents of very low birth weight infants, depression and psychological stress are common among mothers of multiples. These feelings are compounded by fatigue, marital, and financial problems, and a higher risk for child abuse.

REFERENCES

1. Kogan MD, Martin JA, Alexander GR, et al. The changing pattern of prenatal care utilization in the United States, 1981–1995, using different prenatal care indices. *JAMA* 1998;279:1623–1628.
2. Haas JS, Berman S, Goldberg AB, et al. Prenatal hospitalization and compliance with guidelines for prenatal care. *Am J Public Health* 1996;86:815–819.
3. Luke B, Bigger HR, Leurgans S, et al. The cost of prematurity: a case–control study of twins vs singletons. *Am J Public Health* 1996;86:809–814.
4. Bouvier Colle MH, Varnoux N, et al. Case–control study of risk factors for obstetric patients' admission to intensive care units. *Eur J Obstet Gynecol Reprod Biol* 1997;79:173–177.
5. Salanave B, Bouvier-Colle MH. The likely increase in maternal mortality rates in the United Kingdom and in France until 2005. *Paediatr Perinat Epidemiol* 1996;10:418–422.
6. Berkowitz GS, Skovron ML, Lapinski RH, et al. Delayed childbearing and the outcome of pregnancy. *N Engl J Med* 1990;322:659–664.
7. Yasin SY, Beydoun SN. Pregnancy outcome at ≥20 weeks' gestation in women in their 40s: a case–control study. *J Reprod Med* 1988;33:209–213.

8. Edge VL, Laros RK. Pregnancy outcome in nulliparous aged 35 or older. *Am J Obstet Gynecol* 1993;168:1881–188

9. Peipert JF, Bracken MB. Maternal age: an independent risk tor for cesarean delivery. *Obstet Gynecol* 1993;81:200–205.

10. Vercellini P, Zuliani G, Rognoni MT, et al. Pregnancy at for and over: a case–control study. *Eur J Obstet Gynecol Reprod Bio* 1993;48:191–195.

11. Prysak M, Lorenz RP, Kisly A. Pregnancy outcome in nulliparous women 35 years and older. *Obstet Gynecol* 1995;85:65–70.

12. Bianco A, Stone J, Lynch L, et al. Pregnancy outcome at age 40 and older. *Obstet Gynecol* 1996;87:917–922.

13. Dildy GA, Jackson M, Powers GK, et al. Very advanced maternal age: pregnancy after age 45. *Am J Obstet Gynecol* 1996;175:668–674.

14. Zhang J, Savitz DA. Maternal age and placenta previa: a population-based case–control study. *Am J Obstet Gynecol* 1993;168:641–645.

15. Williams MA, Mittendorf R. Increasing maternal age as a determinant of placenta previa: more important than increasing parity? *J Reprod Med* 1993;38:425–428.

16. Forman MR, Meirik O, Berendes HW. Delayed childbearing in Sweden. *JAMA* 1984;252:3135–3139.

17. Kiely JL, Paneth N, Susser M. An assessment of the effects of maternal age and parity in different components of perinatal mortality. *Am J Epidemiol* 1986;123:444–454.

18. Cnattingius S, Forman MR, Berendes HW, et al. Delayed childbearing and risk of adverse perinatal outcome: a population-based study. *JAMA* 1992;268:886–890.

19. Cnattingius S, Berendes HW, Forman MR. Do delayed childbearers face increased risks of adverse pregnancy outcomes after the first birth? *Obstet Gynecol* 1993;81:512–516.

20. Aldous MB, Edmonson MB. Maternal age at first childbirth and risk of low birth weight and preterm delivery in Washington State. *JAMA* 1993;270:2574–2577.

21. Fretts RC, Schmittdiel J, McLean FH, et al. Increased maternal age and the risk of fetal death. *N Engl J Med* 1995;333:953–957.

22. Abma JC, Chandra A, Mosher WD, et al. Fertility, family planning, and women s health: new data from the 1995 National Survey of Family Growth. *Vital Health Stat 23* 1997;(19):1–114.

23. Chandra A, Stephen EH. Impaired fecundity in the United States: 1982–95. *Fam Plann Perspect* 1998;30:34–42.

24. Ventura SJ, Martin JA, Curtin SC, et al. Report of final natality statistics, 1996. *Mon Vital Stat Rep* 1998;46(11 Suppl):1–99.

25. Ventura SJ, Martin JA, Curtin SC, et al. Births: final data for 1998. *Natl Vital Stat Rep* 2000;48(3):1–100.

26. Qasim SM, Karacan M, Corsan GH, et al. High-order oocyte transfer in gamete intrafallopian transfer patients 40 or more years of age. *Fertil Steril* 1995;64:107–110.

27. Widra EA, Gindoff PR, Smotrich DB, et al. Achieving multiple-order embryo transfer identifies women over 40 years of age with improved in vitro fertilization outcome. *Fertil Steril* 1996;65:103–108.

28. Sauer MV, Paulson RJ, Lobo RA. Triplet pregnancy in a 51-year-old woman after oocyte donation. *Am J Obstet Gynecol* 1995;172:1044–1045.

.auer MV, Paulson RJ, Lobo RA. Pregnancy in women 50 or more years of age: outcomes of 22 consecutively established pregnancies from oocyte donation. *Fertil Steril* 1995;64:111–115.

0. Legro RS, Wong IL, Paulson RJ, et al. Recipient's age does not adversely affect pregnancy outcome after oocyte donation. *Am J Obstet Gynecol* 1995;172:96–100.

31. Evans MI, Hume RF, Polak S, et al. The geriatric gravida: multifetal pregnancy reduction, donor eggs, and aggressive infertility treatments. *Am J Obstet Gynecol* 1997;177:875–878.

32. Haning RV Jr, Goldsmith LT, Seifer DB, et al. Relaxin secretion in IVF pregnancies. *Am J Obstet Gynecol* 1996;174:233–240.

33. Tallo CP, Vohr B, Oh W, et al. Maternal and neonatal morbidity associated with in vitro fertilization. *J Pediatr* 1995;127:794–800.

34. Syrop CH, Varner MW. Triplet gestation: maternal and neonatal implications. *Acta Genet Med Gemellol (Roma)* 1985;34:81–88.

35. Pons JC, Mayenga JM, Plu G, et al. Management of triplet pregnancy. *Acta Genet Med Gemellol (Roma)* 1988;37:99–103.

36. Holcberg G, Biale Y, Lewenthal H, et al. Outcome of pregnancy in 31 triplet gestations. *Obstet Gynecol* 1982;59:472–476.

37. Fitzsimmons BP, Bebbington MW, Fluker MR. Perinatal and neonatal outcomes in multiple gestations: assisted reproduction versus spontaneous conception. *Am J Obstet Gynecol* 1998;179:1162–1167.

38. Bell RJ, Eddie LW, Lester AR, et al. Relaxin in human pregnancy serum measured with a homologous radioimmunoassay. *Obstet Gynecol* 1987;69:585–589.

39. Wang JX, Clark AM, Kirby CA, et al. The obstetric outcome of singleton pregnancies following in-vitro fertilization/gamete intra-fallopian transfer. *Hum Reprod* 1994;9:141–146.

40. Tanbo T, Dale PO, Lunde O, et al. Obstetric outcome in singleton pregnancies after assisted reproduction. *Obstet Gynecol* 1995;86:188–192.

41. McClure N, Leya J, Radwanska E, et al. Luteal phase support and severe ovarian hyperstimulation syndrome. *Hum Reprod* 1992;7:758–764.

42. Haning RV Jr, Steinetz B, Weiss G. Elevated serum relaxin levels in multiple pregnancy following menotropin treatment. *Obstet Gynecol* 1985;66:42–45.

43. Luke B, Gillespie B, Min SJ, et al. Critical periods of maternal weight gain: effect on twin birth weight. *Am J Obstet Gynecol* 1997;177:1055–1062.

44. Luke B, Min SJ, Gillespie B, et al. The importance of early weight gain in the intrauterine growth and birthweight of twins. *Am J Obstet Gynecol* 1998;179:1155–1161.

45. Johnson MR, Abbas A, Nicolaides KH. Maternal plasma levels of human chorionic gonadotropin, oestradiol and progesterone before and after fetal reduction. *J Endocrinol* 1994;143:309–312.

46. Abbas A, Johnson M, Chard T, et al. Maternal plasma concentrations of insulin-like growth factor binding protein-1 and placental protein 14 in multifetal pregnancies before and after fetal reduction. *Hum Reprod* 1995;10:207–210.

47. Stone J, Berkowitz RL. Multifetal pregnancy reduction and selective termination. *Semin Perinatol* 1995;19:363–374.

48. Ikeda S, Hasegawa A, Nagai R. Peripartum cardiomyopathy of multiple pregnancy. *Ryoikibetsu Shokogun Shirizu* 1996;14: 170–173.
49. Stones RW, Paterson CM, Saunders NJS. Risk factors for major obstetric haemorrhage *Eur J Obstet Gynecol Reprod Biol* 1993;48: 15–18.
50. McMullen PF, Norman RJ, Marivate M. Pregnancy-induced hypertension in twin pregnancy. *Br J Obstet Gynaecol* 1984;91: 240–248.
51. Spellacy WN, Handler A, Ferre CD. A case-controlled study of 1,253 twin pregnancies from 1982–1987 perinatal database. *Obstet Gynecol* 1990;75:168–171.
52. Coonrod DV, Hickok DE, Zhu K, et al. Risk factors for preeclampsia in twin pregnancies: a population-based cohort study. *Obstet Gynecol* 1995;85:645–650
53. Casele HL, Dooley SL, Metzger BE. Metabolic response to meal eating and extended overnight fast in twin gestation. *Am J Obstet Gynecol* 1996;175:917–921.
54. Sicuranza GB, Weinstein L, Saltzman DH, et al. Incidence of gestational diabetes in multifetal gestations. *J Matern Fetal Invest* 1997;7:115 117.
55. Fisher JE, Smith RS, Lagrandeur R, et al. Gestational diabetes mellitus in women receiving beta-adrenergics and corticosteroids for threatened preterm delivery. *Obstet Gynecol* 1997;90:880–883.
56. Smigaj D, Roman-Drago NM, Amini SB, et al. The effect of oral terbutaline on maternal glucose metabolism and energy expenditure in pregnancy. *Am J Obstet Gynecol* 1998;178: 1041–1047.
57. Garite TJ, Bentley DL, Hamer CA, et al. Uterine activity characteristics in multiple gestations. *Obstet Gynecol* 1990;76:56S–59S.
58. Heffner LJ, Sherman CB, Speizer FE, et al. Clinical and environmental predictors of preterm labor. *Obstet Gynecol* 1993;81: 750–757.
59. Jacobs MM, Knight AB, Arias F. Maternal pulmonary edema resulting from betamimetic and glucocorticoid therapy. *Obstet Gynecol* 1980;56:56–59.
60. Hill WC. Risks and complications of tocolysis. *Clin Obstet Gynecol* 1995;38:725–745.
61. Goldenberg RL, Iams JD, Miodovnik M, et al. The preterm prediction study: risk factors in twin gestations. *Am J Obstet Gynecol* 1996;175:1047–1053.
62. Newman RB, Gill RJ, Wittreich P, et al. Maternal perception of prelabor uterine activity. *Obstet Gynecol* 1986;160:1172–1178.
63. Katz M, Gill PJ, Newman RB. Detection of preterm labor by ambulatory monitoring of uterine activity: a preliminary report. *Obstet Gynecol* 1986;68:773–778.
64. Morrison JC, Martin JN, Martin RW, et al. Prevention of preterm birth by ambulatory assessment of uterine activity: a randomized study. *Am J Obstet Gynecol* 1987;156:536–543.
65. Watson DL, Welch RA, Mariona FG, et al. Management of preterm labor patients at home: does daily uterine activity monitoring and nursing support make a difference? *Obstet Gynecol* 1990;76:32S–35S.

66. Hill WC, Fleming AD, Martin RW, et al. Home uterine activity monitoring is associated with a reduction in preterm birth. *Obstet Gynecol* 1990;76:13S–18S.
67. Mou SM, Sunderji SG, Gall S, et al. Multicenter randomized clinical trial of home uterine activity monitoring for detection of preterm labor. *Am J Obstet Gynecol* 1991;165:858–866.
68. Wapner RJ, Cotton DB, Artal R, et al. A randomized multicenter trial assessing a home uterine activity monitoring device used in the absence of daily nursing contact. *Am J Obstet Gynecol* 1995; 172:1026–1034.
69. Iams JD, Johnson FF, O'Shaughnessy RW, et al. A prospective random trial of home uterine activity monitoring in pregnancies at increased risk of preterm labor. *Am J Obstet Gynecol* 1987;157: 638–643.
70. Iams JD, Johnson FF, O'Shaughnessy RW, et al. A prospective random trial of home uterine activity monitoring in pregnancies at increased risk of preterm labor, II. *Am J Obstet Gynecol* 1988; 159:595–603.
71. Dyson DC, Crites YM, Ray DA, et al. Prevention of preterm birth in high-risk patients: the role of education and provider contact versus home uterine monitoring. *Am J Obstet Gynecol* 1991; 164:756–762.
72. Blondel B, Breart G, Berthoux Y, et al. Home uterine activity monitoring in France: a randomized controlled trial. *Am J Obstet Gynecol* 1992;167:424–429.
73. US Preventive Services Task Force. Home uterine activity monitoring for preterm labor: policy statement. *JAMA* 1993;270: 369–370.
74. US Preventive Services Task Force. Home uterine activity monitoring for preterm labor: review article. *JAMA* 1993;270: 371–376.
75. Colton T, Kayne HL, Zhang Y, et al. A metaanalysis of home uterine activity monitoring. *Am J Obstet Gynecol* 1995;173: 1499–1505.
76. Newman RB, Gill PJ, Campion S, et al. The influence of fetal number on antepartum uterine activity. *Obstet Gynecol* 1989;73: 695–699.
77. Knuppel RA, Lake MF, Watson DL, et al. Preventing preterm birth in twin gestation: home uterine activity monitoring and perinatal nursing support. *Obstet Gynecol* 1990;76:24S–27S.
78. Albrecht JL, Tomich PG. The maternal and neonatal outcome of triplet gestations. *Am J Obstet Gynecol* 1996;174:1551–1556.
79. Elliott JP, Radin TG. Quadruplet pregnancy: contemporary management and outcome. *Obstet Gynecol* 1992;80:421–424.
80. Malone FD, Kaufman GE, Chelmow D, et al. Maternal morbidity associated with triplet pregnancy. *Am J Perinatol* 1998;15: 73–77.
81. Thorp JM, Tumey LA, Bowes WA. Outcome of multifetal gestations: a case–control study. *J Matern Fetal Med* 1994;3:23–26.
82. Peaceman AM, Dooley SL, Tamura RK, et al. Antepartum management of triplet gestations. *Am J Obstet Gynecol* 1992;167: 1117–1120.
83. Papiernik E, Mussy MA, Vial M, et al. A low rate of perinatal deaths for twin births. *Acta Genet Med Gemellol (Roma)* 1985; 34:201–206.

84. Hartikainen-Sorri AL, Jouppila P. Is routine ho. needed in antenatal care of twin pregnancy? *J Pc* 1984;12:31–32.

85. Crowther CA, Neilson JP, Verkuyl DAA, et al. Pretern. in twin pregnancies: can it be prevented by hospital admi. *Br J Obstet Gynaecol* 1989;96:850–853.

86. MacLennan AH, Green RC, O'Shea R, et al. Routine hospi. admission in twin pregnancy between 26 and 30 weeks' gesta tion. *Lancet* 1990;335:267–269.

87. Saunders MC, Dick JS, Brown IM, et al. The effects of hospital admission for bed rest on the duration of twin pregnancy: a randomized trial. *Lancet* 1985;2:793–795.

88. Goshen-Gottstein ER. The mothering of twins, triplets and quadruplets. *Psychiatry* 1980;43:189–204.

89. Singer LT, Salvator A, Guo S, et al. Maternal psychological distress and parenting stress after the birth of a very low-birth-weight infant. *JAMA* 1999;281:799–805.

90. Cronin CMG, Shapiro CR, Casiro OG, et al. The impact of very low-birth-weight infants on the family is long lasting: a matched control study. *Arch Pediatr Adolesc Med* 1995;149:151–158.

91. Garel M, Blondel B. Assessment at 1 year of the psychological consequences of having triplets. *Hum Reprod* 1992;7:729–732.

92. Thorpe K, Golding J, MacGillivray I, et al. Comparison of prevalence of depression in mothers of twins and mothers of singletons. *Br Med J* 1991;302:875–878.

93. Yokoyama Y, Shimizu T, Hayakawa K. Childcare problems and maternal fatigue symptoms in families with twins and triplets. *Jpn J Public Health* 1995;42:187–193.

94. Bryan EM. The consequences to the family of triplets or more. *J Perinat Med* 1991;19 (Suppl 19):24–25.

95. Groothuis JR, Altemeier WA, Robarge JP, et al. Increased child abuse in families with twins. *Pediatrics* 1982;70:769–773.

96. Hansen KK. Twins and child abuse. *Arch Pediatr Adolesc Med* 1994;148:1345–1346.

97. Robarge JP, Reynolds ZB, Groothuis JR. Increased child abuse in families with twins. *Res Nurs Health* 1982;5:199–203.

98. Dhont M, De Sutter P, Ruyssinck G, et al. Perinatal outcome of pregnancies after assisted reproduction: a case–control study. *Am J Obstet Gynecol* 1999;181:688–695.

99. Petersen K, Hornnes PJ, Ellingsen S, et al. Perinatal outcome after in vitro fertilization. *Acta Obstet Gynecol Scand* 1995;74:129–131.

100. Verlaenen H, Cammu H, Derde MP, et al. Singleton pregnancy after in vitro fertilization: expectations and outcome. *Obstet Gynecol* 1995;86:906–910.

101. Gardner MO, Goldenberg RL, Cliver SP, et al. The origin and outcome of preterm twin pregnancies. *Obstet Gynecol* 1995;85:553–557.

102. Schwartz DB, Daoud Y, Gazula P, et al. Gestational diabetes mellitus: metabolic and blood glucose parameters in singleton versus twin pregnancies. *Am J Obstet Gynecol* 1999;181:912–914.

103. Porreco RP, Burke MS, Hendrix ML. Multifetal reduction of triplets and pregnancy outcome. *Obstet Gynecol* 1991;78:335–339.

RK, Helfand BT, Russell TL, et al. Multifetal reduction ...ses the risk of preterm delivery and fetal growth restric- ... in twins: a case–control study. *Fertil Steril* 1997;67:30–33.

...ulot P, Hedon B, Pelliccia G, et al. Effects of selective reduction .n triplet gestation: a comparative study of 80 cases managed with or without this procedure. *Fertil Steril* 1993;60:497–503.

6. Lipitz S, Reichman B, Uval J, et al. A prospective comparison of the outcome of triplet pregnancies managed expectantly or by multifetal reduction to twins. *Am J Obstet Gynecol* 1994;170: 874–879.

107. Lipitz S, Uval J, Achiron R, et al. Outcome of twin pregnancies reduced from triplets compared with nonreduced twin gestations. *Obstet Gynecol* 1996;87:511–514.

108. Seoud MAF, Toner JP, Kruithoff C, et al. Outcome of twin, triplet, and quadruplet in vitro fertilization pregnancies: the Norfolk experience. *Fertil Steril* 1992;57:825–834.

109. Santema JG, Bourdrez P, Wallenberg HCS. Maternal and perinatal complications in triplet compared with twin pregnancy. *Eur J Obstet Gynecol Reprod Biol* 1995;60:143–147.

110. Alexander JM, Hammond KR, Steinkampf MP. Multifetal reduction of high-order multiple pregnancy: comparison of obstetrical outcome with nonreduced twin gestations. *Fertil Steril* 1995;64: 1201–1203.

111. Groutz A, Yovel I, Amit A, et al. Pregnancy outcome after multifetal pregnancy reduction to twins compared with spontaneously conceived twins. *Hum Reprod* 1996;11:1334–1336.

112. Macones GA, Schemmer G, Pritts E, et al. Multifetal reduction of triplets improves perinatal outcome. *Am J Obstet Gynecol* 1993;169:982–986.

113. Sassoon DA, Castro LC, Davis JL, et al. Perinatal outcome in triplet versus twin gestations. *Obstet Gynecol* 1990;75:817–820.

114. Melgar CA, Rosenfeld DL, Rawlinson K, et al. Perinatal outcome after multifetal reduction to twins compared with nonreduced multiple gestations. *Obstet Gynecol* 1991;78:763–767.

115. Smith-Levitan M, Birholz J, Skupski DW, et al. Selective reduction of multifetal pregnancies to twins improves outcome over nonreduced triplet gestations. *Am J Obstet Gynecol* 1996;175: 878–882.

116. Weissman A, Yoffe N, Jakobi P, et al. Management of triplet pregnancies in the 1980s: are we doing better? *Am J Perinatol* 1991;8:333–337.

117. Newman RB, Hamer C, Miller MC. Outpatient triplet management: a contemporary review. *Am J Obstet Gynecol* 1989;161: 547–555.

118. Newman RB, Jones JS, Miller MC. Influence of clinical variables on triplet birth weight. *Acta Genet Med Gemellol (Roma)* 1991; 40:173–179.

119. Bollen N, Camus M, Tournaye H, et al. Embryo reduction in triplet pregnancies after assisted procreation: a comparative study. *Fertil Steril* 1993;60:504–509.

120. Gonen R, Heyman E, Asztalos EV, et al. The outcome of triplet, quadruplet, and quintuplet pregnancies managed in a perinatal unit: obstetric, neonatal, and follow-up data. *Am J Obstet Gynecol* 1990;162:454–459.

121. Kaufman GE, Malone FD, Harvey-Wilkes KB, e
     morbidity and mortality associated with triplet
     Obstet Gynecol 1998;91:342–348.
122. Vervliet J, De Cleyn K, Renier M, et al. Management
     come of 321 triplet and quadruplet pregnancies. *Eur J
     Gynecol Reprod Biol* 1989;33:61–69.
123. Creinin M, Katz M, Laros R. Triplet pregnancy: changes in r.
     bidity and mortality. *J Perinatol* 1991;11:207–212.
124. Collins MS, Bleyl JA. Seventy-one quadruplet pregnancies: man
     agement and outcome. *Am J Obstet Gynecol* 1990;162:1384–1392.
125. Pons JC, Charlemaine C, Dubreuil E, et al. Management and
     outcome of triplet pregnancy. *Eur J Obstet Gynecol Reprod Biol*
     1996;76:131–139.

Management of Triplet and Other High Order Multiples

In a review of 21 triplet births in 1958, Kurtz et al. (1) prefaced their article with the following statement, "Because of the rarity of triplet births, the human interest appeal of such an event is greater than its practical significance." In the four decades since that observation, the issue of high-order multifetal birth has evolved from an obstetrical curiosity to a significant medical and societal concern.

In 1921, Zeleny (2) modified Hellin's law to estimate the naturally occurring rate of triplet and higher-order multiple gestations with the following derivative equation: If the rate for twins is $1/n$, then the rate for triplets is $1/n^2$ and the rate for quadruplets is $1/n^3$. From this equation, it would be estimated that naturally occurring triplets would be born with a frequency of 1 in 6,400 to 7,910 livebirths on the basis of a natural occurrence rate of twins of 1 in 83 to 89 livebirths. Unfortunately, these estimates can no longer be considered accurate because the total number of multifetal gestations now represents the sum of naturally occurring multiples plus the number of iatrogenic multiple pregnancies. Iatrogenic multiple pregnancy is a previously unknown type of multiple birth that is the result of the use of assisted reproductive technology (ART) now available for couples with fertility problems (3).

As of 1990, the frequency of twins had risen to 1 in 43 pregnancies, and triplets were occurring approximately once in every 1,341 deliveries (4). These rates are much higher than would be expected on the basis of the Hellin-Zeleny hypothesis. In absolute numbers, multiple pregnancies had increased to record highs of 101,709 twins, 4,551 triplets, 365 quadruplets, and 57 quintuplets or higher-order births by 1995 (*Monthly Vital Statistics Report,* 1997). Nor do these trends show any sign of slowing. Between 1990 and 1996, rates of triplet birth rose from 861 to 1,361, quadruplets from 45 to 144, and quintuplets and more from 4.2 to 20.8 per million livebirths (5).

Increased rates of high-order multiples are associated with most ART, as follows: clomiphene citrate, 0.5% triplets, 0.3% quadruplets, and 0.13% quintuplets; hMG-hCG, 5% to 10% triplets or more; *in vitro* fertilization (IVF), 6% triplets with replacement of three embryos; and gamete intrafallopian transfer (GIFT), 8.5% triplets with three or more embryos (6–11). It is estimated that 50% to 60% of all triplets, 75% of all quadruplets, and virtually all quintuplet pregnancies are a result of ART.

The rate of naturally occurring high-order multiples also is increasing. Delayed childbirth is one contributor. Births to women older than 30 years in the United States have doubled to more than 30% in the last decade. The frequency of naturally occurring high-order multiples increases at the extremes of reproductive age, with multiparity, or with a family history of multiples (12–15). Approximately one-third of the increase in the triplet birth rate can be attributed to changes in the distribution of maternal ages (16).

The increasing frequency of high-order multip.
nied by high rates of perinatal morbidity, morta.
cost. Composite reviews of older and more contemp.
of triplet births indicate high but improving perinata.
rates, currently estimated to be approximately 100 p
livebirths (Table 10-1).

Collins and Bleyl (17) reported on 71 quadruplets with dat
lected from questionnaires completed by members of a supp
group for parents of high-order multiples (The Triplet Connectior.
The corrected perinatal mortality rate was 67 per 1,000 liveborn
quadruplets. This figure probably is an underestimation because of
ascertainment bias inherent with a questionnaire method. Other
investigators have reported outcomes with variable perinatal mortality rates ranging from as low as 0 to as high as 312 per 1,000
livebirths (Table 10-2).

Perinatal mortality is only the tip of the iceberg. Perinatal morbidity causes significant neonatal suffering, parental anguish, dr
matic expense, and leaves many survivors with long-term disabilities. More than 90% of triplet births are preterm (less than 37
weeks) and more than 40% of the infants are delivered at 32 weeks
or earlier. Almost one-third of triplets have a very low birth weight
(less than 1,500 g) and another third are small for gestational age
(18). The frequency of these morbidities is generally two- to threefold higher than for twin gestations and dramatically higher than
for singletons (Table 10-3). Primarily as a result of prematurity,
60% to 75% of triplets and 75% to 100% of quadruplets are admitted to a neonatal intensive care unit (NICU) for mean durations of
15 to 32 and 24 to 58 days, respectively. Triplets have rates of respiratory distress syndrome (RDS) ranging from 22.8% to 49.7%,
intraventricular hemorrhage (IVH) from 2% to 7.7%, neonatal
necrotizing enterocolitis (NEC) from 1% to 4%, and retinopathy of
prematurity (ROP) from 3% to 6.5% (19–23). The more limited data
available regarding quadruplet pregnancies suggest even higher
rates of morbid neonatal outcome, which is certainly what would
be intuitively expected. These complicated outcomes and prolonged
hospitalizations result in tremendous health care costs associated
with care of higher-order multiples. The total costs per triplet pregnancy may easily exceed $100,000 (24).

Another health care issue engendered by high-order multiples
is the long-term consequences and costs associated with the survivors of extreme prematurity and very low birth weight. It has
been estimated that approximately one-fifth of triplet pregnancies
and one-half of quadruplet pregnancies result in at least one child
with a serious mental or physical disability.

Lipitz et al. (25) provided 1-year follow-up data for 38 triplets
with birth weights less than 1,500 g. Four (11%) had severe
neurologic disabilities, including 1 infant with spastic diplegia
and normal intelligence and 3 infants with spastic quadriplegia
and marked developmental delay. Eight other infants (21%) had
milder developmental problems, such as attention deficit disorder or abnormal muscle tone. In a later report, Lipitz et al. (26)
provided long-term follow-up data on 8 sets of quadruplets, 2 sets
of quintuplets, and 1 set of sextuplets. Three-fourths of the liveborn infants weighed less than 1,500 g, and 30% of the survivors
had neurodevelopmental abnormalities.

(*text continues on page 199*)

Table 10-1. Historical trends in outcomes of triplet pregnancies

Reference	Study Years and Location	Pregnancies (sets)[a]	Weeks' Gestation	Average Birth Weight (g)[b]	Proportion of Deaths			Death Rate per 1,0		
					Stillbirth	Neonatal	Perinatal	Stillbirth	Neonatal	Perinata.
Kurtz et al., 1958 (1)	1931–56 Jersey City, NJ	21	32.7	2,006	5/63	8/58	13/63	79.4	137.9	206.3
Itzkowic, 1979 (35)	1946–76 London, UK	59	34.0	1,829	9/177	32/168	41/177	50.8	190.5	231.6
Michlewitz et al., 1981 (84)	1954–76 Boston	15	34.9	1,823	4/45	15/41	19/45	88.9	365.9	422.2
Daw, 1978 (85)	1958–77 Manchester, UK	14	34.7	1,848	5/42	8/37	13/42	119.0	216.2	309.5
Holcberg et al., 1982 (59)	1960–79 Beer-Sheba, Israel	31	32.1	1,711	9/93	20/84	29/93	96.8	238.1	311.8
Loucopoulos and Jewelewicz, 1982 (28)	1965–81 New York	22	35.8	2,011	3/75	6/72	9/75	40.0	83.3	120.0
Before 1975	6 studies	162 pregnancies (486 triplets)	34.0	1,871	35/495	89/460	124/495	70.7	193.5	250.5
Crowther and Hamilton, 1989 (86)	1975–84 Harare, Zimbabwe	105	32.5	1,651	30/315	73/285	103/315	95.2	256.1	327.0
Pons et al., 1988 (87)	1975–86 Clamart, France	21	36.0	1,710	2/63	5/61	7/63	31.7	82.0	111.1
Thiery et al., 1988 (88)	1975–86 Ghent, Belgium	10	33.9	1,909	1/30	2/29	3/30	33.3	69.0	100.0

Reference	Years & Location	Number								
Lipitz et al., 1989 (25)	1975–88 Tel Hashomer, Israel	78	33.2	1,772	10/225	11/215	21/225	44.4	51.2	93.3
Weissman et al., 1991 (81)	1978–87 Haifa, Israel	29	33.4	1,723	0/87	13/87	13/87	0.0	149.4	149.4
Gonen et al., 1990 (89)	1978–88 Ontario, Canada	24	32.4	1,582	2/72	3/70	5/72	27.8	42.9	69.4
Creinin et al., 1991 (90)	1981–88 San Francisco	16	33.9	1,875	9/48	0/39	9/48	187.5	0.0	187.5
Newman et al., 1989 (19)	1985–88 United States	198	33.6	1,871	13/584	16/571	29/584	22.3	28.0	49.7
Porreco et al., 1991 (91)	Not stated Denver	11	35.7	2,239	0/33	1/33	1/33	0.0	30.3	30.3
Levene et al., 1992 (92)	1989 United Kingdom	139	32.3	Not stated	2/417	3/415	5/417	4.8	7.2	12.0
1970's–1980's	10 studies	631 pregnancies (1,893 triplets)	33.7	1,815	69/1,874	127/1,805	196/1,874	36.8	70.4	104.6
Thorp et al., 1994 (93)	1980–90 Chapel Hill, NC	11	31.1	Not stated	1/33	3/32	4/33	30.3	93.7	121.2
Santema et al., 1995 (94)	1981–91 Rotterdam, The Netherlands	40	32.0	1,478	10/120	14/110	24/120	83.3	127.3	200.0
Seoud et al., 1992 (23)	1982–90 Norfolk, VA	15	31.8	1,666	0/45	0/45	0/45	0.0	0.0	0.0
Lipitz et al., 1994 (95)	1984–92 Tel Aviv, Israel	106	33.5	1,780	5/246	11/241	16/246	20.3	45.6	65.0
Boulot, 1993 (96)	1985–91 Montpellier, France	45	34.4	1,870	2/135	6/133	8/135	14.8	45.1	59.?
Fitzsimmons et al., 1998 (97)	1985–96 Vancouver, Canada	32	32.5	1,689	2/64	4/62	6/64	31.3	64.5	
Melgar et al., 1991 (98)	1987–90 Manhasset, NY	20	33.1	1,925	5/60	2/55	7/60	83.3	36	

Table 10-1. Continued

Reference	Study Years and Location	Pregnancies (sets)[a]	Weeks' Gestation	Average Birth Weight (g)[b]	Proportion of Deaths			Death Rate per 1,000		
					Stillbirth	Neonatal	Perinatal	Stillbirth	Neonatal	Perinatal
Bollen et al., 1993 (99)	1987–92 Brussels	32	32.5	1,668	6/96	16/90	22/96	62.5	177.8	229.2
Peaceman et al., 1992 (29)	1988–91 Chicago	15	34.7	1,957	0/45	1/45	1/45	0.0	22.2	22.2
Macones et al., 1993 (100)	1988–92 Philadelphia	43	31.2	1,593	6/129	21/123	27/129	46.5	170.7	209.3
Albrecht and Tomich, 1996 (20)	1989–94 Maywood, IL	57	33.0	1,820	2/161	5/159	7/161	12.4	31.4	43.5
Kaufman et al., 1998 (21)	1992–96 Boston	55	32.1	1,607	3/165	17/162	20/165	18.2	104.9	121.2
1980's–1990's	12 studies	471 pregnancies (1,413 triplets)	32.7	1,732	42/1,299	100/1,257	142/1,299	32.3	79.6	109.3

[a] Based on nonreduced pregnancies of 20 weeks' or more gestation.
[b] Birth weight is based on liveborn infants only and might have been calculated from presented data or may be the average of the first, second, and third triplets in a set.

Table 10-2. Historical trends in outcomes of quadruplet and quintuplet pregnancies

Reference	Study Years and Location	Pregnancies (sets)[a]	Weeks' Gestation	Average Birth Weight (g)[b]	Proportion of Deaths			Death Rate per 1,000		
					Stillbirth	Neonatal	Perinatal	Stillbirth	Neonatal	Perinatal
Quadruplets										
Pons et al., 1996 (101)	1972–88 Paris, France	65	31.2	1,615	10/460	22/450	32/460	21.7	48.9	69.6
Lipitz et al., 1990 (26)	1975–89 Tel Aviv, Israel	8	31.4	—	9/32	1/23	10/32	281.3	43.5	312.5
Gonen et al., 1990 (89)	1978–88 Toronto, Canada	5	30.0	1,172	0/20	2/20	2/20	0.0	100.0	100.0
Collins and Bleyl, 1990 (17)	1980–89 United States	69	31.4	1,482	10/276	33/266	43/276	36.2	124.1	155.8
Thorp et al., 1994 (93)	1980–90 Chapel Hill, NC	2	31.3	1,512	0/8	0/8	0/8	0.0	0.0	0.0
Seoud et al., 1992 (23)	1982–90 Norfolk, VA	4	31.0	1,414	0/16	0/16	0/16	0.0	0.0	0.0

conti

Table 10-2. Continued

Reference	Study Years and Location	Pregnancies (sets)[a]	Weeks' Gestation	Average Birth Weight (g)[b]	Proportion of Deaths			Death Rate per 1,000		
					Stillbirth	Neonatal	Perinatal	Stillbirth	Neonatal	Perinatal
Elliott and Radin, 1992 (22)	1986–91 Phoenix, AZ	10	32.5	1,536	0/40	0/40	0/40	0.0	0.0	0.0
Melgar et al., 1991 (98)	1987–90 Manhasset, NY	6	24.8	—	—	—	15/24	—	—	625.0
8 studies		169 pregnancies (676 quadruplets)	30.5	1,455	29/852	58/823	102/876	34.0	70.5	116.4
Quintuplets										
Lipitz, 1990 (26)	1975–89 Tel Aviv, Israel	2	29.0	—	0/10	0/10	0/10	—	—	—
Gonen et al., 1990 (89)	1978–88 Toronto, Canada	1	29.0	983	0/5	0/5	0/5	—	—	—

[a]Based on pregnancies of 20 weeks' or more gestation.
[b]Average sibship birth weight based on sets of liveborn infants only.

Table 10-3. Prematurity and low birth wei
U.S. live births: Singletons, twins, triplets 19

	Singletons	Twins	
Mean gestational age (wk)	39.0	35.8	3.
Mean birth weight (g)	3357	2389	17.
Preterm (<37 wk)	9.4	50.7	91.0
Very preterm (<33 wk)	1.7	13.9	41.3
Low birth weight (<2500 g)	6.1	52.2	91.5
Very low birth weight (<1500 g)	1.1	10.1	31.9
Small for gestational age	9.4	35.6	36.6

Note: Values are percentages unless indicated otherwise.

Using vital statistics data and superimposing birth weight–specific rates of infant morbidity, Luke and Keith (27) estimated the risks of moderate and severe intellectual disability among twins and triplets. Compared to singletons, the relative risk of moderate impairment (IQ, 70 to 80) was 1.3-fold higher for twins and 1.7-fold higher for triplets. The relative risk of severe impairment (IQ less than 70) was 1.7-fold higher for twins and 2.9-fold higher for triplets.

DIAGNOSIS AND EARLY DEVELOPMENT

Prior to ultrasonography, most multiple gestations were undetected until late in pregnancy, and in some cases, not until labor and delivery. Ultrasonography allows early diagnosis of multiples, establishment of accurate dating, and determination of placentation.

The most suggestive clinical finding is a fundal height significantly greater than expected for dates. Other findings may include auscultation of different fetal heart rates, unexplained anemia, excessive weight gain, increased fetal activity, unexplained elevation of the maternal serum α-fetoprotein (MSAFP) value, or early onset preeclampsia. First-trimester ultrasonography should be offered to women at increased risk of multiple birth, such as those undergoing ART. Recently, most if not all triplet gestations have been detected during the first or early second trimester (28–30).

Pregnancy with high-order multiples is associated with high rates of first-trimester bleeding, spontaneous resorption, and abortion. Seoud et al. (23) reported the spontaneous loss of all fetuses with previously documented fetal cardiac activity among 17 of 165 twin (10.3%), 2 of 26 triplet (7.7%), and 1 of 5 quadruplet (20%) pregnancies followed through the first trimester after IVF. In addition, 33 twin gestations spontaneously reduced to a singleton, and 9 triplet gestations spontaneously reduced to twins. The overall early pregnancy loss rate considering both spontaneous abortion and reabsorption became 50 of 165 (30.3%) twins, 11 of 26 (30.3%) triplets, and 1 of 5 (20%) quadruplets.

Transabdominal ultrasound for evaluation of fetal anatomy is best performed between 18 and 20 weeks' gestation; however, transvaginal ultrasonography may detect some anomalies as early

...ks. Botting et al. (15) reported a 4.5% anomaly rate ...at was not significantly different from that of a twin ...roup. A relatively low triplet anomaly rate (2.6%) also ...rted by the Norfolk IVF program (23). Others (31,32) ...ported higher rates of congenital malformation (5.8% to ...among triplets. These variable rates may reflect differing ...ortions of spontaneous versus iatrogenic multiple gestations. ...ntical twinning is associated with higher anomaly rates than ...s multiple ovulation.

Unfortunately, the diagnostic accuracy of ultrasound for detection of anomalies among triplets and higher-order multiples has not been reported. Ultrasonographic evaluation of fetal anatomy for high-order multiples would be time consuming and in all likelihood difficult due to intrauterine crowding and the confusion created by the multiple fetuses. However, for 490 consecutively examined sets of twins, 21 of 24 anomalous fetuses were detected for a sensitivity of 88%. The specificity and positive predictive value both were 100%, and the negative predictive value was 99% (33). Detection of anomalies is a prerequisite for interventions such as increased surveillance, change in timing, location, or mode of delivery, consultation with neonatal or surgical subspecialists, and in selected cases, fetal therapy, selective reduction, or termination of pregnancy.

Detection of fetal congenital anomalies among high-order multiples can be enhanced by performing a MSAFP between 15 and 20 weeks' gestation. Median MSAFP levels for triplets are approximately threefold higher than those of singletons. MSAFP levels higher than these tripled norms indicate triplets at increased risk of neural tube and abdominal wall defects. Unfortunately, refinement of the maternal risk of aneuploidy cannot be determined at present with MSAFP testing of high-order multiples. It is important to remember that the MSAFP value always is elevated after multifetal pregnancy reduction and should not be obtained after that procedure (34).

CERCLAGE

Prophylactic

Prophylactic cerclage has been advocated by some obstetricians for high-order multifetal pregnancies (32); however, this procedure has not been shown conclusively to lengthen gestation or improve pregnancy outcome (28,35–37). Two small retrospective, nonrandomized trials have yielded conflicting results. Mordel et al. (38) found no difference in gestational age at delivery between a group of women who underwent elective cerclage ($n = 12$) and a group treated without cerclage ($n = 23$). Goldman et al. (39) reported on 12 women with triplets who underwent elective cerclage and 10 who did not. The women who underwent cerclage had a significant prolongation of their pregnancies (35 weeks) compared with the control group (30.7 weeks). This difference was associated with a concomitant reduction in morbidity and mortality, but a confounding effect of parity favored the cerclage group. Unpublished data from The Triplet Connection revealed a mean gestational age at delivery of 32.7 weeks for 3,140 triplet gestations managed without a cerclage and 32.8 weeks for 58 women who underwent cer-

clage before 16 weeks' gestation. The mean gestationa
was significantly lower (30.7 weeks) for 56 other set
with cerclages placed after 16 weeks. Collins and Bleyl (1
that 14% of the 71 women carrying quadruplets in the
underwent cerclage. The mean gestational age at delive
31.2 weeks for quadruplets whose mothers underwent cerc
which was similar to the overall average of 31.4 weeks. There α
not appear to be any clear benefit to prophylactic cerclage for eithe
triplet or quadruplet pregnancies. This procedure should be reserved for patients with evidence of cervical incompetence.

Rescue

Because of a propensity for premature cervical dilation, high-
order multiples sometimes present the opportunity for rescue
cerclage. Our protocol for rescue cerclage includes perioperative
tocolysis with magnesium sulfate (intravenously 2 to 4 g/hour)
or indomethacin (initial 50 mg rectally then 25 mg orally every
6 hours) or both agents. Specific therapy is provided for diseases
such as gonorrhea, chlamydia, or group B streptococcal infection,
and prophylactic broad-spectrum antibiotics are provided for 7 to
10 days. Reduction of prolapsed membranes frequently is the most
difficult surgical problem. Instillation of 400 to 600 cc sterile water
into the bladder causes the bulging membranes to recede (40).
Once the bulging membranes recede, a ring forceps can be placed
on the anterior and posterior portions of the cervix. With traction
on the cervix, the stitch usually can be placed at a level near the
internal cervical os. Occasionally, a moistened sponge on a ring
clamp or an inflated Foley bulb is necessary to help push the membranes back if bladder filling and traction are not sufficient to clear
the cervical canal. A 5-mm polyester fiber (Mersilene) band is used
because it gives more support and is less likely to tear through a
previously dilated cervix.

Delayed Interval Delivery

The presenting fetus in a high-order multiple occasionally is
delivered at a previable gestation. In this circumstance, delayed
interval delivery may be attempted to prolong the pregnancy for
the remaining fetuses. This technique is described in Chapter 11.
The patient must be informed of a low likelihood of success and
possible risks, which include intrauterine infection, hemorrhage,
loss of the remaining previable or borderline viable infants, and
the need for prolonged hospitalization or bed rest. Informed consent should be carefully documented in the medical record.

Delayed interval delivery has been attempted on three triplet
gestations under our care. Two women had premature rupture of
the membranes (PROM) of triplet A, and the third had premature
cervical dilatation. All fetuses were at previable gestational ages.
Two women underwent rescue cerclage after loss of one fetus, and
the third patient was rescued after losing two of her triplets. In
each case, the rescued fetuses gained significant gestational age
and had positive outcomes (Table 10-4).

NUTRITION

Triplet and higher-order multiples magnify the nutritional requirements of pregnancy. Unfortunately, accumulated knowledge

Table 10-4. Outcome of three triplet pregnancies with delayed.

Patient	Gestational Age at Time of Loss (wk)	Cause of Early Loss	Latency Period (d)	Gestational Age at Delivery (wk)	Reason for Delivery	Weight (g)
1	20 4/7	PROM Triplet A	85	32 3/7	Recurrent PTL Mild preeclampsia Mature lung studies	1,740 1,310
2	19 2/7	PROM Triplet A	85	31 4/7	Recurrent PTL Failed tocolytic therapy	1,235 1,750
3	21[a]	Advanced cervical dilation	112	37	Spontaneous labor after removal of cerclage	2,610

[a] Loss of two fetuses, the first because of intrauterine fetal demise and the second because of PROM after presentation with advanced cervical dilation and prolapsing membranes.
PROM, premature rupture of membranes; PTL, preterm labor.

regarding the effect of nutrition on pregnancy outco
beginning to be extended to the nutritional challenge
twin gestations. Even less information is available
appropriate nutritional interventions in triplet or quadru
nancies. That said, early attention to maternal nutrition a
to be extremely important.

The two most important factors affecting perinatal outcom
high-order multiples are gestational age and birth weight, both
which are affected by nutritional status. Ninety percent of triplets
have a low birth weight (<2,500 g) compared with only 1% of singletons. More than 40% of triplets are delivered before 33 weeks'
gestation as opposed to fewer than 2% of singletons. Twelve percent of triplets have birth weights less than the tenth percentile
by 31 to 34 weeks' gestation; this figure increasing to 64% by 35
to 36 weeks (41). Growth restriction occurs even earlier and with
greater frequency among quadruplets. Premature multiples with
growth retardation receive a double dose of morbidity and fare
worse than preterm infants with normal growth (42,43).

The increased frequency of growth restriction in multifetal gestations has been attributed to the ill-defined concept of uterine
crowding. This concept suggests that fetal competition for maternal nutrients inevitably decreases individual fetal growth (44).
This constrained pattern of growth allows environmental influences such as nutrition to have a greater effect on fetal growth in
multifetal gestations than it does in singleton pregnancies (45).

Most of the literature addressing nutrition in multiples deals
with twin gestations. Studies have demonstrated that progressive
increases in gestational weight gain are paralleled by increases in
mean birth weight and a decline in the incidence of low birth
weight for gestational age (42,46,47). The National Institute of
Medicine and other agencies have suggested a 35 to 45 pound (16
to 20 kg) weight gain for women with term twin pregnancies
(48–51). Luke et al. (47) described the weight gain pattern associated with an average twin birth weight of 2,500 g or more. This
optimal twin birth weight is associated with maternal weight
gains of 40 to 45 pounds (18 to 20 kg). Especially important to opti-
mizing fetal growth in twin gestations is to ensure adequate early
maternal weight gain (52).

Regarding triplet gestations, data from the Multiple Birth Foundation in London, England, indicate that an optimal maternal
weight gain is 1.5 pounds (0.7 kg) per week; 36 pounds (16.2 kg)
before 24 weeks' gestation (41) with a total weight gain between
45 and 55 pounds (20 and 25 kg) for normal or underweight women.
Overweight women with triplets may need to gain only 35 to
45 pounds (16 to 20 kg) to maximize fetal growth. Among the
quadruplet pregnancies reported by Collins and Bleyl (17), the
mean maternal weight gain was 45.8 pounds (20.6 kg) at approximately 31 weeks' gestation. The quadruplet pregnancies reported
by Elliott and Radin (22) averaged a maternal weight gain of
57.4 pounds (25.8 kg) at a mean gestational age of 32.5 weeks. The
importance of early pregnancy weight gain is emphasized by the
incrementally shorter gestational lengths for twins, triplets, and
quadruplets. Patient education, nutritional counseling, emphasis
on early weight gain, and insistence on smoking cessation all should

improved fetal growth in higher-order multiple

...ional Academy of Sciences through its recommended ...llowances has suggested that the average U.S. diet is suf- ...to provide all essential nutrients to meet the demands of a ...eton gestation. The Academy further states that nutrient sup- ...mentation is likely to be necessary in multiple gestations but ...rovides no guidelines for women with twins, triplets, or higher-order multiples. Given the recommendation for increased maternal weight gain and anticipating increased demands for vitamins and nutrients in high-order multiples, it seems reasonable to recommend a 50% to 100% increase in the recommended dietary allowances for singleton pregnancies. To achieve these goals, nutritional counseling should emphasize an iron-enriched, high-protein, high-energy diet. More specific recommendations regarding appropriate nutritional interventions for twin and triplet gestations are detailed in Chapter 6.

PREDICTION OF PRETERM DELIVERY

Between 18 and 24 weeks, there is an excellent window of opportunity to educate patients regarding risk of prematurity and to begin to refine the risk estimate for the specific pregnancy.

Endovaginal Cervical Length

One technique to further define the risk of preterm delivery is endovaginal ultrasonography for objective measurement of cervical length. A prospective study sponsored by the National Institutes of Health evaluated 147 twin gestations for multiple risk factors for spontaneous preterm birth (53). With the exception of urinary tract infection, none of the traditional demographic or obstetrical risk factors for preterm birth, including cervical-vaginal fetal fibronectin, were identified as being significant predictors. However, at 24 weeks' gestation, a short cervix (less than 25 mm) detected by endovaginal ultrasonography was significantly associated with spontaneous preterm birth at less than 32, less than 35, and less than 37 weeks' gestation. Only 5% of women with twins and a cervical length more than 25 mm at 22 to 24 weeks' gestation delivered their infants prior to 32 weeks, whereas 27% delivered before 32 weeks if the cervical length was 25 mm or less (odds ratio [OR], 6.9; 95% confidence interval [CI], 2.0–24.2). The risk of delivery before 35 weeks' gestation increased from 26.5% for women with a cervix longer than 25 mm to 54% (OR, 3.2; 95% CI, 1.3–8.0) for women whose cervix was shorter. In the National Institutes of Health study (53), a cervical length less than 25 mm was twice as common at 24 weeks among women carrying twins (18% versus 9%) and sixfold higher at 28 weeks (33% versus 5%) than among women carrying singletons.

In the single study of ultrasonic assessment of cervical length in triplet pregnancies, Ramin et al. (54) found that mean cervical length was significantly shorter in triplet gestations than in singletons by 25 weeks' gestation (26 versus 35 mm). In addition, at 28, 30, and 32 weeks, mean cervical length was significantly shorter for triplets destined to be delivered before 33 weeks' gestation. Although the current data suggest that cervical length measured

at ultrasound examination is helpful in predicting incr
of preterm delivery, no specific therapeutic interventions ṛ
studied.

Our current practice is to perform endovaginal cervical ṛ
measurement on all women with multifetal gestations betweẹ
and 20 weeks during the fetal anatomic survey to identify any ṣ
nificant cervical shortening or funneling that may represent relạ
tive cervical incompetence. We had a few patients with marked
early cervical shortening attempt strict bed rest and observation,
and the outcomes have not been satisfactory. Subsequently, we
have been more aggressive and recommend cerclage when significant cervical changes are detected. Significant cervical changes are
a length less than 25 mm and the presence of a large cervical fun-
nel. This practice has not been subjected to prospective, randomized testing of its efficacy, nor has the predictive capability of
endovaginal sonography been formally compared with information
obtained by means of digital examination. Assuming that the findings at cervical evaluation are normal at 18 to 20 weeks' gestation,
we repeat endovaginal cervical length measurement at 24 weeks
to help define a patient's risk of premature delivery and to guide
suggestions regarding work or restriction of activity.

Digital Cervical Score

Serial digital cervical examination is also used to assess risk of
preterm delivery. We use a technique first described by Houlton
et al. (55) and called the *cervical score*. A cervical score is calculated
as follows: cervical length (cm) minus cervical dilatation at the
internal os (cm). For example, a cervix that is 3 cm long with a
closed internal os has a score of +3. A cervix that is 1 cm long with
the internal os dilated 1 cm has a score of 0. A cervix that is 1 cm
long with the internal os dilated 3 cm has a score of −2. The cervical score is selected because of its simplicity, capability to be quantified, and its focus on cervical dilatation and effacement. Cervical
position and consistency are subjective by nature, influenced by
plurality, and provide little prognostic information once dilatation
and effacement have been considered (56). The station of the presenting part is significantly affected by parity and by malpresentation, which is common in high-order multiples. Quantification of
the cervical score allows easy communication between examiners,
although evaluation by one examiner is optimal for consistency.

The predictive value of the cervical score for spontaneous preterm
delivery has been studied in a mixed population of twin and triplet
gestations. A cervical score of 0 on or before 34 weeks' gestation was
associated with a sensitivity of 88%, a positive predictive value
of 75%, and a fourfold increase in relative risk of preterm delivery of these multiples (57). The earlier in gestation that a cervical score of 0 is detected, the greater is its positive predictive
value. As the cervical score becomes more negative, the positive
predictive value for subsequent spontaneous preterm delivery
approaches 100% (58). Even though most pregnancies studied
were twins, it is believed that the nature of the relation should
be maintained for triplets. Decisions regarding interventions
such as greater activity restriction, bed rest, hospitalization, prophylactic tocolytic therapy, or home uterine activity monitoring

can be made more rationally with continuous evaluation rvical score.

VENTION OF PRETERM DELIVERY

ork and Activity Restriction

Most obstetricians endorse discontinuation of work, restriction of activity, and bed rest for women with high-order multiples. To have a significant effect on perinatal morbidity or mortality, these restrictions on work and activity have to be instituted between 20 and 24 weeks' gestation. The intensity of these modifications in lifestyle, however, is controversial. Some authors have recommended routine, early hospitalization for triplet gestations; they cite reductions in the frequency of both preterm delivery and delivery of low-birth-weight infants (59,60). Other authors have largely abandoned routine hospitalization for triplet pregnancy without any apparent deterioration in outcome (19,20,28,29). Despite the goal of outpatient management, a large percentage of women with high-order multiples are hospitalized for a variety of indications, including hyperemesis gravidarum, preeclampsia, severe intrauterine growth restriction, advanced cervical dilatation, preterm premature rupture of the membranes, and preterm labor. In one review, 88 of 197 women carrying triplets (44%) needed antepartum hospitalization for indications other than preterm labor (19). In another series, 11 of 15 women with triplets were ultimately admitted to the hospital despite a stated goal of outpatient management (29). Albrecht and Tomich (20) attempted outpatient treatment of all patients but still ended up with an average antepartum maternal hospitalization of 22.0 ± 16.0 days (range, 5 to 65 days).

In a provocative publication, Adams et al. (61) compared the perinatal outcomes of 32 triplet pregnancies in which outpatient bed rest was prescribed (1993 to 1996) with outcomes for a historical cohort of 34 triplets (1985 to 1993) for whom routine hospitalization was used in the third trimester. Outpatient recommendations included the following: (a) lateral recumbent rest (4 to 6 hours/day) beginning at 16 weeks of gestation, (b) increasing rest to 6 to 8 hours/day at 20 weeks, (c) discontinuation of vaginal intercourse at 20 weeks, and (d) complete bed rest beginning at 24 weeks of pregnancy. Not unexpectedly, the number of maternal inpatient hospital days were significantly reduced for the outpatient management group (47.9 ± 22.6 versus 21.2 ± 14.5 days). However, the mean gestational age at delivery was 1 week greater for the hospitalized cohort (33.5 ± 2.8 versus 32.5 ± 2.8 weeks, $p = .16$), and the average birth weight was significantly heavier (1,942 versus 1,718 g; $p < .005$). Maternal and neonatal complications were similar for the two groups, except for preeclampsia, which occurred more frequently among the outpatient group (31.1% versus 8.8%; $p = .02$), and the occurrence of grades I through IV intraventricular hemorrhage (10.4% versus 0.9%; $p = .004$).

The retrospective, nonrandomized nature of the investigation by Adams et al. (61) limits the strength of the conclusions that can be drawn from it. Certainly, the financial savings accrued from a policy of outpatient management cannot be justified if they are achieved at the expense of maternal or fetal well-being. Most intriguing is the positive effect on fetal growth observed in th

hospitalized cohort. If inpatient hospitalization allows mc
plete bed rest, it is possible that the improved uteropla.
blood flow associated with recumbency may enhance fetal gr
(62). Syrop and Varner (60) reported a higher incidence of in.
uterine growth retardation (IUGR) and preterm delivery amoi
triplets whose mothers were prescribed "unrestricted" activity
than among those with "restricted" activity. The effect of elective
bed rest in a hospital on length of twin gestation has been studied
in prospective, randomized trials. These studies did not demonstrate any benefit in terms of reducing the frequency of prematurity or IUGR (63,64). The lower rates of preeclampsia and intraventricular hemorrhage reported by Adams et al (61), all but one
grade I or II, in the hospitalized cohort were novel findings that
will require a randomized, controlled trial.

Although antepartum hospitalization of women with high-order
multiples is not considered routine by most clinicians, the report
by Adams et al. (61) certainly rekindles this issue. Although we
have not adopted routine hospitalization of women with high-order
multiples in our practice, we do believe that the report by Adams
et al. emphasizes the potential benefits of reduced activity and bed
rest. Studies describing the circadian pattern of antepartum uterine activity demonstrate a reduction in the frequency of contractions associated with maternal rest (65).

In our practice, we typically recommend that women with triplets discontinue work between 20 and 24 weeks' gestation. We also
recommend that women with triplets discontinue strenuous exer-
cise other than swimming, household chores, travel, and sexual
intercourse at about the same point in gestation. Initially we recommend rest for at least 2 hours in the morning, 2 hours in the
afternoon, and again for 2 hours in the evening. However, the
degree of restriction of activity advised varies with multiple clinical variables. These variables include obstetric history, symptoms,
digital cervical score, and ultrasound measurement of cervical
length. Maternal symptoms and cervical score are assessed once a
week beginning at approximately 20 weeks' gestation. If the findings suggest increased risk of premature delivery, the degree of
restriction of activity may be advanced to complete bed rest or
even hospitalization. Clinical decision making of this sort cannot
be simplified into an algorithm. It requires the highest level of
experience and informed judgment.

Maternal bed rest also is generally advised for women with
quadruplet pregnancies (17,22). Rest typically begins between 16
and 20 weeks' gestation. Hospitalization is reserved for women
with complications. Our practice and recommendations are not
substantially different for quadruplets, but the patients are
observed with a higher index of suspicion and a lower threshold
for intervention.

Prophylactic Tocolytic Therapy

Prophylactic tocolytic therapy for high-order multifetal gestation is popular in general practice. Of 198 women with triplet pregnancies treated in the United States between 1985 and 1988, 115
(58.1%) were given prophylactic tocolytic therapy, mainly oral
terbutaline sulfate (19). The effectiveness of this therapy, however, remains unproved. There was no difference in gestational

.8 ± 2.8 weeks) or birth weight (1,894 ± 486 g) for the 115
n who received prophylactic tocolytic therapy compared with
33 women who did not (33.2 ± 3.5 weeks and 1,869 ± 518 g).
n-el et al. (36) found no benefits that could be attributed to pro-
hylactic use of β-adrenergic agents. Many reports of management
of triplet or quadruplet pregnancies specifically state that prophylactic tocolytic therapy was not used (20,22,29,61). The lack of
efficacy of prophylactic tocolytic therapy for high-order multifetal
pregnancy might be biased if prophylactic tocolytic therapy was
used more often to treat women perceived to be at greater risk.
The line between prophylactic and therapeutic tocolytic therapy
becomes blurred with extremely intense surveillance for increased
prelabor uterine activity.

Home Uterine Activity Monitoring

Data on triplet gestations indicate that progressive cervical dilation and effacement can occur without significant increases in frequency of prelabor contractions (66). This is reflected in what is
considered to be a higher rate of relative cervical incompetence
among higher-order multifetal pregnancies. If prelabor uterine
activity is not as critical in affecting cervical change in triplet as it
is in twin or singleton pregnancies, the value of HUAM for the
early detection of preterm labor becomes questionable. Although
no results of prospective, randomized, clinical trials are available
for high-order multifetal pregnancies, equivalent clinical outcomes
have been reported by groups that use (19,20,22) and do not use
(29,30,61) HUAM to manage triplet or quadruplet pregnancies.

Triplets demonstrate a marked increase in low-amplitude,
high-frequency contractility (67). Because it affects only localized
segments of the uterus, this contractility is not believed to cause
dilation or effacement of a normal cervix. However, excessive
low-amplitude, high-frequency contractility may be sufficient to
promote dilation and effacement among women with abnormally
compliant cervices or marked uterine distention, as may occur
with high-order multiples.

The use of HUAM should be considered investigational in the
care of women with high-order multifetal pregnancies because of
uncertain efficacy, high cost, and inability to separate its effects
from those of frequent perinatal nursing contact. HUAM is a system designed only to make the earliest possible diagnosis of preterm labor. The ability of HUAM to help prevent preterm birth
requires a coexisting perinatal system and effective tocolytic
therapy.

If it is used, HUAM should be individualized and selective.
Potential candidates for HUAM are women with high-order multiples and cervical scores of 0 or less or cervical length measurements of 25 mm or less before 30 weeks' gestation. Patients with
a prior premature singleton birth or preterm labor in the current
pregnancy also may be candidates. Patients maintaining a cervical score greater than 0 or have a cervical length measurement
more than 35 mm are at relatively low risk of preterm delivery
and do not need additional intervention.

Tocolytic Therapy

Despite a high incidence of preterm labor, tocolytic therapy for
high-order multifetal pregnancy has been described in only a few

reports. Initial reports have been discouraging. Itzkowic (35) attempted tocolytic therapy for 7 of 46 triplet pregnancies and delayed delivery more than 48 hours in only 3 instances. Holcberg et al. (59) used tocolytic therapy for only 5 of 23 triplet pregnancies and successfully delayed delivery more than 48 hours in 4 instances. More encouraging, Newman et al. (19) reported that among 131 women with triplets who had preterm labor, only 29% were not candidates for tocolytic therapy. Of the others, 52% underwent successful tocolytic therapy for more than 7 days. The mean time *in utero* gained for the fetuses was almost 4 weeks.

In the report by Albrecht and Tomich (20), 44 of 57 (86%) women carrying triplets were treated for preterm labor at a mean gestational age of 24.9 ± 3.8 weeks. Thirty-four patients (59.6%) received at least one course of intravenous magnesium sulfate, and 20 patients (35.1%) needed two or more courses. Other tocolytic agents used included oral terbutaline in 41 instances (71.9%), subcutaneous terbutaline infusion pump in 28 (49.1%), indomethacin in 21 (36.8%), and oral nifedipine in 3 instances (6.9%).

Tocolytic therapy for high-order multifetal pregnancy increases the risk of cardiovascular complications such as pulmonary edema, cardiomyopathy, myocardial ischemia, and maternal tachyarrhythmia. Although all these complications are infrequent, high-order multifetal pregnancies should be followed carefully, and intravenous fluid volumes restricted to less than 2,000 mL/day. Tocolytic therapy is generally discontinued between 34 and 35 weeks' gestation for triplets and 32 to 33 weeks' for quadruplets.

Glucocorticoid Administration

A glucocorticoid (betamethasone 12 mg every 24 hours for 2 doses) for induction of fetal lung maturity should be administered to high-order multiples before 32 weeks' gestation if they experience premature labor or premature rupture of the membranes or need delivery for maternal or fetal indications (68). We also administer betamethasone to women before 32 weeks if the cervical score is 0 or less or the endovaginal cervical length measurement is 25 mm or less. Some groups prefer antenatal administration of steroids only when delivery appears to be imminent (20). Others repeat administration weekly when the patient is admitted with an antenatal complication (21). The necessity and safety of repeated steroid dosing is an issue that is still unresolved.

ASSESSMENT OF FETAL GROWTH

Next to prematurity, abnormality of fetal growth is the most important contributor to perinatal morbidity and mortality in multiple gestations. Intrauterine growth nomograms for high-order multiples have not been established. Our preference is to use singleton growth nomograms with an understanding of how multifetal gestations usually deviate from the singleton norms.

Intrauterine growth is independent of the number of fetuses until the third trimester, when the rate of growth slows for multiples. Growth of the multiple fetuses diverges from the fiftieth percentile of singleton growth at progressively earlier gestational ages. Healthy twins grow with the same velocity as singletons until approximately 30 to 31 weeks' gestation. Triplet and quadruplet growth velocity diverges from singleton norms at approximately

27 to 28 and 25 to 26 weeks' gestation, respectively (44). The growth of a singleton fetus typically accelerates after 30 weeks' gestation. Lack of acceleration in growth of multiples in the third trimester is likely the result of suboptimal transfer of nutrients through the uteroplacental circulation to the competing fetuses.

A number of factors have been shown to affect triplet growth. Intrauterine growth and birth weight are higher among male infants and with higher parity independent of gestational age (69). Excellent maternal nutrition with adequate early weight gain and midgestational weight gains of at least 1.5 pounds (0.7 kg) per week have been associated with optimal intrauterine growth (41). Luke et al. (41) found that multiple pregnancy resulting from induced conception was independently associated with less intrauterine growth. However, the sample was relatively small, and numerous potential confounding factors were overrepresented among the induced conceptions, including older maternal age, lower body mass index, smoking, lesser weight gain during pregnancy, and longer gestation. Other investigators found that the apparent effect of ART on triplet birth weight disappeared when parity and fetal sex were controlled (69).

Because of competition for nutrients, the risk of IUGR increases with advancing gestational age. By 35 to 36 weeks, 13% of twins have IUGR. This figure increases to 23% by 37 to 38 weeks and to 38% by 39 to 41 weeks (47). Likewise, 12% of triplets and 24% of quadruplets have IUGR by 32 to 34 weeks, and more than 60% have IUGR by 35 to 36 weeks (26,41). By 36 weeks' gestation, the mean birth weight for triplets is at the tenth percentile for single-tons. Quadruplets are at the tenth percentile for singletons by approximately 32 to 33 weeks.

After 20 weeks' gestation, ultrasound evaluation every 3 to 4 weeks is essential to detect growth abnormalities of high-order multiples. Detection of IUGR is aided by early diagnosis and accurate dating of the pregnancy. IUGR is present when the estimated fetal weight falls below the tenth percentile for singleton pregnancies and is severe when it is below the third percentile. IUGR is more ominous the earlier it is detected.

In addition to use in detecting concordant IUGR, ultrasonography also can be used to detect marked growth discordance. Inter-triplet growth differences are more pronounced than those between twins. The mean intertwin birth-weight difference is approximately 10.3% (70), with 5% of twin pairs displaying 25% or more discordance (71). The mean intertriplet birth-weight difference is 20%. Thirty percent of triplets have a discordance of 25% or more, and 7% of sets of triplets have 40% or greater discordance (72).

The implications of severe discordance or concordant IUGR among high-order multiples in terms of management include increased fetal surveillance and more frequent ultrasound evaluation of fetal growth and amnionic fluid volume. IUGR and discordance may be indications for delivery, depending on severity, gestational age, and the effect on fetal health.

It must be cautioned that antepartum assessment of estimated fetal weight and discordance frequently is erroneous. Given this consideration, it is important to be circumspect in responding to abnormal ultrasound findings at early gestational ages when prematurity may be the greater risk. At later gestational ages,

IUGR and considerable discordance are much more common and these findings would have greater reliability. Suspicion of IUGR or considerable discordance after 34 weeks for triplets or after 32 weeks for quadruplets may be an indication for delivery. In all cases, ultrasound findings should be considered along with the condition of the mother, physical findings, and results of comprehensive fetal testing.

MATERNAL COMPLICATIONS

The incidence of preeclampsia is approximately 19% among triplet pregnancies, 38% for quadruplets, and higher if the patient is nulliparous (73). Preeclampsia with high-order multifetal pregnancy generally occurs earlier and is more severe than with other pregnancies and often is atypical. Hypertension is not always the initial sign, nor is proteinuria universally present. Of the triplet and quadruplet pregnancies described by Hardardottir et al. (73), only 3 of 16 met traditional criteria for preeclampsia. Maternal symptoms typical of severe preeclampsia and laboratory abnormalities such as elevated liver enzyme levels and low platelet counts were the most common presentations. Many women with high-order multifetal pregnancies and preeclampsia eventually have HELLP syndrome (hemolysis, elevated liver function, low platelets).

Albrecht and Tomich (20) and Malone et al. (74) described maternal morbidity associated with triplet pregnancies (57 and 55 sets of triplets, respectively). In both series, preterm labor was the most frequent maternal complication, occurring in 86% and 76% of cases, respectively. Remarkable, however, was the relatively high frequency of potentially life-threatening complications, such as pulmonary edema, pulmonary embolism, peripartum cardiomyopathy, acute fatty liver, and postpartum hemorrhage (Table 10-5).

The complications potentially associated with use of tocolytic agents were emphasized by Albrecht and Tomich (20). One patient had gastrointestinal bleeding after indomethacin therapy, one had pulmonary edema while taking magnesium sulfate, and one had deep venous thrombosis with pulmonary embolism while undertaking prolonged bed rest. Seven women needed blood transfusions because of maternal hemorrhage, including one patient who underwent cesarean hysterectomy.

Other maternal complications encountered with increased frequency as pregnancy progresses include cholestasis, pruritic urticarial plaques and papules of pregnancy, urinary tract infection, acute disc problems, and diastasis of the rectus muscles, which in some cases required surgical correction. Most patients also have a number of somatic problems, including shortness of breath, immobility, loss of balance, varicose veins, pruritic stretch marks, dependent edema, constipation, and hemorrhoids. Although none is particularly threatening, these disorders do weaken the patient's will to comply with continuing efforts to prolong pregnancy. Referral to support groups for women with high-order multifetal pregnancies may be beneficial.

FETAL SURVEILLANCE

Fetal surveillance is routinely begun at 32 weeks' gestation for triplets and 30 weeks for quadruplets unless the pregnancy has

Table 10-5. Maternal morbidity associated with triplet pregnancy

Complication	Albrecht and Tomich (20)	Malone et al. (74)
Number	57	55
Preterm labor	49 (86)	42 (76)
Anemia	28 (58)	15 (27)
Preeclampsia	19 (33)	15 (27)
Preterm PROM	10 (18)	11 (20)
Postpartum hemorrhage	7 (12)	5 (9)
Endometritis	8 (14)	13 (24)
HELLP syndrome	6 (11)	5 (9)
Gestational diabetes	6 (11)	4 (7)
Pulmonary edema	2 (4)	0
Pneumonia	0	2 (4)
Pulmonary embolus	1 (2)	0
Acute fatty liver	1 (2)	4 (7)
Supraventricular tachyarrhythmia	0	2 (4)
Peripartum cardiomyopathy	1 (2)	0
Eclampsia	0	1 (2)

Note: Values in parentheses are percentages.
PROM, premature rupture of membranes; HELLP, hemolysis, elevated liver function, and low platelets.

been complicated by other factors, such as IUGR, markedly discordant growth, preeclampsia, anomalies, abnormal fluid volumes, or monoamnionicity. A nonstress test (75,76) supported by a fetal biophysical profile (77) is reliable for fetal surveillance in high-order multiple gestations. When an ultrasound examination is being performed for other reasons, the biophysical profile can be substituted for the nonstress test. Care always must be taken to ensure that each fetus is individually assessed.

Some obstetricians have questioned the necessity of routine fetal assessment in multiple gestations. However, because of the increasing incidence of IUGR among high-order multiples after 32 weeks' gestation and the low sensitivity of antepartum ultrasonography, it seems appropriate to provide the support of fetal surveillance. We also recommend daily fetal kick counting to our patients with multiples, although we realize it is not always possible to differentiate the fetuses.

Umbilical artery Doppler velocimetry has been reported to have high sensitivity and positive predictive value for stillbirth and IUGR in high-order multifetal pregnancy (78,79). Absent or reversed diastolic flow in the umbilical artery is a possible indication for delivery. More data are needed, however, on the integration of Doppler velocimetry into a fetal surveillance scheme for multiples.

TIMING OF DELIVERY

The issue of elective delivery of high-order multiples because of fear of accelerated postdatism is important. The incidence of IUGR increases throughout the third trimester, and the gestational age at onset is inversely related to the number of fetuses. Studies of large population databases have confirmed that the nadir of fetal mortality occurs at 36 to 38 weeks' gestation for twins with birth weights between 2,500 and 2,800 g. Similar studies for triplets have suggested that the optimal birth weight and gestational age (based on data on 9,523 infants) are 1,900 to 2,200 g at 34 to 35 weeks' gestation (80). For quadruplets, the optimal birth weight and gestational age appear to be 1,400 to 1,500 g at 31 to 33 weeks' gestation (17,22,23).

Prolongation of a twin pregnancy beyond 38 weeks, triplet pregnancy beyond 35 weeks, and quadruplet pregnancy beyond 33 weeks does not necessarily improve outcome and necessitates ultrasound assessment of adequate growth, normal amnionic fluid, and reassuring fetal surveillance. High-order multiples with these gestational ages with IUGR, marked discordance, oligohydramnios, preeclampsia, or other maternal-fetal problems should be delivered. Fetal lung maturity testing may be helpful to individualize the timing of delivery in some cases. However, in well-dated pregnancies without overt or gestational diabetes, we do not hesitate to deliver triplets at 35 weeks or quadruplets beyond 33 weeks without assessing fetal lung maturity when an appropriate indication exists. In most clinical series, triplets reaching 37 weeks' gestation are electively delivered (21,29,61).

MODE OF DELIVERY

Cesarean delivery is the most commonly recommended mode of delivery of triplets. In a nationwide review of triplet management between 1985 and 1988, 94% of the deliveries were cesarean, 4.5% were vaginal, and 1.5% were a combined vaginal-abdominal delivery (19). Triplets are at risk of prematurity, malpresentation, growth discordance, and intrapartum distress and are at the highest risk of being inadequately monitored in labor. Because of these increased intrapartum risks and the degree of manipulation that may be necessary with three or more fetuses, most clinicians prefer cesarean delivery. The best support for this approach is the finding that cesarean delivery eliminates the increased perinatal mortality historically associated with birth order in triplet gestations. Cesarean delivery also is the usual choice for quadruplets and other higher-order fetuses for the same reasons (17).

For preterm triplets, some clinicians advise a low vertical uterine incision, which may be easily extended upward to assist with atraumatic delivery. However for most high-order multifetal gestations, there is excellent development of the lower uterine segment, and a low transverse incision is reasonable in many if not most cases. Weissman et al. (81) reviewed 29 triplet cesareans and found that most had a lower uterine segment transverse incision without untoward effects on neonatal outcome.

In selected cases, vaginal delivery of high-order multiple fetuses can be considered. Dommerques et al. (82) compared neonatal outcomes after 23 uncomplicated vaginal deliveries of triplets with outcomes after 23 control deliveries by cesarean and found no differences. Clark and Roman (83) reported the outcomes for 19 sets of triplets, 7 of which were delivered vaginally. There were no perinatal deaths in the vaginally delivered cohort, although these infants were of greater maturity than those in the cesarean delivery group. If a trial of vaginal delivery is anticipated, it is essential that an experienced obstetric team be available and that malpresentation be anticipated. Optimal cases would be those in which the triplets are 32 weeks gestation or more or 1,500 g each or heavier.

REFERENCES

1. Kurtz GR, Davis LL, Loftus JB. Factors influencing the survival of triplets. *Obstet Gynecol* 1958;12:504–508.
2. Zeleny C. The relative number of twins and triplets. *Science* 1921;53:262–264.
3. Keith L, Oleszczuk JJ. Iatrogenic multiple birth, multiple pregnancy and assisted reproductive technologies. *Int J Obstet Gynecol* 1999;64:11–25.
4. Luke B. The changing pattern of multiple births in the U.S.: maternal and infant characteristics 1973 and 1990. *Obstet Gynecol* 1994;84:101–106.
5. Kiely J. Triplets, quadruplets, and quintuplets (+) in the United States. *Twin Res* 1999;2[Suppl]:518(abst).
6. Caspi E, Ronen J, Schreyer P. The outcome of pregnancy after gonadotrophin therapy. *Br J Obstet Gynaecol* 1976;83:967–973.
7. Schenker JG, Yarkoni S, Branat M. Multiple pregnancies following induction of ovulation. *Fertil Steril* 1981;35:105–123.
8. Andrews MC, Muasher SJ, Levy DL, et al. An analysis of the obstetric outcome of 125 consecutive pregnancies conceived invitro and resulting in 100 deliveries. *Am J Obstet Gynecol* 1986; 154:848–853.
9. Australian In Vitro Fertilisation Collaborative Group. In-vitro fertilisation pregnancies in Australia and New Zealand, 1979–1985. *Med J Aust* 1988;148:429–438.
10. Seibel MM. In vitro fertilization, gamete intrafallopian transfer, and donated gametes and embryos. *N Engl J Med* 1988;318: 828–834.
11. Craft I, Al-Shawaf T, Lewis P, et al. Analysis of 1071 GIFT procedures: the case for a flexible approach to treatment. *Lancet* 1988;1:1094–1099.
12. Guttmacher AF. The incidence of multiple births in man and some of other unipara. *Obstet Gynecol* 1953;2:22–25.
13. Miettinen M. On triplet and quadruplet pregnancies in Finland. *Acta Paediatr Suppl* 1954;99:23–28.
14. Elwood JM. Maternal and environmental factors affecting twin births in Canadian cities. *Br J Obstet Gynaecol* 1985;26:351–356.
15. Botting BJ, MacDonald-Davies I, MacFarlane AJ. Recent trends in the incidence of multiple births and associated mortality. *Arch Dis Child* 1987;62:941–945.
16. Martin JA, MacDorman MF, Mathews TJ. Triplet births: trends and outcomes, 1971–94. *Vital Health Stat 21* 1997;(55):1–20.
17. Collins MS, Bleyl J. Seventy-one quadruplet pregnancies: management and outcome. *Am J Obstet Gynecol* 1990;162:1384–1392.

18. Alexander GR, Kogan M, Martin J, et al. What are the fetal growth patterns of singletons, twins, and triplets in the United States? *Clin Obstet Gynecol* 1998;41:115–25.
19. Newman RB, Hamer C, Miller MC. Outpatient triplet management: a contemporary review. *Am J Obstet Gynecol* 1989;161:547–555.
20. Albrecht JL, Tomich PG. The maternal and neonatal outcome of triplet gestations. *Am J Obstet Gynecol* 1996;174:1551–1556.
21. Kaufman GE, Malone FD, Harvey-Wilkes KB, et al. Neonatal morbidity and mortality associated with triplet pregnancy. *Obstet Gynecol* 1998;91:342–348.
22. Elliott JP, Radin TG. Quadruplet pregnancy: contemporary management and outcome. *Obstet Gynecol* 1992;80:421–428.
23. Seoud MAF, Toner JP, Kruithoff C, et al. Outcome of twin, triplet, and quadruplet in vitro fertilization pregnancies: the Norfolk experience. *Fertil Steril* 1992;57:825–834.
24. Callahan TL, Hall JE, Ettner SL, et al. The economic impact of multiple-gestation pregnancies and the contribution of assisted-reproduction techniques to their incidence. *N Engl J Med* 1994;331:244–249.
25. Lipitz S, Reichman BN, Paret G, et al. The improving outcome of triplet pregnancies. *Am J Obstet Gynecol* 1989;161:1279–1284.
26. Lipitz S, Frenkel Y, Watts C, et al. High order multifetal gestation: management and outcome. *Obstet Gynecol* 1990;65:215–218.
27. Luke B, Keith LG. The contribution of singletons, twins and triplets to low birth weight, infant mortality and handicap in the United States. *J Reprod Med* 1992;37:661–666.
28. Loucopoulos A, Jewelewicz R. Management of multifetal pregnancies: sixteen years' experience at the Sloane Hospital for Women. *Am J Obstet Gynecol* 1982;143:902–905.
29. Peaceman AM, Dooley SL, Tamura RK, et al. Antepartum management of triplet gestations. *Am J Obstet Gynecol* 1992;167:1117–1120.
30. Boulot P, Hedon B, Pelliccia G, et al. Favourable outcome in 33 triplet pregnancies managed between 1985–1990. *Eur J Obstet Gynecol Reprod Biol* 1992;43:123–129.
31. Onyskowova Z, Dolezal A, Jedlicka V. The frequency and the character of malformations in the multiple birth. *Teratology* 1971;4:496–501.
32. Waksman S, Bouchard P, Patey-Savatier P, et al. Les grossesses multifoetales, II: epidemiologie, aspects cliniques. *J Gynecol Obstet Biol Reprod (Paris)* 1990;19:383–389.
33. Edwards MS, Ellings JM, Newman RB, et al. Predictive value of antepartum examination for anomalies in twin gestation. *Ultrasound Obstet Gynecol* 1995;6:43–49.
34. Lynch L, Berkowitz RL. Maternal serum α-fetoprotein and coagulation profiles after multifetal pregnancy reduction. *Am J Obstet Gynecol* 1993;169:987–993.
35. Itzkowic DV. A survey of 59 triplet pregnancies. *Br J Obstet Gynaecol* 1979;86:23–28.
36. Ron-el R, Caspi E, Schreyer P, et al. Triplet and quadruplet pregnancies and management. *Obstet Gynecol* 1981;57:458–463.
37. Rush RW, Isaacs S, McTerhon K, et al. Randomized controlled trial of cervical cerclage in women at high risk of spontaneous preterm delivery. *Br J Obstet Gynaecol* 1984;91:742–730.

38. Mordel N, Zajicek G, Benshusham A, et al. Elective suture of the uterine cervix in triplets. *Am J Perinatol* 1993;10:14–16.

39. Goldman GA, Dicker D, Peleg D, et al. Is elective cerclage justified in the management of triplet and quadruplet pregnancy? *Aust N Z J Obstet Gynaecol* 1989;29:9–12.

40. Scheerer LJ, Lam F, Bartolucci L, et al. A new technique for reduction of prolapsed fetal membranes for emergency cervical cerclage. *Obstet Gynecol* 1989;74:408–410.

41. Luke B, Bryan E, Sweetland C, et al. Prenatal weight gain and the birthweight of triplets. *Acta Genet Med Gemellol (Roma)* 1995;44:93–101.

42. Luke B, Minoque J, Witter FR. The role of fetal growth restriction and gestational age on length of hospital stay in twin infants. *Obstet Gynecol* 1993a;81:949–953.

43. Kilpatrick SJ, Jackson R, Croughan-Minihane MS. Perinatal mortality in twins and singletons matched for gestational age at delivery at 30 weeks. *Am J Obstet Gynecol* 1996;174:66–71.

44. McKeown T, Record RG. Observations on foetal growth in multiple pregnancy in man. *J Endocrinol* 1952;8:386–400.

45. Gluckman PD, Breier GH, Oliver M, et al. Fetal growth in late gestation: a constrained pattern of growth. *Acta Paediatr Scand Suppl* 1990;367:105–110.

46. Luke B, Minoque J, Abbey H, et al. The association between maternal weight gain and the birthweight of twins. *J Matern Fetal Med* 1992;1:267–276.

47. Luke B, Minoque J, Witter FR, et al. The ideal twin pregnancy: patterns of weight gain, discordancy and length of gestation. *Am J Obstet Gynecol* 1993;169:588–597.

48. Pederson AL, Worthington-Roberts B, Hickok PE. Weight gain during twin gestation. *J Am Diet Assoc* 1989;89:642–646.

49. Eller DP, Newman RB, Ellings JM, et al. Modifiable determinants of birth weight variability in twins. *J Matern Fetal Med* 1993;2:254–259.

50. Brown JE, Schloesser PT. Prepregnancy weight status, prenatal weight gain, and the outcome of term twin gestations. *Am J Obstet Gynecol* 1990;162:182–186.

51. Subcommittee on Nutritional Status and Weight Gain During Pregnancy. Weight gain in twin pregnancies. In: *Nutrition During Pregnancy*. Washington, DC: National Academy Press, 1990: 212–221.

52. Luke B, Min SJ, Gillespie B, et al. The importance of early weight gain in the intrauterine growth and birth weight of twins. *Am J Obstet Gynecol* 1998;179:1155–1161.

53. Goldenberg RL, Iams JD, Miodovnik M, et al., and the National Institute of Child Health and Human Development Maternal-Fetal Medicine Unit Network. The preterm prediction study: risk factors in twin gestations. *Am J Obstet Gynecol* 1996;175: 1047–1053.

54. Ramin KD, Ogburn PL, Mulholland TA, et al. Ultrasonic assessment of cervical length in triplet pregnancies. *Am J Obstet Gynecol* 1999;180:1442–1445.

55. Houlton MCC, Marivate M, Philpott RH. Factors associated with preterm labor and changes in the cervix before labour in twin pregnancy. *Br J Obstet Gynaecol* 1982;89:190–194.

56. Lange JP, Zecher NJ, Westergaard JG, et al. Prelabor evaluation of inducibility. *Obstet Gynecol* 1982;60:137–146.
57. Newman RB, Godsey RK, Ellings JM, et al. Quantification of cervical change: relationship to preterm delivery in the multifetal gestation. *Am J Obstet Gynecol* 1991a;165:264–269.
58. Neilson JP, Verkuyl DAA, Crowther CA, et al. Preterm labor in twin pregnancies: prediction by cervical assessment. *Obstet Gynecol* 1988;72:719–723.
59. Holcberg G, Biale Y, Lewenthal H, et al. Outcome of pregnancy in 31 triplet gestations. *Obstet Gynecol* 1982;59:472–476.
60. Syrop CH, Varner MW. Triplet gestation: maternal and neonatal implications. *Acta Genet Med Gemellol (Roma)* 1985;34:81–88.
61. Adams DM, Sholl JS, Haney EI, et al. Perinatal outcome associated with outpatient management of triplet pregnancy. *Am J Obstet Gynecol* 1998;178:843–847.
62. Manshande JP, Eeckels R, Manshande-Desmet V, et al. Rest versus heavy work during the last weeks of pregnancy: influence on fetal growth. *Br J Obstet Gynaecol* 1987;94:1059–1067.
63. Saunders MC, Dick JS, Brown IM. The effects of hospital admission for bedrest on the duration of twin pregnancy: a randomized trial. *Lancet* 1985;2:793–795.
64. Hartikarnen-Sorri AL, Jouppila P. Is routine hospitalization needed in antenatal care of twin pregnancy? *J Perinat Med* 1984; 12:31–32.
65. Moore TR, Iams JD, Creasy RK, et al., and The Uterine Activity in Pregnancy Working Group. Diurnal and gestational patterns of uterine activity in normal human pregnancy. *Obstet Gynecol* 1994;83:517–523.
66. Newman RB, Gill PJ, Campion S, et al. The influence of fetal number on antepartum uterine activity. *Obstet Gynecol* 1989b; 73:695–699.
67. Newman, RB, Gill PJ, Campion S, Katz M. Antepartum ambulatory tocodynamometry: the significance of low-amplitude, high frequency contractions. *Obstet Gynecol* 1987;70:701–705.
68. Pons JC, Fernandez H, Diochin P, et al. Prise en charge des grossesses triples. *J Gynecol Obstet Biol Reprod (Paris)* 1989; 18:72–78.
69. Newman RB, Jones JS, Miller MC. Influence of clinical variables on triplet birth weight. *Acta Genet Med Gemellol (Roma)* 1991; 40:173–179.
70. Yarkoni S, Reece A, Holford T, et al. Estimated fetal weight in the evaluation of growth in twin gestations: a prospective longitudinal study. *Obstet Gynecol* 1987;69:636–639.
71. Carlson N. Discordant twin pregnancy: a challenging condition. *Contemp Ob/Gyn* 1989;34:100–116.
72. Jones JS, Newman RB, Miller MC. Cross-sectional analysis of triplet birth weight. *Am J Obstet Gynecol* 1991;168:135–140.
73. Hardardottir H, Kelly K, Bork MD, et al. Atypical presentation of preeclampsia in high-order multifetal gestations. *Obstet Gynecol* 1996;87:370–374.
74. Malone FD, Kaufman GE, Chelmow D, et al. Maternal morbidity associated with triplet pregnancy. *Am J Perinatol* 1998;15:73–77.
75. Lenstrup C. Predictive value of antepartum nonstress testing in multiple pregnancies. *Acta Obstet Gynecol Scand* 1984;63: 597–601.

76. Lodeiro JG, Vintzileos AM, Feinstein SJ, et al. Fetal biophysical profile in twin gestations. *Obstet Gynecol* 1986;67:824–827.

77. Elliott JP, Finberg HJ. Fetal biophysical profile testing as an indicator of fetal well-being in high-order multiple gestation. *Am J Obstet Gynecol* 1995;172:508–512.

78. Rafla NM. Surveillance of triplets with umbilical artery velocimetry waveforms. *Acta Genet Med Gemellol (Roma)* 1989;38: 301–307.

79. Giles WB, Trudinger BJ, Cook CM, et al. Umbilical artery waveforms in triplet pregnancy. *Obstet Gynecol* 1990;75:813–818.

80. Luke B. Reducing fetal deaths in multiple gestations: optimal birth weights and gestational ages for infants of twin and triplet births. *Acta Genet Med Gemellol (Roma)* 1996;45:333–348.

81. Weissman A, Yoffe N, Jakobi P, et al. Management of triplet pregnancies in the 1980s: are we doing better? *Am J Perinatol* 1991; 8:333–337.

82. Dommerques M, Mahieu-Caputo D, Mandelbrot L, et al. Delivery of uncomplicated triplet pregnancies: is the vaginal route safer? *Am J Obstet Gynecol* 1995;172:513–517.

83. Clark JP, Roman JD. A review of 19 sets of triplets: the positive results of vaginal delivery. *Aust N Z J Obstet Gynaecol* 1994; 34:50–53.

84. Michlewitz H, Kennedy J, Kawada C, et al. Triplet pregnancies. *J Reprod Med* 1981;26:243–246.

85. Daw E. Triplet pregnancy. *Br J Obstet Gynaecol* 1978;85:505–509.

86. Crowther CA, Hamilton RA. Triplet pregnancy: a 10-year review of 105 cases at Harare Maternity Hospital, Zimbabwe. *Acta Genet Med Gemellol (Roma)* 1989;38:271–278.

87. Pons JC, Mayenga JM, Plu G, et al. Management of triplet pregnancy. *Acta Genet Med Gemellol (Roma)* 1988;37:99–103.

88. Thiery M, Kermans G, Derom R. Triplet and higher-order births: what is the optimal delivery route? *Acta Genet Med Gemellol (Roma)* 1988;37:89–98.

89. Gonen R, Heyman E, Asztalos EV, et al. The outcome of triplet, quadruplet and quintuplet pregnancies managed in a perinatal unit: obstetric, neonatal, and follow-up data. *Am J Obstet Gynecol* 1990;162:454–459.

90. Creinin M, Katz M, Laros R. Triplet pregnancy: changes in morbidity and mortality. *J Perinatol* 1991;11:207–212.

91. Porreco RP, Burke MS, Hendrix ML. Multifetal reduction of triplets and pregnancy outcome. *Obstet Gynecol* 1991;78:335–339.

92. Levene MI, Wild J, Steer P. Higher multiple births and the modern management of infertility in Britain. *Br J Obstet Gynaecol* 1992;99:607–613.

93. Thorp JM, Tumey LA, Bowes WA Jr. Outcome of multifetal gestations: a case–control study. *J Matern Fetal Med* 1994;3:23–26.

94. Santema JG, Bourdrez P, Wallenberg HCS. Maternal and perinatal complications in triplet compared with twin pregnancy. *Eur J Obstet Gynecol Reprod Biol* 1995;60:143–147.

95. Lipitz S, Reichman B, Uval J, et al. A prospective comparison of the outcome of triplet pregnancies managed expectantly or by multifetal reduction to twins. *Am J Obstet Gynecol* 1994;170: 874–879.

96. Boulot P, Hedron B, Pelliccia G, et al. Effects of selective reduction in triplet gestation: a comparative study of 80 cases managed with or without this procedure. *Fertil Steril* 1993;60:497–503.

97. Fitzsimmons BP, Bebbington MW, Fluker MR. Perinatal and neonatal outcomes in multiple gestations: assisted reproduction versus spontaneous conception. *Am J Obstet Gynecol* 1998;179: 1162–1167.

98. Melgar CA, Rosenfeld DL, Rawlinson K, et al. Perinatal outcome after multifetal reduction to twins compared with nonreduced multiple gestations. *Obstet Gynecol* 1991;78:763–767.

99. Bollen N, Camus M, Tournaye H, et al. Embryo reduction in triplet pregnancies after assisted procreation: a comparative study. *Fertil Steril* 1993;60:504–509.

100. Macones GA, Schemmer G, Pritts E, et al. Multifetal reduction of triplets improves perinatal outcome. *Am J Obstet Gynecol* 1993:169:982–986.

101. Pons JC, Charlemaine C, Dubreuil E, et al. Management and outcome of triplet pregnancy. *Eur J Obstet Gynecol Reprod Biol* 1996;76:131–139.

11

Intrapartum Management of Multiples

GENERAL PRINCIPLES OF INTRAPARTUM MANAGEMENT

Successful intrapartum management of multiple gestations requires careful preparation and attention to several important general principles (Table 11-1). First and foremost is an assemblage of experienced and skilled personnel. The obstetrical team should be familiar with the risks posed by multiple gestations and a team leader should be designated. The team leader should be experienced with both operative and manipulative delivery techniques. The team should include another physician or nurse capable of monitoring the progress of labor, assisting with delivery, and performing intrapartum ultrasound examinations. Other necessary personnel include nursing staff, an anesthetist, and a neonatal team sufficient to resuscitate two or more infants.

A second principle of intrapartum management is to ascertain presentation and estimate the weight of each fetus on admission to the labor and delivery unit. The conceptual framework most commonly used to categorize the intrapartum management of twin gestations is based on their relative presentations. These categories include both twins in a vertex presentation, the first twin vertex and the second nonvertex, and the first twin in a nonvertex presentation. These categories are distributed as approximately two-fifths, two-fifths, and one-fifth, respectively (1). Repeating the ultrasound assessment after delivery of the first twin is important, because the second twin may change position after delivery of the first twin in as many as 20% of cases (2).

Successful intrapartum management of multiple gestations also requires continuous and simultaneous monitoring of both fetuses during labor. This is most efficiently achieved with electronic fetal heart rate monitoring. Multiple gestations are at increased risk of several intrapartum complications that can manifest as an abnormal fetal heart rate pattern. These include dysfunctional uterine contractility, premature separation of the placenta, especially after birth of the first twin, prolapse of the umbilical cord, cord entanglement, and uteroplacental insufficiency. These complications are most common when the twins have intrauterine growth retardation (IUGR) or there is significant growth discordance. Although external monitoring of both fetuses is acceptable, care must be taken to ensure that the same twin is not being simultaneously monitored by both cardiographs. When the membranes of the first twin have ruptured, that twin may be monitored directly with a fetal scalp electrode while the second is monitored externally.

Ready availability of anesthetic services is critical for consistently successful intrapartum management. Due to the frequent and sometimes emergency need for operative or manipulative obstetrical procedures, continuous epidural analgesia has proven highly effective for both labor and delivery in multiple gestations,

Table 11-1.   General principles of intrapartum management of multiple gestations

Presence of two skilled obstetric attendants for labor and delivery
Anesthesiologist available at delivery
Neonatal care personnel sufficient for resuscitation of all newborns
Portable ultrasound scanner
Reliable intravenous access (16–18 gauge)
Cardiotocograph with dual monitoring capability
Delivery bed with lithotomy stirrups
Obstetric forceps (Piper's if breech delivery planned) or vacuum
   apparatus
Premixed oxytocin infusion
Tocolytic agent of choice for uterine relaxation
Methergine, 15-methyl prostaglandin $F_{2\alpha}$, or both
Immediate availability of blood
Capabilities and staff for emergency cesarean section

and is considered the anesthetic approach of choice (3). Less desirable alternatives to epidural analgesia include intravenous narcotic analgesia for labor and pudendal block with perineal infiltration of local anesthetic for delivery. If intrauterine manipulation is needed unexpectedly, general anesthesia with a halogenated agent may be necessary to achieve uterine relaxation. Both conduction and general anesthesia are appropriate for the cesarean delivery of multiple gestations.

A final principle of intrapartum management is to ensure the availability of blood. Women with multiple gestation have greater average blood loss with delivery and are at higher risk of postpartum hemorrhage due to uterine atony. Women carrying multiples also are at increased risk of abruptio placentae, placenta previa, and needing cesarean section. These risks may be superimposed on maternal anemia, which is one of the most common complications associated with multiple gestations.

LABOR

Compared to singleton gestations, women with multiples have increased baseline frequency of uterine contractions during the latter half of gestation (4). This increased baseline uterine contractility leads to advanced prelabor cervical changes. Almost 40% of nulliparous and 60% of parous women with multiple gestations present in labor with a cervix dilated more than 3 cm. The respective figures for women with singleton pregnancies are 7% and 23% (5). As a result of this prelabor cervical change, the latent phase is typically shorter in multiple than in singleton gestation. However, the active phase of labor for multiples is longer than singleton norms particularly for nulliparous women. This relative uterine inertia during the active phase usually is ascribed to uterine overdistention and an increased frequency of malpresentation. Uterine overdistention causes an increased frequency of contractions that typically are of a lesser intensity (6). This pattern of uterine activity is referred to as *hypotonic uterine dysfunction* and is not uncommon in multiple gestations.

Oxytocin induction or augmentation of labor is acceptable in the care of women with multiples, although oxytocin should be used judiciously, as is always the case when there is uterine overdistention. The longer active phase in multiples counterbalances the shorter latent phase; the result is a similar overall duration of labor for single and multiple gestations (5).

Multiple factors influence the duration of the descent phase. Overall, this phase is slightly lengthened due to the presence of multiple fetuses. The smaller size of multifetal gestations should allow for a more rapid descent phase, although other factors, such as malpresentation and the possibility of collision, may offset this advantage.

There is often a period of hypocontractility after delivery of the first infant. The laxity of the uterine wall caused by reduced intrauterine volume must be taken up by aggressive retraction of the uterine muscle before effective uterine contractility can resume. To shorten this lag time, a previously prepared oxytocin infusion can be started. A typical preparation may be 40 units of oxytocin in 1,000 mL of physiologic saline solution. The infusion is begun at 1 to 2 mL/minute. The dosage can then be escalated at 5-minute intervals until adequate uterine contractility is achieved.

In the third stage of labor, women with multiple gestations are at increased risk of postpartum hemorrhage due to uterine atony. In anticipation of a possible hemorrhage, oxytocin should be started immediately after delivery of the second twin if administration has not already begun. Twenty to 40 units of oxytocin can be added to 1,000 mL of intravenous crystalloid solution and infused at 100 to 200 cc an hour. If bleeding persists, 0.2 mg methylergonovine maleate (Methergine) can be given intramuscularly or by means of transabdominal intramyometrial injection. Chronic or pregnancy-induced hypertension is a not uncommon contraindication to the use of methylergonovine maleate. Another effective alternative is intramuscular or intramyometrial injection of 0.25 mg of 15-methyl prostaglandin F2α. Administration of 15-methyl prostaglandin F2α can be repeated a second time in 10 to 15 minutes if the bleeding has not abated. Consideration should be given to continuing the oxytocin infusion for several hours after delivery to help reduce postpartum bleeding.

DELIVERY

Intrapartum management of multiple gestations requires the anticipation of unpredictable events and the need to consider at least three separate patients. It is a tremendous challenge to deliver multiples in such a way as to ensure the best possible outcome for mother and babies. Unfortunately, there is a conspicuous absence of strong clinical evidence to guide decision making. With the exception of one randomized, controlled trial conducted by Rabinovici et al. (7), to our knowledge all the literature addressing the intrapartum management of multiple gestations describes either observational or nonrandomized comparative trials. Although a tremendous amount of clinical experience is cataloged in these studies, they may ultimately create a false impression. Such studies suffer from numerous methodological deficiencies, including the difficulties inherent in retrospective data collection, selection bias, and unconsidered confounding variables. It is conceivable that differences in outcomes may more likely reflect the clinical differences on which the mode of delivery was chosen rather than on the efficacy of the approach.

Vertex–Vertex

It is generally agreed that in the 40% of instances in which both twins are in a vertex presentation, delivery can be vaginal with a high likelihood of success (1,8–10). Despite speculation, there is no evidence that vertex vaginal delivery of a very low birth weight twin (less than 1,500 g) is associated with any increased risk of perinatal mortality or interventricular hemorrhage (11).

After delivery of the first twin, the presenting part of the second twin should be confirmed by means of pelvic examination or real-time ultrasonography. If labor has not resumed within 10 minutes of the delivery of the first twin, administration of oxytocin should be initiated. As throughout labor, it is important that continuous heart rate monitoring of the second twin be assured. The infant's head should be identified within the pelvic inlet with special attention to excluding either a compound or funic presentation. Once effective uterine contractions are reestablished, the woman is encouraged to bear down in order to achieve further descent. Amniotomy should be performed during a contraction and with moderate fundal pressure applied to help fix the vertex within the pelvis. The amniotic sac can be grossly ruptured if the infant's head is well applied, or a leak can be produced with a spinal needle if the vertex is not well applied.

Previous data suggested that the time between deliveries of twins should not exceed 30 minutes. This recommendation has been obviated by the development of electronic fetal monitoring, intrapartum ultrasound, and intensive neonatal support. Much of the data suggesting higher perinatal morbidity and mortality associated with long delays between deliveries describe an era in which the second twin frequently was not recognized until after delivery of the first (12). Jouppila et al. (13) in 1975 began to question the wisdom of an arbitrary time limit for the interval between the delivery of the first and second twin. Rayburn et al. (14) in 1984 reviewed the cases of 115 twin pairs and reported that the mean time between delivery of the twins was 21 minutes with a range of 1 minute to more than 2 hours. Delivery of the second twin occurred in 15 minutes or less in almost two-thirds of the cases. When the time interval was more than 15 minutes, there was no excess trauma or fetal compromise. Rayburn et al. concluded that expectancy between the delivery of the two twins was associated with the lowest risk of perinatal morbidity. Delays of greater than 1 hour have not been associated with adverse outcomes for the second twin as long as fetal heart rate was continuously monitored (15).

In some cases, deterioration of the fetal condition may occur before a safe vaginal delivery is possible. Some complications, such as premature placental separation or prolapse of the umbilical cord, are clinically apparent. In other cases, deterioration of the fetal heart rate tracing may be indecipherable. Acute and severe distress of the second twin should usually be managed with prompt operative vaginal delivery or cesarean delivery. High vacuum or forceps delivery should be avoided except in the most severe of emergencies. Even then these techniques should be considered only during preparation for emergency cesarean delivery. Likewise, internal podalic version should be considered only when emergency delivery is mandated and cesarean delivery cannot be performed immediately. There are no results of current series to document the safety of internal podalic version in cases of fetal distress. Because of the possibility of intrapartum fetal distress and the limited options for effectively dealing with that situation, access to immediate cesarean delivery should be considered the standard of care for multiple gestations.

Internal podalic version and breech extraction of the second twin should probably not be considered unless (a) there is a clear and emergent obstetrical indication, (b) the fetus has an estimated fetal weight of 1,500 g or more, (c) the operator is experienced in the performance of internal podalic version and breech extraction, (d) anesthesia is available for effective uterine relaxation, and (e) simultaneous preparation is being made for emergency cesarean delivery should the attempted internal podalic version fail.

Vertex–Nonvertex

Opinions diverge regarding the optimal mode of delivery of twins in a vertex–nonvertex presentation. In the late 1970's and early 1980's, cesarean delivery was advocated by many obstetricians as the optimal management of vertex–nonvertex twin gestation. Farooqui et al. (12) reported that the breech second twin appeared to be at increased risk of mortality if delivered vaginally. Other advocates of cesarean delivery pointed to reports of depressed Apgar scores and increased rates of perinatal morbidity for the vaginally delivered nonvertex second twin (16–19). As a result, Taylor (20) editorially recommended that if either twin had a malpresentation cesarean delivery would be the best method of intrapartum management. Cetrulo et al. (21) in 1980 reviewed pertinent obstetric and pediatric literature and concluded that if the second twin is in a breech or transverse position cesarean delivery is associated with the lowest rate of neonatal morbidity and mortality. In 1986, Cetrulo (8) reviewed his own experience at St. Margaret's Hospital, Boston, where virtually all vertex–nonvertex twins were delivered by cesarean. This practice eliminated any differences in morbidity and mortality between twin A and twin B.

Since the early 1980's, however, there has been a significant accumulation of primarily observational, nonrandomized clinical experiences that show there is no increased risk of adverse neonatal outcome when the nonvertex second twin is delivered vaginally. In 1982, Acker et al. (22) compared outcomes for 76 breech second twins weighing 1,500 g or more extracted vaginally with outcomes for 74 nonvertex second twins delivered by cesarean section. There was no perinatal mortality in either group, nor were there any significant differences in the frequency of low 5-minute Apgar scores. In 1985, Chervenak et al. (1) reported similar findings for 93 vertex–breech and 42 vertex–transverse twin gestations. The nonvertex second twins delivered vaginally (78% of the breech and 53% of the transverse lies) did as well as the first twins delivered from a vertex presentation. There were no neonatal deaths or instances of interventricular hemorrhage among any of the newborns weighing more than 1,500 g and delivered vaginally. In an earlier article, Chervenak et al. (10) reviewed the perinatal outcomes of 385 consecutive twin deliveries and found no association between the occurrence of birth trauma and mode of delivery. In the series, there were only four cases of serious birth trauma, two of which involved a vertex-presenting twin A delivered by means of midforceps and vacuum extraction, respectively. One infant was a 3,420-g twin B delivered by means of total breech extraction who had a greenstick fracture of the right clavicle and a nondisplaced fracture of the right humerus. The only neonatal death related to birth trauma was that of a a 1,000-g breech twin B delivered by cesarean through a low vertical uterine incision. This infant had perinatal asphyxia and died 12 hours after birth.

In the only prospective, randomized clinical trial addressing this issue, Rabinovici et al. (7) in Israel found no difference in neonatal outcome among 60 nonvertex second twins randomly assigned to vaginal or cesarean delivery after 35 weeks of gestation (Table 11-2). Adam et al. (23), in Halifax, Nova Scotia, reviewed 397 vertex–nonvertex twin sets in which both twins weighed more than 1,000 g and had no lethal anomalies. There were no significant increases in either perinatal morbidity or mortality when the nonvertex second twins delivered vaginally were compared with those delivered by cesarean section. Of 99 nonvertex twin Bs weighing 1,500 g or more and delivered by either assisted or total breech extraction, there was only one instance of intraventricular hemorrhage. That infant had an uncomplicated total breech extraction with Piper forceps applied to the aftercoming head. The infant also had moderate respiratory distress syndrome (RDS), which may have contributed to the intraventricular bleeding. Fishman et al. (24), in Southern California, analyzed 390 vaginally delivered second twins—207 delivered vertex and 183 delivered breech. No significant differences in neonatal outcome could be found between the vertex- and breech-delivered second twins even when stratified by birth weight. Although the authors found no excessive morbidity or mortality associated with total breech extraction of the second twin, the sample size was too small to draw any conclusions regarding infants weighing less than 1,500 g. Greig et al. (25) reported on the effect of presentation on neonatal outcome for 457 sets of twins, 76 of whom had a mean birth weight less than 1,500 g. These investigations failed to find any significant differences in neonatal morbidity between the nonvertex second twins delivered vaginally and those delivered by cesarean section. Greig et al. concluded that their experience would not support routine cesarean delivery of nonvertex second twins at any birth weight.

Anticipatory planning for a vertex–nonvertex vaginal twin delivery requires consideration of several important issues. First, the operator must be experienced in vaginal breech delivery. In the absence of an experienced operator, cesarean delivery should be performed. Prior to delivery, there should be a sonographic assessment of the size of each fetus. If twin B is more than 500 g heavier than twin A, a vaginal breech extraction of twin B is best avoided. Epidural analgesia also is advisable so as to make intrauterine manipulation easier and to enhance the patient's cooperation and effort. After delivery of the first infant, vaginal examination should be immediately performed to determine the presentation of twin B.

Table 11-2. Prospective, randomized comparison of vaginal or cesarean delivery of term (>35 weeks), nonvertex second twins

Variable	First Twin		Second Twin	
	Vaginal	Cesarean	Vaginal	Cesarean
Number	27	27	27	27
Maternal age (yr, mean ± SD)	30.3 ± 4.3	29.8 ± 5.2		
Nulliparity (no.)	6 (22.2%)	7 (26.9%)		
Maternal fever (no.)	3 (11.1%)	11 (40.7%)[a]		
Maternal anemia (no.)	2	3		
Postpartum hospitalization (d, mean ± SD)	4.9 ± 2.9	8.0 ± 2.0[b]		
Gestation (wk, mean ± SD)	37.7 ± 1.6	37.5 ± 1.5		
Birth weight (g, mean ± SD)	2,477 ± 370	2,533 ± 423	2,459 ± 510	2,484 ± 632
Transient tachypnea (no.)	1	2	0	2
Apnea (no.)	0	0	2	0
Neonatal hypoglycemia (no.)	1	2	2	3
Neonatal hyperbilirubinemia (no.)	3	4	5	5
Neonatal hospitalization (d, mean ± SD)	7.6 ± 8.6	10.1 ± 6.3[c]	8.0 ± 8.1	13.1 ± 12.1[c]

[a] $p = .01$.
[b] $p < .0001$.
[c] $p < .0001$.

From Rabinovici J, Barkai G, Rechman B, et al. Randomized management of the second non-vertex twin: vaginal delivery or cesarean section. *Am J Obstet Gynecol* 1987;156:52–56, with permission.

If twin B is in a frank breech presentation and engaged in the birth canal, gentle fundal pressure should be applied and artificial rupture of the membranes performed with a uterine contraction. With spontaneous delivery of the breech-presenting infant to the umbilicus, an assisted breech extraction can be performed using a technique identical to that for singleton breech delivery. With a transverse lie, complete, or footling breech presentation, a total breech extraction is performed. The operator places his or her hand into the uterine cavity, grasps both of the infant's feet, and brings the infant into the birth canal. Care should be taken to ensure that both feet are grasped rather than the hands or a hand and a foot. If possible, the membranes should not be ruptured until the feet are brought well down into the birth canal. Relaxation of the lower uterine segment to assist with the breech extraction can be achieved with either the intravenous administration of 50 to 100 µg nitroglycerin or subcutaneous administration of 0.25 to 0.5 mg of terbutaline sulfate. The success rate for second twin vaginal breech delivery should exceed 95% (24,26).

Emergency complications such as abruptio placentae or fetal bradycardia may in some cases be amenable to emergency total breech extraction. However, complications such as prolapse of the umbilical cord or compound presentation may be aggravated by an attempt at breech extraction, and emergency cesarean delivery would be preferable. In a review of 510 twin gestations, Samra et al. (27) reported that 184 (36%) were cesarean deliveries. Of those delivered by cesarean, 22 (12%) were combined vaginal-abdominal deliveries. Bider et al. (28) reviewed all available reports describing combined vaginal-abdominal delivery. They identified 137 such cases among 2,691 twin deliveries (5%). Although this figure is probably an overestimation due to reporting bias, most authors conclude that this form of delivery is increasingly more common. The main reasons cited for combined delivery were persistent transverse lie, prolapsed cord, failed external version with retraction of the cervix, and the absence of an experienced operator. As previously stated, in the absence of an experienced obstetrical attendant, cesarean section of both twins at the outset would seem to be preferable to a combined vaginal-abdominal delivery.

Intrapartum External Cephalic Version

External cephalic version has been recommended as part of the intrapartum management of a nonvertex second twin. Chervenak et al. (29) initially reported on the use of external cephalic version in 11 breech and 14 transverse presentations of twin B. Intrapartum version was successful and allowed vaginal delivery of more than 70% of infants in breech or transverse lies. Success was not influenced by gestational age, birth weight, or parity. Success appeared to be enhanced with the use of epidural analgesia and to be hindered by a birth weight disparity of more than 500 g. In another small study, Tchabo and Tomai (30) achieved successful version and vertex vaginal delivery of 28 of 30 nonvertex second twins—12 transverse and 18 breech. In a larger study, Kaplan et al. (31) achieved a 75% success rate with external cephalic version of 100 nonvertex second twins. Kaplan et al. concluded that intrapartum external cephalic version is a safe and effective alternative to routine cesarean delivery of vertex–nonvertex twins.

Alternatively, Gocke et al. (26) analyzed the outcomes for 136 sets of vertex–nonvertex twins who had birth weights of 1,500 g or more. Of this cohort, 41 patients had undergone attempts at external cephalic version, 55 underwent a primary attempt at breech extraction, and 40 had a primary cesarean section. There were no differences in either neonatal morbidity or mortality among the three groups. Successful vaginal delivery was achieved by only 46% of the patients undergoing external cephalic version as opposed to all but 2 (96%) of those patients undergoing a primary attempt at breech extraction. Part of the reason for this difference was that one-third of the patients who had undergone successful conversion to a cephalic presentation underwent emergency cesarean delivery due to fetal distress, cord prolapse, or compound presentation. Similar results were reported by Wells et al. (32), who reviewed a cohort of vertex–nonvertex twins whose mothers had undergone primary cesarean section, breech extraction, and external cephalic version. The external version group was more likely to require emergency anesthesia and undergo abdominal delivery of the second twin than was the breech extraction group.

Chauhan et al. (33) reported on their experience with external cephalic version of the second twin and reviewed the literature to assemble 118 cases that could be evaluated (Table 11-3). They found that the rate of successful vaginal delivery of the second twin after version was highly variable between reports (46% to 80%); the overall success rate was only 58% (69 of 118). Chauhan et al. also

Table 11-3. Literature review of the comparative efficacy and safety of external cephalic version (singleton or non-vertex second twin) and second twin breech extraction

	External Cephalic Version		Breech Extraction
	Singleton	Nonvertex	Second Twin
No. of series reviewed	13	5	11
Sample size range	10–304	15–41	11–183
No. of evaluable patients	1,339	118	683
No. of successful vaginal deliveries	857 (64%)	69 (58%)	568 (98%)[a]
No. of combined complications	19 (1.4%)	12 (10%)	7 (1%)
No. of instances of cord prolapse	NA	6 (5%)	2 (0.3%)

[a] 558 of 568. Two reports excluded for not including the total number of attempted breech extractions.
NA, not available.
From Zhang J, Bowes WA, Fortney JA. Efficacy of external cephalic version: a review. *Obstet Gynecol* 1993;82:306–312 and Chauhan SP, Roberts WE, McLaren RA, et al. Delivery of the non-vertex second twin: breech extraction versus external cephalic version. *Am J Obstet Gynecol* 1995;173:1015–1020.

found a complication rate of 10% (12 of 118) associated with external version of the second twin. The reported complications included 6 instances of cord prolapse, 4 episodes of fetal distress, 1 instance of abruptio placentae, and 1 compound presentation. For comparison, Chauhan et al. (33) also reviewed published reports of breech extraction of a nonvertex second twin. The authors accumulated 683 cases of breech extraction in 11 published reports, including their own. Excluding two reports that did not provide the total number of attempted deliveries, Chauhan et al. described 568 attempted second twin breech extractions, 558 (98%) of which were successful. The overall complication rate was only 1% (7 instances of complications in 683 deliveries). They included 3 fractured humeri, 2 episodes of fetal distress, and 2 instances of cord prolapse. Neonatal complications such as intraventricular hemorrhage, respiratory distress syndrome, and perinatal asphyxial syndrome were not considered due to incomplete reporting and the fact that they are not specifically related to the mode of delivery.

Decisions regarding the route delivery of vertex–nonvertex twins often are dictated by physicians' comfort or experience; neonatal outcomes appear to be similar with either breech extraction, external cephalic version, or cesarean delivery. However, the costs associated with these various delivery modes are infrequently considered. Mauldin et al. (34) reported on both the obstetric and neonatal outcomes and maternal and neonatal hospital charges for 84 vertex–nonvertex twin gestations (Fig. 11-1). Comparison groups included 41 twin pairs delivered by spontaneous vaginal delivery and breech extraction (Group A), 19 twin pairs delivered by spontaneous vaginal delivery and external cephalic version (Group B), and 24 twin pairs delivered by means of primary cesarean delivery (Group C). The three groups did not differ with

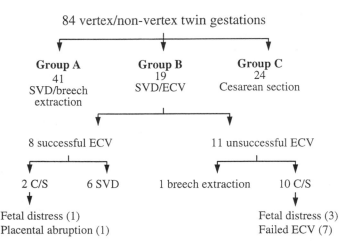

Figure 11-1. Clinical outcomes of 84 vertex–nonvertex twin gestations. **A:** Spontaneous vaginal delivery, breech extraction. **B:** Spontaneous vaginal delivery, external cephalic version. **C:** Primary cesarean section.

respect to maternal demographics, medical complications, gestational age, birth weight, fetal sex, or intrauterine growth restriction. Maternal charges were significantly lower in the breech extraction Group A ($5,890 ± $2,304) compared to either the external version Group B ($8,638 ± $4,175) or the cesarean delivery Group C ($7,608 ± $3,256). Although maternal morbidity was similar among the groups, the length of stay was significantly shorter for women in the breech extraction group (3.4 days versus 6.3 and 7.0 days respectively). Even more remarkable were the significantly lower neonatal hospital charges found for the breech extraction Group A (Table 11-4). The difference in hospital charges was, at least in part, a result of decreased rates of neonatal morbidity, less frequent ventilator use, reduced level II or neonatal intensive care unit admission, and shorter hospital stays for the infants delivered by means of spontaneous vaginal delivery and breech extraction. Mauldin et al. (34) concluded that analysis of the cost-effectiveness of various delivery options for a vertex–nonvertex twin favors breech extraction of the second twin.

The aim of analyzing costs and outcomes is to provide insight into the medical decision making process. If any procedure or technique provides better outcomes at lower costs, the decision is clear; particularly if the measured outcome is clinically compelling. If a given technique provides better outcomes at higher costs, then the decision depends on the ability of society, the patient, or both to accept this cost for the degree of improvement in outcome. The results of the retrospective analysis by Mauldin et al. (34) suggest that vaginal breech extraction of a nonvertex second twin provides equivalent, if not superior, outcomes at a lower cost. Efforts should continue to be made to offer breech extraction to suitable twin pairs with vertex–nonvertex presentations so that clinical outcomes can be improved while use of resources is minimized.

External cephalic version is certainly an alternative for obstetricians not comfortable with total breech extraction or for those cases in which the fetus is not a candidate for vaginal breech delivery due to either very low birth weight (less than 1,500 g) or considerable birth-weight disparity (more than 500 g). In these cases, the patient should be counseled about the possible need for cesarean delivery of the second twin if the attempt at external cephalic version is unsuccessful or if complications develop. As always, the capabilities for immediate cesarean delivery should be kept close at hand.

Attempts at intrapartum external cephalic version should be directed by an experienced operator. Epidural analgesia is advisable both for patient comfort and abdominal wall relaxation. The position of the second twin should be identified sonographically prior to the delivery of the first twin. This allows the attempt at external cephalic version to be initiated without delay following delivery of the first twin. Ultrasound confirms the fetal lie and the transducer itself can be used to apply pressure to the fetal vertex and assist in the external version attempt even as the first twin is being delivered (Fig. 11-2). This is particularly applicable to the transverse lie, which can often be induced into a vertex-presenting longitudinal position with transducer pressure alone. After the first twin has been delivered, the primary operator immediately

Table 11-4. Neonatal outcomes of vertex and nonvertex twin gestations delivered by means of spontaneous vaginal delivery and breech extraction (group A), spontaneous vaginal delivery and external cephalic version (group B), and primary cesarean delivery (group C)

Variable	Group A	Group B	Group C	Significance
No. of sets	41	19	24	
Birth weight (g, mean ± SD)				
Twin A	2,270 ± 741	2,233 ± 561	2,169 ± 680	NS
Twin B	2,167 ± 728	2,295 ± 702	2,116 ± 739	NS
VLBW, <1,500 g (no.)	12	4	8	NS
IUGR (%)	12	11	10	NS
Mean discordancy (%)	10	10	12	NS
Ventilator requirement (%)	5	12	24	$p = .02$
Healthy newborn (%)	71	51	50	$p = .04$
Length of stay in neonatal nursery (d, mean ± SD)	4.8 ± 8.9	12.4 ± 12.7	16.8 ± 21.8	$p = .0002$
Charges (US$, mean ± SD)				
Overall	$3,526 ± 5,017	$11,754 ± 15,457	$36,994 ± 54,318	$p = .0001$
Twin A	$4,128 ± 6,260	$9,569 ± 12,832	$29,080 ± 48,095	
Twin B	$2,800 ± 2,863	$14,535 ± 18,554	$44,909 ± 60,987	

NS, not significant; VLBW, very low birth weight; IUGR, intrauterine growth retardation.

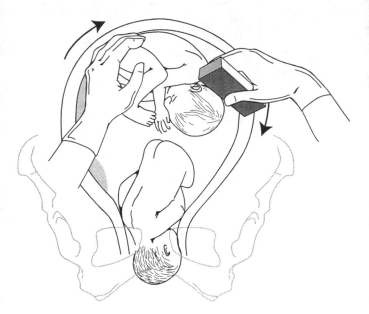

Figure 11-2. External cephalic version of twin B (transverse lie) is initiated even before the delivery of twin A is completed. An assistant uses the pressure of the ultrasound transducer to guide the fetal vertex into the pelvis while the other hand is used to push the fetal breech upward to establish a longitudinal lie.

assumes responsibility for the version of the second twin, especially when it is in a breech presentation.

Version attempts can be performed either as a forward or backward roll using the shortest arc between the vertex and the pelvic inlet. Generally the version can be accomplished by a single operator, although occasionally the assistance of a second operator is necessary (Fig. 11-3). Once the vertex has been guided into the pelvis, it frequently remains at a relatively high station. Gentle fundal pressure, oxytocin augmentation, and maternal expulsive efforts may be used at that point to achieve descent of the fetal vertex. Once the vertex is within the pelvis, vaginal examination should be performed to rule out compound or funic presentation. That done, artificial rupture of the membranes can then be performed with a contraction, and maternal expulsive efforts can be intensified.

Nonvertex First Twin

In fewer than 20% of cases, the first twin is in a nonvertex presentation. When that presentation is transverse, cesarean section is obviously indicated. When twin A presents as a breech, most clinicians choose cesarean delivery. Data on which to base this recommendation are limited. Kelsick and Minkoff (16) reported a 4.5% perinatal loss rate when vaginal delivery was attempted with twin A in a breech presentation as opposed to only a 2.4% loss rate when

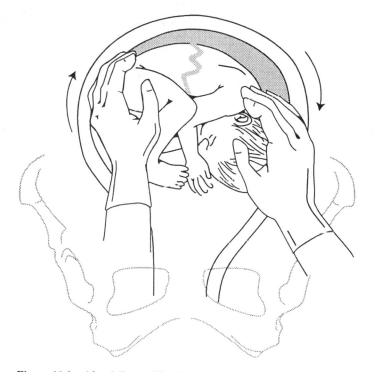

Figure 11-3. After delivery of the first twin, the primary operator assumes responsibility for external cephalic version of twin B. The fetal breech is elevated from the pelvis and replaced into the uterine fundus while the fetal vertex is guided from the fundus into the pelvic inlet. Once the fetal vertex overlies the pelvic inlet, the mother can continue pushing, and amniotomy can be performed.

delivery was cesarean. Similar findings were reported by Cheng and Hannah (35), who reviewed the literature in 1993. On the other hand, Blickstein et al. (36) found no significant differences in perinatal outcome between 24 breech–vertex twins delivered vaginally and 35 similar gestations delivered abdominally.

Interlocking of the fetal heads is an extremely rare but potentially disastrous complication associated with the vaginal delivery of breech–vertex twins. When the twin in breech presentation descends, its chin can become locked into the neck and chin of the vertex second twin (Fig. 11-4). Although the report is dated, Cohen et al. (37) encountered interlocking twins only once in 817 twin deliveries. Similarly, Oettinger et al. (38) did not encounter any interlocking among 36 breech–vertex twin pairs delivered vaginally. They also reported no increase in neonatal morbidity or mortality compared to 46 other sets of breech–vertex twins delivered by cesarean. When interlocking twins are encountered, successful outcomes can be achieved with emergency cesarean

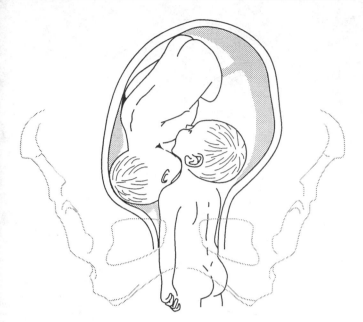

Figure 11-4.   Chin to chin locking of breech–vertex twins.

section or, as was found in at least one case report, the Zavenelli maneuver (39).

Whereas interlocking twins are extremely rare, a potentially more common problem is subtle interference of the second twin on the descent of the first. Deflection of the head of twin A during delivery due to the interference of the second twin can increase the risk of head entrapment and cervical spine injury, as has been reported (39a,39b) for singleton breech gestations delivered with a hyperextended head. Collision or impaction of the twins can increase the risk of labor abnormality or cord prolapse. In addition, because many twins have a low birth weight, there is concern that the extremities and torso may be delivered through a cervix that is inadequately dilated or effaced to allow easy delivery of the after-coming head.

Due to a lack of information documenting the safety of vaginal delivery of a nonvertex-presenting first twin, the American College of Obstetricians and Gynecologists recommends cesarean delivery. If vaginal delivery of the breech-presenting twin is planned, the risks and benefits of vaginal delivery should be fully discussed with the patient, and consent must be obtained.

Cesarean Delivery

The decision to deliver by cesarean does not eliminate the possibility of a technically difficult or traumatic birth. Among the 385 twin deliveries reported by Chervenak et al. (10), the only neonatal death related to birth trauma was that of a 1,000-g second twin extracted with difficulty during a low vertical cesarean. Successful abdominal delivery of twins requires much the same careful preparation, decision making, and technical skill that would be required of a vaginal twin birth. There should be neonatal resuscitation teams appropriate to the number of fetuses being delivered. There also should be adequate nursing staff to support both the obstetrical and neonatal teams. Due to the oftentimes significantly increased size of the uterus, exaggerated left lateral displacement may be necessary to prevent aortocaval compression. The anesthesiologist should be prepared to offer assistance with uterine relaxation if that should be necessary during the operation. Uterine relaxation with 50 to 100 μg intravenous nitroglycerin or subcutaneous injection of 0.25 to 0.50 mg terbutaline sulfate both provide rapid onset tocolysis. Both the anesthesiologist and the nursing staff should be prepared to assist with the control of postpartum hemorrhage. An oxytocin infusion should be prepared in advance and other uterotonic agents, such as 15-methyl prostaglandin F2α and methylergonovine maleate (Methergine) should be available. Some obstetricians also advise that either a vacuum extractor or Piper forceps be available for assistance in delivery of the second twin, depending on its presentation.

The type of uterine incision should be based on the size and weight of the twins, the skill of the operator, and the degree of development of the lower uterine segment. A lower uterine segment transverse incision can be used safely in most instances, particularly when the infants weigh more than 1,500 g and the lower uterine segment is well developed.

There is always the risk that the upper uterine segment will clamp down and entrap the second twin. A contraction ring may develop between the upper and lower uterine segments making either vertex or breech delivery of the second twin extremely difficult. In addition, contraction of the uterus also can trap the aftercoming head of a breech second twin. Because of this possibility, some obstetricians prefer a vertical uterine incision. This incision should be strongly considered when the lower uterine segment is thick and when the second twin is malpresenting and is anticipated to have a very low birth weight. A vertical incision also should be considered when there is no fetal pole or only a footling presentation in the lower uterine segment.

In addition to consideration of a vertical uterine incision, other techniques that help reduce the risk of uterine contraction and entrapment of the second twin are to keep the membranes intact until commencement of delivery and to minimize the delay between the delivery of the first and second twin. Tocolytic therapy may also be used during cesarean section; either therapeutically if difficulties occur during delivery of the second twin or prophylactically to help avoid entrapment, particularly of very low birth weight infants. Both intravenous nitroglycerin and subcutaneous terbutaline have the advantages of rapid onset without high risk of subsequent uterine atony. If uterine relaxation is unsuccessful, it may be necessary to extend the uterine incision. If a transverse lower uterine segment incision has been used, it is preferable to extend one edge of the incision creating a "J" incision rather than extending the incision in the midline, creating a weaker "I" incision.

SPECIAL CONSIDERATIONS

Premature Twins

There is no clear evidence that very low birth weight twins with a vertex–vertex presentation are compromised by allowing vaginal delivery. Most obstetricians, however, would agree that a very low birth weight first twin with a breech presentation would likely do better delivered by cesarean. However, there is no consensus regarding the most appropriate route of delivery of very low birth weight twins when twin A is vertex and twin B is nonvertex.

Data already presented would not seem to justify the routine cesarean delivery of vertex–nonvertex twins; however, there is concern regarding the safety of vaginal breech delivery of nonvertex second twins weighing less than 1,500 g. There are reports of an increased frequency of perinatal asphyxia and birth trauma associated with the vaginal breech delivery of very low birth weight second twins, although, admittedly, the databases are small (11,23).

Davison et al. (40) compared the outcomes for 54 breech-extracted second twins weighing between 750 and 2,000 g with those for the vertex-presenting first twin sibling and for 43 sets of twins delivered by cesarean. The mean birth weight was 1,415 ± 334 g for the vaginally delivered twin sets and 1,394 ± 328 g for those delivered by cesarean. The authors could find no significant difference in survival rate or frequency of respiratory distress syndrome, necrotizing enterocolitis, intracranial hemorrhage, use of mechanical ventilation, need for oxygen therapy, or length of hospitalization between the breech-extracted second twins and the second twins delivered by cesarean. They concluded that routine cesarean delivery was not justified for nonvertex second twins weighing less than 2,000 g.

Greig et al. (25) also concluded that there was no evidence to support routine cesarean delivery of low or very low birth weight twins based on their series of 457 twin sets. It must be noted, however, that despite the large size of this series, only 9 nonvertex second twins weighing less than 1,500 g were delivered vaginally. Although many obstetricians have adopted cesarean delivery of very low birth weight nonvertex second twins, there are few data to support conclusively this shift in management. Rydhstrom (41) presented an interesting historical perspective comparing the outcome of twin deliveries from 1973 to 1976 with those from 1981 to 1983. Between these time periods, the cesarean section rate increased from 7.7% to almost 70% for low birth weight twins. Rydhstrom concluded that the "analysis failed to reveal any significant impact of abdominal birth on the fetal outcome for low birth weight twins, even when fetal presentation was taken into account." The issue remains unresolved. Given the existing controversy, the American College of Obstetricians and Gynecologists has concluded that cesarean delivery of nonvertex second twins weighing less than 1,500 to 2,000 g is an appropriate management option.

Prior Cesarean

Previous cesarean should not be considered an absolute contraindication to vaginal delivery of twin gestation. Most of the landmark studies regarding vaginal delivery after cesarean excluded twin gestations due to concerns that uterine overdistention may increase the risk of uterine rupture. Despite these reasonable concerns, small studies have not identified an increased risk of uterine rupture during labor in twin gestations when the uterus has a scar (42,43). Strong et al. (44) described 56 women with twins and a prior cesarean who underwent a trial of labor with a 72% success rate. In that series, two patients had uterine scar dehiscence but no symptomatic uterine rupture. There was no increase in maternal or neonatal morbidity among patients undergoing a trial of labor. The investigators concluded that a trial of labor for properly selected patients is reasonable as long as the usual safeguards for attempted vaginal birth after cesarean are followed.

In the largest series reported to date, Miller et al. (45) reviewed the outcomes of 210 women with a twin pregnancy and one or more prior cesarean births. Ninety-two of these women undertook a trial of labor, and 64 delivered both twins vaginally. One patient had uterine scar dehiscence, but there were no symptomatic uterine ruptures. The perinatal outcome was identical for those women undertaking a trial of labor and those who did not after correction for previously existing risk factors. There was a single maternal death resulting from a pulmonary embolus following a cesarean without a trial of labor. Obviously, larger studies will be needed to ultimately confirm the safety of a trial of labor in selected twin pregnancies. At present, however, a trial of labor appears to be an acceptable alternative to routine elective repeat cesarean delivery. Certainly as a result of the uterine overdistention, patient selection should be very careful, and the commonly accepted exclusion criteria should be used: women with a known vertical uterine scar, a previous uterine rupture, an unrepaired previous dehiscence, or obstetrical contraindications to labor.

Delayed Interval Delivery

Because of the propensity for premature cervical dilation and previable delivery, multiple gestations sometimes present the opportunity for delayed interval delivery. Life-saving prolongation of multiple gestation has been described in case reports and small series (46–50). The optimal situation occurs in a diamniotic-dichorionic twin gestation in which loss of the first fetus is the result of extrusion caused by preterm premature rupture of the membranes or true cervical incompetence. Delayed interval delivery also can be attempted when there are separate implantations associated with uterine abnormalities such as didelphic uterus (51,52). A less favorable circumstance is delivery complicated by advanced preterm labor or bleeding. Obvious contraindications to delayed interval delivery include profuse hemorrhage, hemodynamic instability, or intraamniotic infection. Monochorionic placentation also is a relative contraindication to delayed interval delivery because of uncertainty about the effect of shared but interrupted placental circulation. Before this procedure is performed, the patient should be informed of a low likelihood of success and possible risks, including intrauterine infection, hemorrhage, subsequent loss of the remaining previable or borderline viable fetus or fetuses and the need for prolonged hospitalization or bed rest (51).

With consent and if the delivery situation is stable, the patient can be considered for delayed interval delivery. Delayed interval delivery has been successfully achieved without the use of a rescue cerclage (46,50); however, in our experience, we have not found this approach to be as successful. We found in a review of case reports that use of adjunctive rescue cerclage affords a better chance of greatly prolonging the interval between deliveries.

Our protocol includes perioperative tocolysis using intravenous magnesium sulfate (2 to 4 g/hour) and oral indomethacin (25 mg every 6 to 8 hours), which are initiated immediately after delivery of the first fetus. Prophylactic broad-spectrum antibiotics are begun and continued for 7 to 10 days. Not all clinicians agree with the use of either tocolysis or prophylactic antibiotics. There are no data to establish the necessity or efficacy of use of these agents. Sakala and Branson (53) reported a case of pseudomembranous colitis caused by *Clostridium difficile* in which prophylactic antibiotics were used to prolong the interval between deliveries. There is general agreement that pathogens such as gonorrhea, chlamydia, and group B streptococcal infection should be specifically identified and treated when present.

After delivery of the first fetus, the umbilical cord is tied, cut short, and allowed to retract back into the uterus. Prolapse of the membranes of the second fetus causes a difficult operative problem and reduces the likelihood of a successful procedure. If the membranes are prolapsed, we instill 400 to 600 mL sterile water into the bladder to induce the bulging membranes to recede (54). At that point, ring forceps are placed on the anterior and posterior portions of the cervix. With traction, rescue cerclage is performed with 5-mm polyester fiber (Mersilene) placed by means of the McDonald technique. As the cerclage is placed and then tightened, a moistened sponge on a ring clamp may be helpful in pushing the membranes back if bladder filling and traction are not sufficient. The 5-mm polyester fiber band is preferred because it gives more support and is less likely to tear through a previously dilated cervix. For the next 7 to 10 days, tocolysis, antibiotics, and hospitalized observation are continued. Beyond that point, strict bed rest either in the hospital or at home is advised but tocolysis and antibiotics are discontinued.

SUMMARY

The intrapartum management of multiple gestations presents numerous challenges to obstetric care providers because of the multiple variations in presentation. Successfully managing these pregnancies requires a high level of preparedness and skill. Unfortunately, the literature is not definitive in its conclusions about the best intrapartum strategies to follow. This chapter outlines these controversies and defines the options available for intrapartum care. The recommendations in Fig. 11-5, which are based on a review of the literature, are offered as the preferred methods of intrapartum management of multiple gestation.

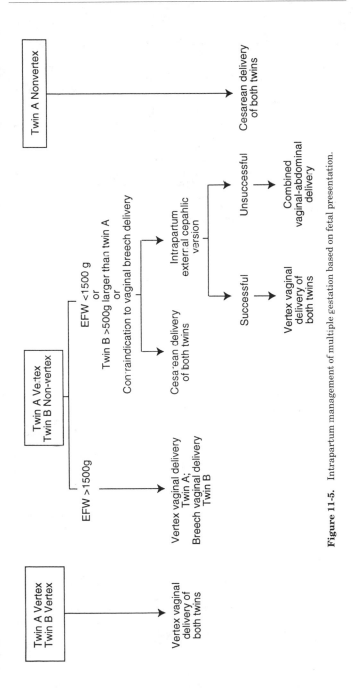

Figure 11-5. Intrapartum management of multiple gestation based on fetal presentation.

REFERENCES

1. Chervenak FA, Johnson RE, Youcha S, et al. Intrapartum management of twin gestations. *Obstet Gynecol* 1985;65:119–124.
2. Trofatter K. Twin pregnancy: the management of delivery. *Clin Perinatol* 1988;15:93–106.
3. Crawford JS. A prospective study of 200 consecutive twin deliveries. *Anaesthesia* 1987;42:33–43.
4. Newman RB, Gill PJ, Katz M. Uterine activity during pregnancy in ambulatory patients: comparison of singleton and twin gestations. *Am J Obstet Gynecol* 1986;154:530–531.
5. Friedman EA, Sachtleben MR. The effect of uterine overdistention on labor, I: multiple pregnancy. *Obstet Gynecol* 1964;23:164–171.
6. Alvarez H, Caldeyro R. Contractility of human uterus recorded by new methods. *Surg Gynecol Obstet* 1950;91:1.
7. Rabinovici J, Barkai G, Rechman B, et al. Randomized management of the second non-vertex twin: vaginal delivery or cesarean section. *Am J Obstet Gynecol* 1987;156:52–56.
8. Cetrulo CL. The controversy of mode of delivery in twins: the intrapartum management of twin gestations, I. *Semin Perinatol* 1986;10:39–43.
9. Laros RK, Dattel BJ. Management of twin pregnancy: the vaginal route is still safe. *Am J Obstet Gynecol* 1988;158:1330–1338.
10. Chervenak FA, Youcha S, Johnson RE, et al. Antenatal diagnosis and perinatal outcome in a series of 385 consecutive twin pregnancies. *J Reprod Med* 1984;29:727–731.
11. Morales WJ, O'Brien WF, Knuppel RA, et al. The effect of mode of delivery on the risk of intraventricular hemorrhage in nondiscordant twin gestations under 1,500 g. *Obstet Gynecol* 1989;73:107–110.
12. Farooqui MO, Grossman JH, Shannon RA. A review of twin pregnancy and perinatal mortality. *Obstet Gynecol Surv* 1973;28:144–152.
13. Jouppila P, Kauppila A, Koivisto M, et al. Twin pregnancy: the role of active management during pregnancy—the role of active management during pregnancy and delivery. *Acta Obstet Gynecol Scand Suppl* 1975;54:13–19.
14. Rayburn WF, Lavin JP Jr, Miodovnik M, et al. Multiple gestation: time interval between delivery of the first and second twins. *Obstet Gynecol* 1984;63:502–506.
15. Feng TI, Swindle RE Jr, Huddleston JF. A lack of adverse effect of prolonged delivery interval between twins. *J Matern Fetal Med* 1995;5:222–225.
16. Kelsick F, Minkoff H. Management of the breech second twin. *Am J Obstet Gynecol* 1982;144:783–786.
17. Ho SK, Wu PYK. Perinatal factors in neonatal morbidity in twin pregnancy. *Am J Obstet Gynecol* 1975;122:979–987.
18. Ware HH. The second twin. *Am J Obstet Gynecol* 1971;110:865.
19. Kaupilla A, Joupilla P, Coivisto M, et al. Twin pregnancy: a clinical study of 335 cases. *Acta Obstet Gynecol Scand Suppl* 1975;54:5–11.
20. Taylor ES: Editorial. *Obstet Gynecol Surv* 1976;31:535–536.
21. Cetrulo CL, Ingradia CJ, Sbarra AJ. Management of multiple gestation. *Clin Obstet Gynecol* 1980;23:(2):533–548.
22. Acker D, Leiberman M, Holbrook H, et al. Delivery of the second twin. *Obstet Gynecol* 1982;59:710–711.
23. Adam C, Allen AC, Baskett TF. Twin delivery: influence of the presentation and method of delivery on the second twin. *Am J Obstet Gynecol* 1991;165:23–27.

24. Fishman A, Grub DK, Kovacs BW. Vaginal delivery of the non-vertex second twin. *Am J Obstet Gynecol* 1993;168:861–864.
25. Greig PC, Veille JC, Morgan T, et al. The effects of presentation and mode of delivery on neonatal outcome in the second twin. *Am J Obstet Gynecol* 1992;167:901–906.
26. Gocke SE, Nageotte MP, Garite T, et al. Management of the non-vertex second twin: primary cesarean section, external version, or primary breech extraction. *Am J Obstet Gynecol* 1989;161:111–114.
27. Samra JS, Spillane H, Mukoyoko J, et al. Cesarean section for the birth of the second twin. *Br J Obstet Gynecol* 1990;97:234–236.
28. Bider D, Korach J, Hourvitz A, et al. Combined vaginal-abdominal delivery of twins. *J Reprod Med* 1995;40:131–134.
29. Chervenak FA, Johnson RE, Berkowitz RL, et al. Intrapartum external version of the second twin. *Obstet Gynecol* 1983;62:160–165.
30. Tchabo JG, Tomai T. Selected intrapartum external cephalic version of the second twin. *Obstet Gynecol* 1992;79:421–423.
31. Kaplan B, Peled Y, Rabinerson E, et al. Successful external version of B-twin after birth of A-twin for vertex-nonvertex twins. *Eur J Obstet Gynecol Reprod Biol* 1995;58:157–160.
32. Wells SR, Thorp JM Jr, Bowes WA Jr. Management of the non-vertex second twin. *Surg Gynecol Obstet* 1991;172:383–385.
33. Chauhan SP, Roberts WE, McLaren RA, et al. Delivery of the non-vertex second twin: breech extraction versus external cephalic version. *Am J Obstet Gynecol* 1995;173:1015–1020.
34. Mauldin JG, Newman RB, Mauldin PD. Cost effective delivery and management of the vertex and non-vertex twin gestation. *Am J Obstet Gynecol* 1998;179:864–869.
35. Cheng M, Hannah M. Breech delivery at term: a critical review of the literature. *Obstet Gynecol* 1993;82:605–618.
36. Blickstein I, Shohamz-Schwartz Z, Lancet MD, et al. Vaginal delivery of the second twin in breech presentation. *Obstet Gynecol* 1987; 69:774–776.
37. Cohen M, Kohl SG, Rosenthal AH. Fetal interlocking complicating twin gestation. *Am J Obstet Gynecol* 1965;91:407–412.
38. Oettinger M, Ophir E, Markovitz J, et al. Is cesarean section necessary for delivery of a breech first twin? *Gynecol Obstet Invest* 1993;35:38–43.
39. Swartjes JM, Bleker OP, Schutte MF. The Zavanelli maneuver applied to locked twins. *Am J Obstet Gynecol* 1992;166:532.
40. Davidson L, Easterling T, Jackson JC, et al. Breech extraction of low birth weight second twins: can cesarean section be justified? *Am J Obstet Gynecol* 1992;166:497–502.
41. Rydhstrom H. Prognosis for twins with birth weight <1,500 g: the impact of cesarean section in relation to fetal presentation. *Am J Obstet Gynecol* 1990;163:528–533.
42. Gilbert L, Saunders N, Sharp F. The management of multiple pregnancy in women with a lower segment cesarean scar. Is a repeat cesarean section really a safe option? *Br J Obstet Gynaecol* 1988;95:1312–1316.
43. Brady K, Read JA. Vaginal delivery of twins after previous cesarean section. *N Engl J Med* 1988;319:118–119.
44. Strong TH Jr, Phelan JP, Ahn MO, et al. Vaginal delivery after cesarean section in the twin gestation. *Am J Obstet Gynecol* 1989; 61:29–32.
45. Miller DA, Mullin P, Hou D, et al. Vaginal birth after cesarean section in twin gestation. *Am J Obstet Gynecol* 1996;175:194–198.

46. Wittmann BK, Farquharson D, Wong GP, et al. Delayed delivery of second twin: report of four cases and review of the literature. *Obstet Gynecol* 1992;79:260–263.

47. Poeschmann PP, Van Oppen CAC, Bruinse HW. Delayed interval delivery in multiple pregnancies: report of three cases and review of the literature. *Obstet Gynecol Surv* 1992;47:139.

48. Simpson CW, Olatunbosun OA, Baldwin UJ. Delayed interval delivery in triplet pregnancy: report of a single case and review of the literature. *Obstet Gynecol* 1984;64:85–115.

49. Banchi MT. Triplet pregnancy with second trimester abortion and delivery of twins at 35 weeks gestation. *Obstet Gynecol* 1984; 64:728–730.

50. Woolfson J, Fay T, Bates A. Twins with 54 days between delivery: case report. *Br J Obstet Gynaecol* 1983;90:685–686.

51. Lavery JP, Austin RJ, Schaefer DS, et al. Asynchronous multiple birth syndrome. *Am J Obstet Gynecol* 1992;166:396(abst).

52. Long MG, Gibb DMF, Kempley S, et al. Retention of the second twin: a viable option? *Br J Obstet Gynaecol* 1991;98:1295–1299.

53. Sakala EP, Branson BC. Prolonged delivery abortion interval in twin and triplet pregnancies. *J Reprod Med* 1987;32:79–81.

54. Scheerer LJ, Lam F, Bartolucci L, et al. A new technique for reduction of prolapsed fetal membranes for emergency cervical cerclage. *Obstet Gynecol* 1989;74:408–410.

55. Zhang J, Bowes WA, Fortney JA. Efficacy of external cephalic version: A review. *Obstet Gynecol* 1993;82:306–312.

12

Neonatal and Postneonatal Considerations in Multifetal Pregnancies

PERINATAL RISKS

Low Birth Weight and Prematurity

Infants of multiple pregnancy are disproportionately represented among the low birth weight (LBW) and premature infant populations. The average birth weight and gestational age for singletons is 3,358 g at 39.3 weeks, compared to 2,500 g at 36.2 weeks for twins, and 1,698 g at 32.2 weeks for triplets (1,2). Children of a multiple pregnancy are much more likely than singletons to be born LBW (less than 2,500 g) or very low birth weight (VLBW, less than 1,500 g) and preterm (PT, before 37 weeks' gestation) or early preterm (EPT, before 32 weeks' gestation). Although multiples comprise only 3% of all livebirths, they account for 16% of preterm births, 21% of LBW infants, and 25% of VLBW infants (1–4) (Fig. 12-1).

Neonatal Morbidity and Mortality

Because of their higher incidence of growth retardation and prematurity, infants of multiple births are at greater risk for neonatal morbidity, and fetal, neonatal, and postneonatal mortality. Survivors are at continued higher risk of postneonatal morbidity and subsequent perinatally-related disability (5–10). Despite the frequent use of home uterine monitoring to detect preterm contractions (11,12), prophylactic or emergency administration of tocolytics to limit their frequency (11–13) and the increasing antenatal use of corticosteroids to accelerate fetal lung maturity (12–16), neonatal morbidity among infants of multiple births is substantially higher than among singletons, proportional to the number of fetuses in the set of sibship. Based on a summary of the current literature, the incidence of a variety of neonatal complications, as well as rates of stillbirths, neonatal deaths, and perinatal deaths by plurality are presented in Table 12-1. The incidence of these complications and rates of death are presented as risks (odds ratio) compared with that for singletons in Table 12-2 and as risks compared with that among twins in Table 12-3.

As shown in Table 12-1, admission to a neonatal intensive care unit (NICU) is necessary for about one-fourth of all twins and as many as three-fourths of all triplets and quadruplets, with an average length of stay of 18 days, 30 days, and 58 days, respectively. The incidence of respiratory distress syndrome, one of the most costly complications of prematurity, is reported to occur among as many as 14% of twins, 41% of triplets, and 64% of quadruplets. Triplets and other infants of higher-order births are at significantly increased risk compared to singletons and twins for intraventricular hemorrhage and retinopathy of prematurity (17). Infants of multiple gestation account for 20% of all NICU

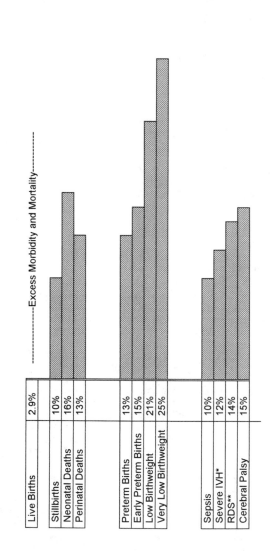

Live Births	2.9%
Stillbirths	10%
Neonatal Deaths	16%
Perinatal Deaths	13%
Preterm Births	13%
Early Preterm Births	15%
Low Birthweight	21%
Very Low Birthweight	25%
Sepsis	10%
Severe IVH*	12%
RDS**	14%
Cerebral Palsy	15%

—————————Excess Morbidity and Mortality—————————

*IVH is intraventricular hemorrhage
**RDS is respiratory distress syndrome

Figure 12-1.   Contribution of multiple births to perinatal and postneonatal morbidity and mortality.

Table 12-1. Neonatal complications by plurality

	Singletons	Twins	Triplets	Quadruplets
No. of pregnancies	112,820	2,632	542	165
No. of infants	112,456	5,264	1,593	657
Gestation (wk, range of mean)	38–40	31–37	27–35.7	24.8–32.5
Birth weight (g, range of mean)	3,268–3,594	1,837–2,510	895–2,239	1,172–1,645
Admission to neonatal intensive care unit (%)	11	19	79	84
Newborn length of stay per infant (d)	3	8.5–24	11.7–82	24–66
Hyperbilirubinemia (%)	5	22	48	75
Respiratory distress syndrome (%)	2	14	41	64
Intraventricular hemorrhage (%)	0.2	3	8	5
Patent ductus arteriosus (%)	0.8	5	11	55
Necrotizing enterocolitis (%)	0.4	1	2	4
Sepsis (%)	0.9	2	5	4
Bronchopulmonary dysplasia (%)		4	5	18
Mechanical ventilation (%)		19	34	69
Stillbirth rate	11.0/1,000	34.2/1,000	63.9/1,000	51.4/1,000
Neonatal death rate	9.0/1,000	38.0/1,000	67.4/1,000	102.9/1,000
Perinatal death rate	19.9/1,000	71.0/1,000	126.9/1,000	150/1,000

Data from

Singletons: Gardner et al., 1995 (18); Robertson et al., 1992 (121); Tallo et al., 1995 (122); Ross et al., 1999 (123).

Twins: Gardner et al., 1995 (18); Tallo et al., 1995 (122); Ross et al., 1999 (123); Lynch et al., 1996 (124); Porreco et al., 1991 (125); Silver et al., 1997 (126); Boulot et al., 1993 (127); Lipitz et al., 1994, 1996 (128, 129); Seoud et al., 1992 (130); Fitzsimmons et al., 1998 (131); Santema et al., 1995 (132); Alexander et al., 1995 (133); Groutz et al., 1996 (134); Macones et al., 1993 (135); Thorp et al., 1994 (136); Sassoon et al., 1990 (137); Melgar et al., 1991 (138).

Triplets: Kaufman et al., 1998 (17); Weissman et al., 1991 (65); Tallo et al., 1995 (122); Ross et al., 1999 (123); Porreco et al., 1991 (125); Boulot et al., 1993 (127); Lipitz et al., 1994 (128); Seoud et al., 1992 (130); Fitzsimmons et al., 1998 (131); Santema et al., 1995 (132); Macones et al., 1993 (135); Thorp et al., 1994 (136); Sassoon et al., 1990 (137); Melgar et al., 1991 (138); Peaceman et al., 1992 (140); Gonen et al., 1990 (141).

Quadruplets: Collins and Bleyl, 1990 (11); Elliott and Radin, 1992 (15); Ross et al., 1999 (123); Seoud et al., 1992 (130); Thorp et al., 1994 (136); Melgar et al., 1991 (138); Gonen et al., 1990 (141); Pons et al., 1996 (142).

Table 12-2. Risk of neonatal complications among twins, triplets, and quadruplets versus singletons as odds ratio and 95% confidence intervals

	Singletons	Twins	Triplets	Quadruplets
No. of pregnancies	112,820	2,632	542	165
No. of infants	112,456	5,264	1,593	657
Admission to neonatal intensive care unit	1.0	2.0 (1.9–2.1)	30.5 (27.0–34.5)	42.7 (34.5–52.8)
Hyperbilirubinemia	1.0	5.6 (4.3–7.4)	18.4 (14.5–23.3)	60.3 (18.1–221.6)
Patent ductus arteriosus	1.0	7.1 (4.0–12.2)	14.6 (9.8–21.5)	149.2 (56.6–396.8)
Necrotizing enterocolitis	1.0	4.1 (1.3–11.5)	6.3 (3.4–11.3)	10.4 (5.1–20.3)
Sepsis	1.0	2.4 (0.9–6.1)	6.0 (4.1–8.6)	5.0 (2.6–9.4)
Respiratory distress syndrome	1.0	7.5 (5.6–9.9)	31.3 (27.1–36.3)	79.3 (38.4–165.6)
Intraventricular hemorrhage	1.0	20.2 (10.1–39.2)	47.6 (33.8–67.0)	28.2 (11.1–121.8)
Stillbirth	1.0	3.2 (2.4–4.2)	6.1 (4.8–7.9)	4.9 (3.3–7.2)
Neonatal death	1.0	4.3 (3.3–5.7)	7.9 (6.1–10.3)	12.6 (9.3–17.1)
Perinatal death	1.0	3.8 (3.1–4.5)	7.2 (6.0–8.6)	8.6 (6.7–11.0)

Data: Same as Table 12-1.

Table 12-3. Risk of neonatal complications among triplets and quadruplets versus twins as odds ratio and 95% confidence interval

	Twins	Triplets	Quadruplets
No. of pregnancies	2,632	542	165
No. of infants	5,264	1,593	657
Admission to neonatal intensive care unit	1.0	15.4 (13.4–17.7)	21.5 (17.2–26.9)
Hyperbilirubinemia	1.0	3.3 (2.3–4.7)	10.7 (3.1–40.7)
Patent ductus arteriosus	1.0	2.2 (1.1–4.2)	21.1 (6.9–66.2)
Necrotizing enterocolitis	1.0	1.5 (0.5–5.6)	2.5 (0.7–9.7)
Sepsis	1.0	2.5 (0.9–7.2)	2.0 (0.6–6.9)
Respiratory distress syndrome	1.0	4.2 (3.1–5.7)	10.6 (4.8–23.6)
Bronchopulmonary dysplasia	1.0	1.2 (0.5–3.3)	4.8 (1.3–17.7)
Mechanical ventilation	1.0	2.1 (1.6–3.0)	9.3 (2.9–31.7)
Intraventricular hemorrhage	1.0	2.4 (1.2–4.8)	1.4 (0.3–7.1)
Stillbirth	1.0	1.9 (1.4–2.7)	1.5 (1.0–2.4)
Neonatal death	1.0	1.8 (1.3–2.6)	2.9 (2.0–4.2)
Perinatal death	1.0	1.9 (1.5–2.4)	2.3 (1.7–3.1)

Data: Same as Table 12-1.

admissions, 16% of all neonatal deaths, and 26% of all perinatal deaths (18–20) (Fig. 12-1). Compared to singletons, the risk of dying before their first birthday is nearly 7 times greater for twins and almost 20 times greater for triplets and higher-order multiples (5,10,21,22). Among survivors, the relative risk of severe disability related to birth weight and gestational age is 1.7 (95% CI, 1.6–2.0) for twins and 2.9 (95% CI, 1.5–5.5) for triplets (8). Compared to singletons of the same gestational age, infants of multiple births have significantly lower physical and mental indexes in early childhood (7), cognitive outcome by school age has been related to medical complications, such as chronic lung disease, and social risk factors (23).

Intrauterine growth retardation (IUGR) is a major factor in neonatal morbidity and mortality for all neonates, but particularly for multiples. Chen et al. (24) reported that although gestational age at birth was the most significant contributor to mortality, infants with IUGR were at significantly increased risk of sepsis as well as mortality. Growth-retarded premature infants, regardless of their plurality, have a significantly higher risk of morbidity and mortality than do appropriately grown infants (25–27), and the survivors have a high rate of developmental problems and learning and growth deficits during childhood (28,29). The rate of major developmental disabilities has been reported to be 25% at 1 year of age among twins with birth weights of 1,000 g or less (18). When matched for gestational age, appropriately grown twins and singletons do not differ in morbidity or associated costs (25,26,30,31), and at lower birth weights, multiples consistently have a survival advantage (5,10,21,31).

Risks Unique to Multiples

The risk of death or disability among infants of multiple births is magnified not only by the higher incidence of IUGR and prematurity, but also by a constellation of interrelated factors, some unique to the twinning or tripling process. These factors include gender effects and zygosity, discordancy, and fetal demise of siblings. Gender effects—being part of a like-gender or unlike-gender sibling set—are a useful proxy when zygosity has not been determined (see Chapter 2). Like-gender twin pairs, particularly males, are at higher risk of mortality; all monozygotic (identical) twins are included in this group. Monozygotic twins are known to be at increased risk of placental and cord complications, and congenital anomalies. Although it has been reported that males generally have an intrauterine growth pattern different from that of females and weigh more at birth, they also tend to have a shorter length of gestation. Several studies have demonstrated that male–male twin gestations are significantly shorter than either female twins or discordant gender twins (24,32). Male gender, though, also is significantly associated with an increased incidence of pulmonary disease, even after controlling for length of gestation, because surfactant is produced earlier by female fetuses (24,33,34).

Discordancy, another unique factor among infants of multiple gestations, is a measure of the difference between sibling birth weights. Most researchers have defined this factor as the percentage difference between the birth weights divided by the birth weight of the larger twin (8,26,35–41). Less frequently it has been defined as the ratio of the smaller to the larger twin, with the larger assigned 100% (42,43), or defined as the birth-weight difference divided by the average of the twin pair (9). Birth-weight discordancy of 20% or more is associated with significant increases in morbidity. Birth weight and discordancy are typically assessed together because the effect of the latter is minimal in the absence of IUGR (40,41).

The third unique factor among infants of multiple gestations is the fetal demise of a sibling or siblings and the resultant increased postnatal risk of morbidity, mortality, or disability for the survivor. If the intrauterine death occurs during the first or early second trimester, the dead fetus usually becomes a fetus papyraceus, which subsequently dehydrates and innocuously decomposes, partially or completely; the development of the surviving sibling usually is unaffected. First-trimester bleeding with the spontaneous death of one or more siblings has been reported to occur in as many as 30% to 35% of multiple gestations. This phenomenon is estimated to occur much more frequently than previously believed, suggesting that as many as 1 in 8 pregnancies begins as twins, and that for every liveborn twin pair, 10 to 12 twin conceptions result in singleton births. As discussed in Chapter 4, the first-trimester death of a sibling that reduces a quadruplet to a triplet pregnancy or a triplet to a twin pregnancy can have the therapeutic effect of increasing the mean birth weight of surviving siblings and increasing length of gestation.

Twin–Twin Transfusion Syndrome

Another complication unique to multiples is the twin–twin transfusion syndrome (see Chapter 8). First characterized by Herlitz in 1941 (44), the twin–twin transfusion syndrome is a complication resulting from imbalanced blood flow through vascular communications in the placenta, resulting in the favoring of one twin and the compromise of the other. The prognosis is very poor, with a perinatal mortality rate of 60% to 100% for both twins (45–47). Vascular communications occur in nearly all monochorionic placentas, but rarely occur in dichorionic placentas, although it has been reported in some fused dichorionic placentas. The twin–twin transfusion syndrome therefore is found almost exclusively in monochorionic twin pregnancies, occurring in 5% to 15% of cases (46,48).

Ultrasonographic criteria for the diagnosis of twin–twin transfusion syndrome include (49,50): (a) significant size disparity in fetuses of the same sex; (b) disparity in size between two amniotic sacs; (c) disparity in size of the umbilical cords; (d) single placenta; and (e) evidence of hydrops in either fetus or findings of congestive heart failure in the recipient. In some instances, the discordance in amniotic fluid volume is so great that the amnion adheres to the smaller baby so that it appears stuck to the wall of the uterus. It becomes very difficult to visualize the dividing membrane between the twins. Not pathognomonic for the twin–twin transfusion syndrome, the stuck twin phenomenon may also result from structural fetal anomalies, congenital infection, chromosomal abnormalities, or rupture of the membranes. Neonatal criteria for the diagnosis of twin–twin transfusion syndrome include: (46,51) (a) demonstration of a hemoglobin difference of greater than 5 g/dL and (b) birthweight difference greater than 20%. Birth weight and hematological discordance is common among monochorionic twins, and in itself is not sufficient for a diagnosis.

Many different types of treatments for twin–twin transfusion syndrome have been reported, including medical therapy with indomethacin or digoxin, repeated amniocentesis, selective feticide, hysterotomy with removal of one fetus, and laser obliteration of placental anastomoses. The treatment is usually dependent on the gestational age at presentation. In some cases, one fetus may die, which is then associated with increased neurologic morbidity for the survivor. With fetal demise, the polyhydramnios and hydrops fetalis both resolve, although resolution may take as long as 6 weeks.

Congenital Anomalies

The type and frequency of congenital anomalies among multiples is influenced by gender, race, and zygosity of the infant. As observed in singletons, male twins have a higher frequency of congenital anomalies than females overall, as well as a higher frequency of major malformations. Among twins, monozygotic (identical) twins have a higher frequency of and concordance (i.e., both twins have the same anomaly) for congenital anomalies than do dizygotic (fraternal) twins. The effect of zygosity on the incidence of congenital anaomlies can be inferred by using gender as an imperfect surrogate and comparing incidence among like-gender multiples (approximately half of whom are monozygotic) and unlike-gender multiples (all of whom are dizygotic). It has been consistently demonstrated that the excess incidence of congenital anomalies is caused entirely by an increase from monozygotic twins; dizygotic twins have rates similar to those of singletons, except for a higher rate of temporary positional anomalies due to crowding.

Congenital anomalies among monozygotic twins have been categorized based on three presumed etiologies: 1) early, localized defects in morphogenesis; 2) disruption of normal blood flow due to placental vascular anastomoses; and 3) temporary deformations imposed late in gestation by limited uterine space. Structural anomalies as a consequence of uterine constraint, such as aberrant foot positioning, occur among both monozygotic and dizygotic twins and are usually temporary, returning to normal form and growth after birth.

Twins have higher frequencies of congenital anomalies of the central nervous system, the cardiovascular system, and the gastrointestinal tract than do singletons. Twins have a more than twofold increase in cardiovascular and alimentary tract anomalies and smaller increases in anomalies of the central nervous system, musculoskeletal system, ear, and respiratory tract than do singletons. Significantly increased specific anomalies include macrocephaly, encephalocele, cleft lip and palate, anomalies of the diaphragm, cardiac septal defects, tracheoesophageal fistula, malformations of the alimentary tract, inguinal and umbilical hernia, and cystic kidney. Multiples also are susceptible to congenital anomalies as the toxic result of the fetal demise of a sibling (see Chapter 4).

The rates of congenital anomalies are higher among whites than blacks, males than females, and multiples than singletons. The highest rates occur among infants born to women in the oldest age categories and infants with birth weights less than 2,000 g. Two major studies have examined race-specific rates of congenital anomalies among multiples and singletons on a national basis. One study analyzed data derived from certificates of livebirths for the years 1973 and 1974 (1). The investigators found an overall incidence of congenital anomalies of 821 per 100,000 births, with rates of 829.8 per 100,000 for whites and 732.4 per 100,000 for blacks. When stratified by both race and plurality, these differences widened, with multiples having an 18% higher rate. The incidence of congenital anomalies among single livebirths was 817.8, with a rate of 826.5 for whites and 731.7 for blacks. Among plural livebirths, the rate was 965.7, with a rate of 1,010.7 for whites and 764.1 for blacks.

BIRTH RISKS

Twin Pregnancies

Second-born twins are at increased risk of birth asphyxia caused by malpresentation, prolapsed cord, placental separation, and operative delivery. These neonates have lower Apgar scores, lower oxygen and higher carbon dioxide umbilical venous and arterial pressures, and a higher incidence of cord blood acidemia at birth (52–54), with resultant higher neonatal mortality (55,56). Contemporary studies have shown little or no difference in acid-base status at birth, credited to continuous electronic fetal surveillance (24).

Triplet Pregnancies

Birth order has long been known to be an important factor in vaginal delivery of triplets, with the second and particularly the third neonates suffering the highest morbidity and mortality (57–62). Among triplets born vaginally rather than by cesarean, the third-born has a significantly higher risk of having low 1- and 5-minute Apgar scores (relative risk [RR], 5.5; 95% CI, 2.4–12.8 and RR, 13.5; 95% CI, 3.0–61.0) and respiratory disorders (RR, 2.3; 95% CI, 1.0–5.3) (63). Holcberg et al. (64) reported an increased incidence of neonatal death and perinatal death with birth order, increasing from 27% to 30% to 53%, and 26% to 26% to 42%, respectively.

Among vaginal deliveries of triplets, birth order has an important predictive value on infant outcome because (a) the second and third neonates are usually malpresented; (b) the second and third neonates are exposed to more obstetric maneuvers (i.e., breech extraction and forceps delivery); (c) there is a prolonged interval between delivery of infants; and (d) abrupt hemodynamic changes are caused by the reduction in uterine capacity after delivery of the first and second neonates (62). Problems with malpresentation and changes in presentation that can occur during active labor and delivery increase the risk of umbilical cord prolapse and complicate assessment of fetal heart rate during labor. Weissman et al. (65), in a study of 29 triplet pregnancies, reported that most of the perinatal deaths occurred among malpresented or second and third born neonates. Cesarean birth is associated with good acid-base status in newborns of triplet pregnancies (66,67).

INFANT AND CHILDHOOD RISKS

Physical Development

Numerous studies have shown that infants with LBW are more likely to remain shorter and lighter throughout early childhood. This is especially true of children who had IUGR rather than shortened gestation alone (68). Extremely LBW children (500 to 999 g) demonstrate the most severe continued growth retardation after birth; they have slower growth in height and weight by 8 years of age (69). Studies have demonstrated that children who had IUGR not only remain shorter and lighter than normal birth weight children but they also are weaker in physical performance by adolescence (70), which may represent a long-term deficit in muscle development. Because of the higher rates of LBW and prematurity, children of multiple gestations are at greater risk of having lower physical and mental indexes during childhood compared to singletons (7,71). In a cross-sectional study of twins 2 to 12 years of age, boys with severe IUGR at birth (birth weight z score less than –2.0) had a significantly increased risk of moderate stunting (z score between –2.0 and –1.2) in their current weight (odds ratio [OR], 2.67; 95% CI, 1.55–4.58), while girls with severe IUGR at birth had significantly increased risk of moderate stunting in their current height (OR, 4.09; 95% CI, 1.49–10.99) (71).

Studies comparing the childhood growth of twins versus single-tons generally indicate rapid recovery in weight deficit within the first 3 months, recovery in height deficit within the first year, with smaller subsequent incremental gains and parity with singletons by 6 to 8 years of age (72,73). Twins with growth retardation, whether small for gestational age (SGA, below the singleton tenth percentile) or both SGA and premature, are slower to recover. Twin children of taller mothers achieve a more complete recovery of birth weight and length deficits. Although most twins appear to recover from birth weight and length deficits by 8 years of age, twins from monozygotic pairs who weigh less than 1,750 g at birth are more likely to have a residual weight deficit (72).

Mental development of twins follows a similar pattern to that of growth. An initial deficit is generally recovered by 6 to 8 years of age (72,74–78). VLBW and very premature twins, though, have significantly lower mental scores on the Bayley Scales of Infant Development at 24 months and lower IQ scores on the Stanford Binet Intelligence Scale at 36 months (79). The smaller child from a monozygotic pair is at additional increased risk of poor mental development, particularly among males with birth weight discor-dancy of more than 25% (80).

Immunologic Development

Before birth, immature infants, whether from a multiple or a singleton pregnancy, are much more susceptible to the adverse effects of intrauterine infection. After birth, the greater the imma-turity at birth, the more impaired is immunocompetence. Although there is improvement in immune response as these infants age, some children will continue to exhibit impaired immune responses throughout childhood. Immature infants have fewer mature thymo-cytes and less clear demarcation between the cortex and medulla of the thymus. Impairment of the lymphocyte response to mito-genic stimulation and IgG production *in vitro* is more likely to occur among infants with growth retardation than among term infants with normal birth weights. Reduced levels of IgG occur among pre-term infants because of the shortened time period of passage from mother to infant during the third trimester.

An analysis of the Child Health Supplement of the National Health Interview Survey, a national probability sample of children from birth to 17 years of age, reported that LBW children have sig-nificantly more chronic conditions, hospitalizations, days in bed because of illness, limitations of activity, and school days lost be-cause of illness (81). Among all children younger than 6 years, com-pared to normal birth weight children, those who were LBW had a higher risk of two or more hospitalizations (RR, 2.2; 95% CI, 1.4–3.0), 8 or more days sick in bed (RR, 2.0; 95% CI, 1.4–2.5), and poor or fair health status as perceived by their parents (RR, 2.4; 95% CI, 1.3–3.5). VLBW children are at even higher risk of multi-ple health problems during early childhood (82).

Neurologic Development

Mental Retardation

Children who were born growth-retarded or premature are at increased risk of mental retardation later in childhood. In a population-based study, the Centers for Disease Control and Prevention found that children born LBW are at increased risk of mental retardation (IQ 70 or less) at 10 years of age (OR, 2.8; 95% CI, 1.9–4.2)(83). The magnitude of the association varied both with the degree of the LBW and the severity of mental retardation. The strongest association was between VLBW (birth weight less than 1,500 g) and severe mental retardation (IQ less than 50) (OR, 29.4; 95% CI, 5.8–148.2), whereas the weakest association was between moderate LBW (1,500 to 2,499 g) and mild mental retardation (IQ, 50 to 70) (OR, 2.0; 95% CI, 1.3–3.2). A surprising finding in this study was the twofold increase in risk of mild mental retardation among children who had been preterm and of normal birth weight (OR, 2.2; 95% CI, 1.2–4.0).

The risk of mild mental retardation (IQ, 50 to 70) increases among children who had been LBW infants. Among 5-year-old children in the Child Health and Development Studies of the Kaiser Health Plan in Oakland, California, the relative risk of mild mental retardation for children with LBW was 3.4 (95% CI, 1.2–5.4) compared with children of normal birth weight (more than 2,955 g) (84). The association between impaired cognitive development is inversely related to birth weight, with risks of IQ less than 85 for school-aged children with birth weights of 1,501 to 2,500 g (OR, 1.98; 95% CI, 0.93–4.29), 1,001 to 1,500 g (OR, 2.20; 95% CI, 1.12–4.42), and less than 1,000 g (OR, 5.23; 95% CI, 2.62–10.6). In addition, some researchers have found the risk of impaired cognitive performance to be greater among males than among females (85).

Cerebral Palsy

The overall prevalence of cerebral palsy is estimated to be 2.4 per 1,000 children (86,87); however, this disorder occurs much more frequently among a rapidly growing, high-risk group—children of multiple pregnancies (Table 12-4). Estimates of the prevalence of cerebral palsy among twins range from 6.7 to 12.6 per 1,000 children (88–91); among triplets, the risk estimates soar to 28.0 to 44.8 per 1,000 children (89,91). The increased rate of cerebral palsy among children of multiple gestations is in part related to the elevated risk of preterm birth and LBW (92). Half of all twins and 9 out of 10 triplets are born prematurely (less than 37 completed weeks' gestation) (93), and infants of multiple births account for one-fifth of all instances of LBW (less than 2,500 g) and one-fourth of all instances of VLBW (less than 1,500 g) (4,94). LBW babies are disproportionately represented among children with cerebral palsy; VLBW infants have rates of cerebral palsy 25 to 31 times those of normal birth weight children (95). Several factors have been linked to the increased risk of disability among multiples, including preeclampsia, infection, preterm premature rupture of membranes (PPROM), and delivery before 32 weeks' gestation (96–98).

Table 12-4.   The risk of cerebral palsy by plurality

	Survivors to 1 Year	Survivors to 3 Years
Triplets	28/1,000 (11–63)	6.7/1,000 (4.2–11)
Twins	7.3/1,000 (5.2–10)	1.1/1,000 (0.97–1.3)
Singletons	1.6/1,000 (1.4–1.8)	
>2,500 g		
Twins	4.2/1,000 (2.2–7.7)	2.4/1,000 (0.8–6.5)
Singletons	1.1/1,000 (1.0–1.3)	0.7/1,000 (0.5–0.8)
Twins		
Fetal death of co-twin	96/1,000 (36–218)	121/1,000 (40–291)
Both twins survived	12/1,000 (8.2–17)	9.3/1,000 (5.3–16)
Triplets		
Fetal death of co-triplet	154/1,000 (27–463)	
All triplets survived	29/1,000 (9.3–77)	

Risk of producing a child with cerebral palsy

Singleton	0.2%	with fetal death	0.1%	with fetal death
Twins	1.3%	10%	1.2%	12.1%
Triplets	7.6%	29%		

Note: Values in parentheses are range.
Adapted from Petterson B, Nelson KB, Watson L, Stanley F. Twins, triplets, and cerebral palsy in births in Western Australia in the 1980s. *Br Med J* 1993;307:1239–1243. Grether JK, Nelson KB, Cummins SK. Twinning and cerebral palsy: experience in four Northern California counties, births 1983 through 1985. *Pediatrics* 1993;92:854–858, with permission.

Although being preterm or LBW may predispose multiples to developing cerebral palsy, these factors alone do not completely account for the increased prevalence among multiples. Even at normal birth weights (more than 2,500 g), twin children have rates of cerebral palsy three to five times the rate among singletons (88–91). The reasons for this increased risk among twins with normal growth is not clear. Grether et al. (88) found an increased incidence of cerebral palsy among twins born at 2,500 g in association with intrauterine death of a co-twin. These investigators speculated that vascular anastomoses in the placentas of monozygous twins might be a contributing factor in some cases. More generally, Williams and O'Brien (99) studied asymmetric growth restriction among twins, as indexed by a low weight to length ratio. They found that such growth restriction became increasingly more common among twins as gestational age at birth advanced, and was significantly associated with the subsequent development of cerebral palsy. These authors attributed this altered pattern of intrauterine growth to increased competition for maternal nutritional resources in multiple gestations, resulting in decreased maternal fat stores, and increased rates of nutritional deprivation among these infants.

Another factor contributing to the development of cerebral palsy among normal birth weight multiples may be alterations in maternal metabolism adversely affecting neurologic development *in utero*. For example, in a study of singleton pregnancies comparing diabetic and nondiabetic pregnant women and the mental development of their children, Rizzo et al. (100) reported a significant association between gestational ketonemia in the mother and subsequent lower IQ of the child. These researchers found a significant inverse association between the mother's third-trimester plasma β-hydroxybutyrate levels and both the mental development index scores of the Bayley Scales of Infant Development and average Stanford-Binet scores at the age of 2 years. Women pregnant with twins have significantly lower fasting blood glucose and insulin levels (101) and are more prone to developing ketonemia than are women with singleton pregnancies (102). The state of accelerated starvation that occurs with singleton pregnancy is magnified in multiple pregnancy, resulting in potentially chronic *in utero* exposure to the toxic by-products of lipid metabolism.

VLBW infants account for more than one-fourth of all new cases of cerebral palsy (103–105). Although medical technology has improved survival rates among VLBW neonates, improvements in neurological outcomes have lagged behind survival in this high-risk group. As a consequence, the proportion of all cases of cerebral palsy in this birth weight group has increased (103–107). A population-based study (88) showed that 10% of all cases of cerebral palsy occurred among twins, and 22% of cases of cerebral palsy among VLBW infants occurred among twins. Twins of normal birth weight (more than 2,500 g) had a greater than threefold increased risk of cerebral palsy compared to singletons of similar birth weight (RR, 3.6; 95% CI, 1.3–9.7). This risk was related to monozygosity and the intrauterine death of the co-twin. Among children who survived the fetal death of a twin, cerebral palsy was more than 100-fold more prevalent (RR, 108; 95% CI, 42–273). Twin pregnancies produce a child with cerebral palsy 12 times more often than do singleton pregnancies (88). The likelihood per pregnancy of long-term neurologic disability compared to a singleton pregnancy is eight times higher for twins and 47 times higher for triplets (89).

Prenatal maternal infection, such as chorioamnionitis, among VLBW neonates further increases the risk of neurologic damage and cerebral palsy (98,108). Several studies have provided evidence linking perinatal infection and neonatal brain injury among both term and preterm infants. Leviton et al. (109,110) reported that cerebral white matter abnormality among neonates is associated with maternal urinary tract infection and neonatal sepsis. Bejar et al. (111) reported that amnionitis is associated with intracerebral echodensity, a cranial ultrasound finding that is predictive of cerebral palsy. Several other investigators have reported an association between neonatal sepsis and intracerebral echodensity (112,113). Grether and Nelson (114) reported an increased risk of cerebral palsy among normal birth weight infants exposed to maternal infection (OR, 9.3; 95% CI, 3.7–23.0).

There is substantial clinical and laboratory evidence for the relationship between chorioamnionitis and neurologic injury. Based on findings for both humans and laboratory animals, Yoon et al. (115)

proposed the following pathogenic theory: during the course of an intrauterine infection, microbial products stimulate circulating fetal mononuclear cells to produce interleukin 1-β and tumor necrosis factor, which may increase the permeability of the blood-brain barrier and allow passage of microbial products and cytokines into the nervous system. These products may stimulate fetal microglia (the central nervous system macrophage) to produce tumor necrosis factor, interleukin 1-β and interleukin 1-6. These cytokines may have a direct cytotoxic effect on oligodendrocytes, which are the cells responsible for myelinogenesis. Fetal infection and inflammatory cytokine production may lead to injury at the most vulnerable period of myelinogenesis, at its peak between 28 to 32 weeks' gestation.

SOCIAL ISSUES

Multiple births present a unique challenge to family dynamics. Mothers have reported feeling shock, ambivalence, depression, and anger at the diagnosis of multiple pregnancy, and at birth many of these feeling may resurface and intensify (116). Many women feel overwhelmed by the birth of multiples and lack the ability and resources to nurture two or more infants at the same time. Mothers of multiples often resort to compromises in child care, such as propping bottles and confining children to cribs or playpens, to maximize their efficiency, but such practices undermine the mother-child relationship.

Infants of multiple births present many factors that predispose them to child abuse: they are more likely to be born LBW and premature, require prolonged and repeated hospitalizations, and have feeding and developmental problems. In addition, multiples incorporate known factors for abuse—larger families and inadequate spacing of children. Because of these factors, children of multiple pregnancies and their siblings are at increased risk of child abuse. Studies have shown that even after controlling for other perinatal factors, the stress of rearing multiples is a significant risk for abuse (117–120). Health care providers should be cognizant of the stress associated with the birth of multiples and the burden such care places on the family. Preparation for the physical and economic demands of caring for multiples should begin long before their birth, including establishing support systems to help the parents.

CLINICAL CONSIDERATIONS AND KEY POINTS

- Half of all twins and 9 out of 10 triplets are born prematurely.
- Infants of multiple births account for one-fifth of all LBW infants and one-fourth of all VLBW infants.
- Children born with growth retardation or prematurely, regardless of plurality, are at increased risk of mental retardation later in childhood.
- It is estimated that twin pregnancies produce a child with cerebral palsy 12 times more often than do singleton pregnancies.
- Even at normal birth weights (more than 2,500 g), twin children have rates of cerebral palsy three to five times higher than those of singletons.
- It is estimated that one-fifth of all triplet pregnancies and one-half of all quadruplet pregnancies result in at least one child with a major disability.

- Several factors have been linked to the increased risk of disability among multiples, including preeclampsia, chorioamnionitis, preterm premature rupture of the membranes, and delivery at less than 32 weeks' gestation.
- Fetal infection and inflammatory cytokine production may lead to injury at the most vulnerable period of myelinogenesis, at its peak between 28 to 32 weeks' gestation.
- During the first postnatal year there is rapid catch-up growth in weight and height deficits. There are smaller incremental gains during early childhood such that by 6 to 8 years of age most twins will have reached growth parity with singletons.

REFERENCES

1. Taffel SM. Health and demographic characteristics of twin births: United States, 1988. National Center for Health Statistics. *Vital Health Stat 21* 1992;(50):1–17.
2. Martin JA, MacDorman MF, Mathews TJ. Triplet births: trends and outcomes, 1971–94. National Center for Health Statistics *Vital Health Stat 21* 1997;(55):1–20.
3. Ventura SJ, Martin JA, Curtin SC, et al. Births: final data for 1998. *National Vital Statistics Report* 2000;48(3):1–100.
4. Ventura SJ, Martin JA, Curtin SC, et al. Report of final natality statistics, 1996. *Mon Vital Stat Rep* 1998;46(11 Suppl)1–99.
5. Luke B, Minogue J. The contribution of gestational age and birthweight to perinatal viability in singletons versus twins. *J Matern Fetal Med* 1994;3:263–274.
6. Kiely JL. The epidemiology of perinatal mortality in multiple births. *Bull N Y Acad Med* 1990;66:618–637.
7. Brandes JM, Scher A, Itzkovits J, et al. Growth and development of children conceived by in vitro fertilization. *Pediatrics* 1992;90:424–429.
8. Luke B, Keith LG. The contribution of singletons, twins, and triplets to low birth weight, infant mortality, and handicap in the United States. *J Reprod Med* 1992;37:661–666.
9. Fowler MG, Kleinman JC, Kiely JL, et al. Double jeopardy: twin infant mortality in the United States, 1983–84. *Am J Obstet Gynecol* 1991;165:15–22.
10. Kiely JL, Kleinman JC, Kiely M. Triplets and higher-order multiple births: time trends and infant mortality. *Am J Dis Child* 1992;146:862–868.
11. Collins MS, Bleyl JA. Seventy-one quadruplet pregnancies: management and outcome. *Am J Obstet Gynecol* 1990;162:1384–1392.
12. Newman RB, Hamer C, Miller MC. Outpatient triplet management: a contemporary review. *Am J Obstet Gynecol* 1989;161: 547–555.
13. Chelmow D, Penzial AS, Kaufman G, et al. Costs of triplet pregnancy. *Am J Obstet Gynecol* 1995;172:677–682.
14. Elliott JP, Radin TG. Quadruplet pregnancy: contemporary management and outcome. *Obstet Gynecol* 1992;80:421–424.
15. Elliott JP, Radin TG. The effect of corticosteroid administration on uterine activity and preterm labor in high-order multiple gestations. *Obstet Gynecol* 1995;85:250–254.
16. National Institutes of Health Consensus Development Conference Statement. Effect of corticosteroids for fetal maturation on perinatal outcomes. *Am J Obstet Gynecol* 1995;173:246–252.

17. Kaufman GE, Malone FD, Harvey-Wilkes KB, et al. Neonatal morbidity and mortality associated with triplet pregnancy. *Obstet Gynecol* 1998;91:342–348.
18. Gardner MO, Goldenberg RL, Cliver SP, et al. The origin and outcome of preterm twin pregnancies. *Obstet Gynecol* 1995;85: 553–557.
19. Donovan EF, Ehrenkranz RA, Shankaran S, et al. Outcomes of very low birth weight twins cared for in the National Institute of Child Health and Human Development Neonatal Research Network's intensive care units. *Am J Obstet Gynecol* 1998;179: 742–749.
20. Stevenson DK, Wright LL, Lemons JA, et al. Very low birth weight outcomes of the National Institute of Child Health and Human Development Neonatal Research Network, January 1993 through December 1994. *Am J Obstet Gynecol* 1998; 179:1632–1639.
21. Luke B. Reducing fetal deaths in multiple gestations: optimal birthweights and gestational ages for infants of twin and triplet births. *Acta Genet Med Gemellol (Roma)* 1996;45:333–348.
22. Martin JA, Park MM. Trends in twin and triplet births: 1980–97. Natl Vital Stat Rep 1999;47(24):1–20.
23. Leonard CH, Piecuch RE, Ballard RA, et al. Outcome of very low birth weight infants: multiple gestation versus singletons. *Pediatrics* 1994;93:611–615.
24. Chen SJ, Vohr BR, Oh W. Effects of birth order, gender, and intrauterine growth retardation on the outcome of very low birth weight in twins. *J Pediatr* 1993;123:132–136.
25. Kilpatrick J, Jackson R, Croughan-Minihane MS. Perinatal mortality in twins and singletons matched for gestational age at delivery at ≥30 weeks. *Am J Obstet Gynecol* 1996;174:66–71.
26. Luke B, Minogue J, Witter FR. The role of fetal growth restriction and gestational age on length of hospital stay in twin infants. *Obstet Gynecol* 1993;81:949–953.
27. Piper JM, Xenakis EMJ, McFarland M, et al. Do growth-retarded premature infants have different rates of perinatal morbidity and mortality than appropriately grown premature infants? *Obstet Gynecol* 1996;87:169–174.
28. Ackerman BA, Thomassen PA. The fate of "small twins:" a four-year follow-up study of low birthweight and prematurely born twins. *Acta Genet Med Gemellol (Roma)* 1992;41:97–104.
29. Low JA, Handley-Derry MH, Burke SO, et al. Association of intrauterine fetal growth retardation and learning deficits at age 9 to 11 years. *Am J Obstet Gynecol* 1992;167:1499–1505.
30. Luke B, Bigger H, Leurgans S, et al. The costs of prematurity: a case-control study of twins versus singletons. *Am J Public Health* 1996;86:809–814.
31. Wolf E, Vintzileos AM, Rosenkrantz TS, et al. A comparison of pre-discharge survival and morbidity in singleton and twin very low birth weight infants. *Obstet Gynecol* 1992;80:436–439.
32. Newton W, Keith L, Keith D. The Northwestern University multi-hospital twin study, IV: duration of gestation according to fetal sex. *Am J Obstet Gynecol* 1984;149:655–658.
33. Collins JW, David RJ, Boehm JJ. RDS explains sex but not race differences in birth weight-specific mortality. *Pediatr Res* 1987; 21:393A(abst).

34. Torday JS, Nielsen HC, Fencl MDM, et al. Sex differences in fetal lung maturation. *Am Rev Respir Dis* 1981;123:205–208.
35. Babson SG, Phillips DS. Growth and development of twins dissimilar in size at birth. *N Engl J Med* 1973;289:937–940.
36. Ylitalo V, Kero P, Erkkola R. Neurological outcome of twins dissimilar in size at birth. *Early Hum Dev* 1988;17:245–255.
37. Erkkola R, Ala-Mello S, Piiroinen O, et al. Growth discordancy in twin pregnancies. *Obstet Gynecol* 1985;66:203–206.
38. O'Brien WF, Knuppel RA, Scerbo JC, et al. Birth weight in twins: an analysis of discordancy and growth retardation. *Obstet Gynecol* 1986;67:483–486.
39. Crane J, Tomich P, Kapta M. Ultrasonic growth patterns in normal and discordant twins. *Obstet Gynecol* 1980;55:678–683.
40. Fraser D, Picard R, Picard E, et al. Birth weight discordance, intrauterine growth retardation and perinatal outcomes in twins. *J Reprod Med* 1994;39:504–508.
41. Bronsteen R, Goyert G, Bottoms S. Classification of twins and neonatal morbidity. *Obstet Gynecol* 1989;74:98–101.
42. Blickstein I, Shoham-Schwartz Z, Lancet M, et al. Characterization of the growth-discordant twin. *Obstet Gynecol* 1987;70:11–14.
43. Blickstein I, Shoham-Schwartz Z, Lancet M. Growth discordancy in appropriate for gestational age, term twins. *Obstet Gynecol* 1988;72:582–584.
44. Herlitz G. Zur kenntnis der anämischen und polyzytämischen Zustände bei Neugeborenen sowie des Icterus gravis neonatorum. *Acta Paediatr* 1941;29:211–219.
45. Cheschier NC, Seeds JW. Polyhydramnios and oligohydramnios in twin gestations. *Obstet Gynecol* 1988;71:882–884.
46. Rausen AR, Seki M, Strauss L. Twin transfusion syndrome. *J Pediatr* 1965;66:613–628.
47. Gonsoulin W, Moise KJ, Kirshon B, et al. Outcome of twin-twin transfusion diagnosed before 28 weeks of gestation. *Obstet Gynecol* 1990;73:214–216.
48. Benirschke K, Kim CK. Multiple pregnancy, I. *N Engl J Med* 1973;288:1276–1284.
49. Brennan JN, Diwan RJ, Rosen MG, et al. Fetofetal transfusion syndrome: prenatal ultrasonographic diagnosis. *Radiology* 1982;143:535–536.
50. Wittmann BK, Baldwin VJ, Nichol F. Antenatal diagnosis of twin transfusion syndrome by ultrasound. *Obstet Gynecol* 1981;58:123–127.
51. Tan KL, Tan R, Tan SH, et al. The twin transfusion syndrome: clinical observations on 35 affected pairs. *Clin Pediatr (Phila)* 1979;18:111–114.
52. Nakano R, Takemura H. Birth order in delivery of twins. *Gynecol Obstet Invest* 1988;25:217–222.
53. Young BK, Suidan J, Antoine C, et al. Differences in twins: the importance of birth order. *Am J Obstet Gynecol* 1985;151:915–921.
54. Eskes TKAB, Timmer H, Kollée L, et al. The second twin. *Eur J Obstet Gynecol Reprod Biol* 1985;19:159–166.
55. Puissant F, Leroy F. The fate of the second twin. *Eur J Obstet Gynecol Reprod Biol* 1984;15:275–277.
56. Fakeye O. Perinatal factors in twin mortality in Nigeria. *Int J Gynaecol Obstet* 1986;24:309–314.

57. Syrop CH, Varner MW. Triplet gestation: maternal and neonatal implications. *Acta Genet Med Gemellol (Roma)* 1985;34:81–88.

58. Crowther CA, Hamilton RA. Triplet pregnancy: a 10-year review of 105 cases at Harare Maternity Hospital, Zimbabwe. *Acta Genet Med Gemellol (Roma)* 1989;38:271–278.

59. Pons JC, Mayenga JM, Plu G, et al. Management of triplet pregnancy. *Acta Genet Med Gemellol (Roma)* 1988;37:99–103.

60. Kurtz GR, Davis LL, Loftus JB. Factors influencing the survival of triplets. *Obstet Gynecol* 1958;12:504–508.

61. Itzkowic D. A survey of 59 triplet pregnancies. *Br J Obstet Gynaecol* 1979;86:23–28.

62. Michlewitz H, Kennedy J, Kawada C, et al. Triplet pregnancies. *J Reprod Med* 1981;26:243–246.

63. Lipitz S, Reichman B, Paret G, et al. The improving outcome of triplet pregnancies. *Am J Obstet Gynecol* 1989;161:1279–1284.

64. Holcberg G, Biale Y, Lewenthal H, et al. Outcome of pregnancy in 31 triplet gestations. *Obstet Gynecol* 1982;59:472–476.

65. Weissman A, Yoffe N, Jakobi P, et al. Management of triplet pregnancies in the 1980s: are we doing better? *Am J Perinatol* 1991;8:333–337.

66. Creinin M, MacGregor S, Socol M, et al. The Northwestern University triplet study, IV. *Am J Obstet Gynecol* 1988;159:1140–1143.

67. Antoine C, Kirshenbaum NW, Young BK. Biochemical differences related to birth order in triplets. *J Reprod Med* 1986;31:330–332.

68. Binkin NJ, Yip R, Fleshood L, et al. Birth weight and childhood growth. *Pediatrics* 1988;82:828–834.

69. Kitchen WH, Doyle LW, Ford GW, et al. Very low birth weight and growth to age 8 years. *Am J Dis Child* 1992;146:40–45.

70. Martorell R, Ramakrishnan U, Schroeder DG, et al. Intrauterine growth retardation, body size, body composition and physical performance in adolescence. *Eur J Clin Nutr* 1998;52:S43–S53.

71. Luke B, Leurgans S, Keith L, et al. The childhood growth of twin children. *Acta Genet Med Gemellol (Roma)* 1995;44:169–178.

72. Wilson RS. Growth and development of human twins. In: Falkner F, Tanner JM, eds. *Human growth: a comprehensive treatise,* 2d ed. vol. 3. *Methodology, ecological, genetic, and nutritional effects on growth.* New York: Plenum Press, 1986:197–211.

73. Ooki S, Asaka A. Physical growth of Japanese twins. *Acta Genet Med Gemellol (Roma)* 1993;42:275–287.

74. Dezoete JA, MacArthur BA. Cognitive development and behaviour in very low birthweight twins at four years. *Acta Genet Med Gemellol (Roma)* 1996;45:325–332.

75. McDiarmid JM, Silva PA. Three-year-old twins and singletons: a comparison of some perinatal, environmental, experiential, and developmental characteristics. *Aust Paediatr J* 1979;15:243–247.

76. Silva PA, McGee RO, Powell J. Growth and development of twins compared with singletons at ages five and seven: a follow–up report from the Dunedin Multidisciplinary Child Development Study. *Aust Paediatr J* 1982;18:35–36.

77. Silva PA, Crosado B. The growth and development of twins compared with singletons at ages 9 and 11. *Aust Paediatr J* 1985;21:265–267.

78. Morley R, Cole TJ, Powell R, et al. Growth and development in premature twins. *Arch Dis Child* 1989;64:1042–1045.
79. Stauffer A, Burns WJ, Burns KA, et al. Early developmental progress of preterm twins discordant for birthweight and risk. *Acta Genet Med Gemellol (Roma)* 1988;37:81–87.
80. O'Brien PJ, Hay DA. Birthweight differences, the transfusion syndrome and the cognitive development of monozygotic twins. *Acta Genet Med Gemellol (Roma)* 1987;36:181–196.
81. Overpeck MD, Moss AJ, Hoffman HJ, et al. A comparison of the childhood health status of normal birth weight and low birth weight infants. *Public Health Rep* 1989;104:58–70.
82. McCormick MC, Brooks-Gunn J, Workman-Daniels K, et al. The health and developmental status of very low-birth-weight children at school age. *JAMA* 1992;267:2204–2208.
83. Mervis CA, Decouflé P, Murphy CC, et al. Low birthweight and the risk for mental retardation later in childhood. *Paediatr Perinat Epidemiol* 1995;9:455–468.
84. McDermott S, Coker AL, McKeown RE. Low birthweight and risk of mild mental retardation by ages 5 and 9 to 11. *Paediatr Perinat Epidemiol* 1993;7:195–204.
85. Seidman DS, Laor A, Gale R, et al. Birth weight and intellectual performance in late adolescence. *Obstet Gynecol* 1992;79:543–546.
86. Boyle CA, Yeargin-Allsopp M, Doernberg NS, et al. Prevalence of selected developmental disabilities in children 3–10 years of age: the Metropolitan Atlanta Developmental Disabilities Surveillance Program. *MMWR Morb Mortal Wkly Rep* 1991;45:1–14.
87. Robertson CM, Svenson LW, Joffres MR. Prevalence of cerebral palsy in Alberts. *Can J Neurol Sci* 1998;25:117–122.
88. Grether JK, Nelson KB, Cummins SK. Twinning and cerebral palsy: experience in four northern California counties, births 1983 through 1985. *Pediatrics* 1993;92:854–858.
89. Petterson B, Nelson KB, Watson L, et al. Twins, triplets, and cerebral palsy in births in Western Australia in the 1980s. *Br Med J* 1993;307:1239–1243.
90. Williams K, Hennessey E, Alberman E. Cerebral palsy: effects of twinning, birthweight, and gestational age. *Arch Dis Child* 1996;75:F178–F182.
91. Pharoah POD, Cooke T. Cerebral palsy and multiple births. *Arch Dis Child* 1996;75:F174–F177.
92. Scheller JM, Nelson KB. Twinning and neurologic morbidity. *Am J Dis Child* 1992;146:1110–1113.
93. Kiely JL. What is the population-based risk of preterm birth among twins and other multiples? *Clin Obstet Gynecol* 1998; 41:3–11.
94. Alexander GR, Kogan M, Artin J, et al. What are the fetal growth patterns of singletons, twins, and triplets in the United States? *Clin Obstet Gynecol* 1998;41:115–125.
95. Kuban KCK, Leviton A. Cerebral palsy. *N Engl J Med* 1994; 30:188–195.
96. Yokoyama Y, Shimizu T, Hayakawa K. Incidence of handicaps in multiple births and associated factors. *Acta Genet Med Gemellol (Roma)* 1995a;44:81–91.
97. Yokoyama Y, Shimizu T, Hayakawa K. Handicaps in twins and triplets. *Jpn J Hyg* 1995b;49:1013–1018.

98. O'Shea TM, Klinepeter KL, Meis PJ, et al. Intrauterine infection and the risk of cerebral palsy in very low-birthweight infants. *Paediatr Perinat Epidemiol* 1998;12:72–83.

99. Williams MC, O'Brien WF. Low weight/length ratio to assess risk of cerebral palsy and perinatal mortality in twins. *Am J Perinatol* 1998;15:225–228.

100. Rizzo T, Metzger BE, Burns WJ, et al. Correlations between antepartum maternal metabolism and intelligence of offspring. *N Engl J Med* 1991;325:911–916.

101. Spellacy WN, Buhi WC, Birk SA. Carbohydrate metabolism in women with a twin pregnancy. *Obstet Gynecol* 1980;55:688–691.

102. Casele H, Dooley S, Metzger B. Metabolic response to meal eating and extended overnight fast in twin gestation. *Am J Obstet Gynecol* 1996;174:375(abst).

103. Stanley FJ. Survival and cerebral palsy in low birthweight infants: implications for perinatal care. *Paediatr Perinatal Epidemiol* 1992;6:298–310.

104. Cummins SK, Nelson KB, Grether JK, et al. Cerebral palsy in four northern California counties, births 1983 through 1985. *J Pediatr* 1993;123:230–237.

105. Bhushan V, Paneth N, Kiely JL. Impact of improved survival of very low birthweight infants on recent secular trends in the prevalence of cerebral palsy. *Pediatrics* 1993;91:1094–1100.

106. Hagberg B, Hagberg G, Olow I, et al. The changing panorama of cerebral palsy in Sweden, VII: prevalence and origin in the birth year period 1987–90. *Acta Paediatr Scand* 1996;85:954–960.

107. Mutch L, Alberman E, Hagberg B, et al. Cerebral palsy epidemiology: where are we now and where are we going? *Dev Med Child Neurol* 1992;34:547–555.

108. Alexander JM, Gilstrap LC, Cox SM, et al. Clinical chorioamnionitis and the prognosis for very low birth weight infants. *Obstet Gynecol* 1998;91:725–729.

109. Leviton A, Gilles F, Neff R, et al. Multivariate analysis of risk of perinatal telencephalic leucoencephalopathy. *Am J Epidemiol* 1976;104:621–626.

110. Leviton A, Gilles FH. Acquired perinatal leukoencephalopathy. *Ann Neurol* 1984;16:1–8.

111. Bejar R, Wozniak P, Allard M, et al. Antenatal origin and neurologic damage in newborn infants, I: preterm infants. *Am J Obstet Gynecol* 1988;159:357–363.

112. Sinha SK, Davies JM, Sims DG, et al. Relationship between periventricular haemorrhage and ischaemic brain lesions diagnosed by ultrasound in very preterm infants. *Lancet* 1985;2:1154–1156.

113. Faix RG, Donn SM. Association of septic shock caused by early onset group B streptococcal sepsis and periventricular leukomalacia in preterm infants. *Pediatrics* 1985;76:415–419.

114. Grether JK, Nelson KB. Maternal infection and cerebral palsy in infants of normal birth weight. *JAMA* 1997;278:207–211.

115. Yoon BH, Romero R, Kim CJ, et al. High expression of tumor necrosis factor-α and interleukin-6 in periventricular leukomalacia. *Am J Obstet Gynecol* 1997;177:406–411.

116. Goshen-Gottstein ER. The mothering of twins, triplets, and quadruplets. *Psychiatry* 1980;43:189–204.

117. Groothuis JR, Altemeier WA, Robarge JP, et al. Increased child abuse in families with twins. *Pediatrics* 1982;70:769–773.
118. Tanimura M, Matsui I, Kobayashi N. Child abuse of one of a pair of twins in Japan. *Lancet* 1990;336:1298–1299.
119. Hansen KK. Twins and child abuse. *Arch Pediatr Adolesc Med* 1994;148:1345–1346.
120. Robarge JP, Reynolds ZB, Groothuis JR. Increased child abuse in families with twins. *Res Nurs Health* 1982;5:199–203.
121. Robertson PA, Sniderman SH, Laros RK, et al. Neonatal morbidity according to gestational age and birth weight from five tertiary care centers in the United States, 1983 through 1986. *Am J Obstet Gynecol* 1992;166:1629–1645.
122. Tallo CP, Vohr B, Oh W, et al. Maternal and neonatal morbidity associated with in vitro fertilization. *J Pediatr* 1995;127:794–800.
123. Ross MG, Downey CA, Bemis-Heys R, et al. Prediction by maternal risk factors of neonatal intensive care admissions: evaluation of >59,000 women in national managed care program. *Am J Obstet Gynecol* 1999;181:835–842.
124. Lynch L, Berkowitz RL, Stone J, et al. Preterm delivery after selective termination in twin pregnancies. *Obstet Gynecol* 1996; 87:366–369.
125. Porreco RP, Burke MS, Hendrix ML. Multifetal reduction of triplets and pregnancy outcome. *Obstet Gynecol* 1991;78:335–339.
126. Silver RK, Helfand BT, Russell TL, et al. Multifetal reduction increases the risk of preterm delivery and fetal growth restriction in twins: a case–control study. *Fertil Steril* 1997;67:30–33.
127. Boulot P, Hedon B, Pelliccia G, et al. Effects of selective reduction in triplet gestation: a comparative study of 80 cases managed with or without this procedure. *Fertil Steril* 1993;60:497–503.
128. Lipitz S, Reichman B, Uval J, et al. A prospective comparison of the outcome of triplet pregnancies managed expectantly or by multifetal reduction to twins. *Am J Obstet Gynecol* 1994;170: 874–879.
129. Lipitz S, Uval J, Achiron R, et al. Outcome of twin pregnancies reduced from triplets compared with nonreduced twin gestations. *Obstet Gynecol* 1996;87:511–514.
130. Seoud MAF, Toner JP, Kruithoff C, et al. Outcome of twin, triplet, and quadruplet in vitro fertilization pregnancies: the Norfolk experience. *Fertil Steril* 1992;57:825–834.
131. Fitzsimmons BP, Bebbington MW, Fluker MR. Perinatal and neonatal outcomes in multiple gestations: assisted reproduction versus spontaneous conception. *Am J Obstet Gynecol* 1998;179: 1162–1167.
132. Santema JG, Bourdrez P, Wallenberg HCS. Maternal and perinatal complications in triplet compared with twin pregnancy. *Eur J Obstet Gynecol Reprod Biol* 1995;60:143–147.
133. Alexander JM, Hammond KR, Steinkampf MP. Multifetal reduction of high-order multiple pregnancy: comparison of obstetrical outcome with nonreduced twin gestations. *Fertil Steril* 1995;64: 1201–1203.
134. Groutz A, Yovel I, Amit A, et al. Pregnancy outcome after multifetal pregnancy reduction to twins compared with spontaneously conceived twins. *Hum Reprod* 1996;11:1334–1336.

135. Macones GA, Schemmer G, Pritts E, et al. Multifetal reduction of triplets improves perinatal outcome. *Am J Obstet Gynecol* 1993;169:982–986.

136. Thorp JM, Tumey LA, Bowes WA Jr. Outcome of multifetal gestations: a case–control study. *J Matern Fetal Med* 1994;3:23–26.

137. Sassoon DA, Castro LC, Davis JL, et al. Perinatal outcome in triplet versus twin gestations. *Obstet Gynecol* 1990;75:817–820.

138. Melgar CA, Rosenfeld DL, Rawlinson K, et al. Perinatal outcome after multifetal reduction to twins compared with nonreduced multiple gestations. *Obstet Gynecol* 1991;78:763–767.

139. Albrecht JL, Tomich PG. The maternal and neonatal outcome of triplet gestations. *Am J Obstet Gynecol* 1996;174:1551–1556.

140. Peaceman AM, Dooley SL, Tamura RK, et al. Antepartum management of triplet gestations. *Am J Obstet Gynecol* 1992;167:1117–1120.

141. Gonen R, Heyman E, Asztalos EV, et al. The outcome of triplet, quadruplet, and quintuplet pregnancies managed in a perinatal unit: Obstetric, neonatal, and follow-up data. *Am J Obstet Gynecol* 1990;162:454–459.

142. Pons JC, Nekhlyudov L, Dephot N, et al. Management and outcomes of 65 quadruplet pregnancies: sixteen years' experience in France. *Acta Genet Med Gemellol (Roma)* 1996;45:367–375.

UNIVERSITY OF CHESTER, BACHE EDUCATION CENTRE

Subject Index

References followed by "f" indicate figures; those followed by "t" denote tables.

LIBRARY, UNIVERSITY OF CHESTER

LIBRARY, UNIVERSITY OF CHESTER